Recent Research in Liver Diseases

Recent Research in Liver Diseases

Edited by Tucker Banks

hayle
medical

New York

Hayle Medical,
750 Third Avenue, 9th Floor,
New York, NY 10017, USA

Visit us on the World Wide Web at:
www.haylemedical.com

ISBN: 978-1-63241-640-7

Cataloging-in-Publication Data

Recent research in liver diseases / edited by Tucker Banks.
p. cm.
Includes bibliographical references and index.
ISBN 978-1-63241-640-7
1. Liver--Diseases. 2. Liver--Diseases--Research. I. Banks, Tucker.
RC845 .R43 2019
616.362--dc23

Table of Contents

Permissions

List of Contributors

Index

Preface

Every book is initially just a concept; it takes months of research and hard work to give it the final shape in which the readers receive it. In its early stages, this book also went through rigorous reviewing. The notable contributions made by experts from across the globe were first molded into patterned chapters and then arranged in a sensibly sequential manner to bring out the best results.

The human liver is susceptible to a number of diseases and infections. Hepatitis is a common condition affecting the liver. Chronic hepatitis B or C is the leading cause of liver cancer. Globally, hepatitis B virus infects around 248 million people, while hepatitis C virus infects nearly 142 million people. Hepatitis A and E generally resolve and do not become chronic. Hepatitis D infects only in the presence of hepatitis B, and afflicts around 20 million people globally. Any blockage of the hepatic veins causes Budd-Chiari syndrome, which causes ascites, liver enlargement and abdominal pain. Many liver diseases, such as progressive familial intrahepatic cholestasis, alpha-1 antitrypsin deficiency, biliary atresia, alagille syndrome, Langerhans cell histiocytosis, etc., affect babies and young children. This book brings forth some of the most innovative concepts and elucidates the unexplored aspects of liver diseases. It includes some of the vital pieces of work being conducted across the world, on liver diseases. Those in search of information to further their knowledge will be greatly assisted by this book.

It has been my immense pleasure to be a part of this project and to contribute my years of learning in such a meaningful form. I would like to take this opportunity to thank all the people who have been associated with the completion of this book at any step.

Editor

Liver Transplantation in Acute Liver Failure: Indications and Outcome

Rocío González Grande and Miguel Jiménez Pérez

Abstract

The term acute liver failure (ALF) refers to the acute (<26 weeks) and severe worsening in liver function associated with encephalopathy in a person with no underlying chronic liver disease. ALF constitutes a critical clinical syndrome that is potentially reversible but has a very variable prognosis. No specific treatment is available, and liver transplantation (LT) is the treatment of choice in many cases. However, the challenge remains of identifying those patients with a poor likelihood of spontaneous recovery of liver function and for whom the indication and time of LT in order to guarantee survival (based on identification of prognostic factors) need to be established. In Europe, 8% of LT are due to ALF. Although the results of LT due to ALF have improved over recent years, they are still far from those seen after elective LT.

Keywords: liver transplant, acute liver failure, prognostic score, outcome

1. Introduction

Acute liver failure (ALF) is defined as the presence of acute liver injury, that is, a rise in transaminases at least three times the upper limit of normal, jaundice, and coagulopathy, together with the onset of encephalopathy in a person with no previous liver disease [1]. Exceptions to this definition include the acute onset of Wilson disease, autoimmune hepatitis, and the Budd-Chiari syndrome, as well as reactivation of the hepatitis B virus (HBV) [2].

Though no consensus exists on the severity of the coagulopathy or the encephalopathy marking the transition from acute liver injury to ALF, an INR ≥1.5 and any degree of encephalopathy are generally accepted [3]. Clinically, ALF is classified according to the interval between the onset of jaundice, considered as the initial symptom, and the encephalopathy. The ALF is considered to be hyperacute if the encephalopathy appears within

7 days of the jaundice, acute if it appears between 8 and 28 days, and subacute when it appears beyond 28 days [4]. The disease is considered chronic if it has a history of more than 26 weeks.

Table 1 summarizes the causes of ALF. Worldwide, infection is the most common cause, though in developed countries drug-induced hepatic injury is responsible for up to 50% of cases. As many as 30% of cases are of unknown etiology [5].

The main causes of death due to ALF are infection and decerebration from cerebral edema. The medical management of patients is based on support measures, early identification, and treatment of complications until spontaneous recovery of liver function or liver transplantation (LT) [6].

Establishing the indication for and time of LT in a patient with ALF should be as precise as possible in order to avoid, on one hand, unnecessary risks for a recoverable patient and on the other an increased likelihood of death associated with a delay in transplantation.

Viral
HAV, HBV, HCV, HEV
CMV, EBV, HSV, VZV, dengue
Pharmacologic/toxic
Paracetamol (acetaminophen)
Idiosyncratic drug reaction
Amanita phalloides
Vascular
Budd-Chiari
Ischemic hepatitis
Pregnancy
Preeclampsia
HELLP
Fatty liver of pregnancy
Others
Wilson disease
Autoimmune hepatitis
Lymphomas and other neoplastic diseases
Hemophagocytic lymphohistiocytosis
Cryptogenic

Table 1. Etiology of the acute liver failure.

2. Indication for liver transplantation in acute liver failure

Liver transplantation in ALF has represented an inflection point in the survival of affected patients, who previously suffered a mortality rate of almost 85% in the pretransplant era [7].

Indicating LT too soon involves the possibility of performing the transplant in patients who may still experience spontaneous recovery with complete liver function, thereby adding the risks associated with an urgent transplant and lifelong immunosuppression, in addition to the waste of a valuable organ. However, delaying the decision to transplant in patients with ALF can increase the risk of infection, irreversible brain damage, multiorgan failure, or even death. Accordingly, selection of ALF patients who need LT should be based on the early identification of factors predicting a poor clinical outcome, as well as application of prognostic models combining different parameters. Unfortunately, the prognostic models available have certain limitations, low sensitivity and specificity, and worse predictive value than desired [8].

2.1. Predictive factors

The etiology is considered a predictive factor. Around 60% of patients with ALF due to paracetamol intoxication, hepatitis A, ischemic hepatitis, or pregnancy may survive with no need for transplantation, whereas only 30% of cases with drug-induced liver injury, autoimmune hepatitis, and various cases of unknown etiology achieve spontaneous recovery [9].

The duration of symptoms has traditionally had a prognostic value. The subacute presentation of ALF is associated with a worse prognosis than acute and hyperacute ALF, though these differences are probably conditioned by the etiology of the subacute failure [10].

Encephalopathy, although it forms part of the definition of ALF, should also be classified. Patients with grades 1–2 encephalopathy have an excellent prognosis, whereas grades 3–4 encephalopathy is associated with a low likelihood of spontaneous resolution [11] and is thus criteria for admission to the intensive care unit, with a recommendation to measure the intracranial pressure as a marker of the preservation of brain perfusion [12]. Coagulopathy, as a direct indicator of liver function, is considered to predict the severity. Generally measured using the prothrombin time (PT) or the International Normalized Ratio (INR), a PT over 90 s or an INR >4 is associated with a mortality rate above 90% [13]. Factor V levels <20% in patients younger than 30 years and levels <30% in those older than 30 years indicate a worse prognosis.

The histologic findings have also been proposed as predictors of the outcome and the likelihood of spontaneous recovery. Though some series have related the risk of death with the presence of >50% hepatocyte necrosis, the little representativity of the samples together with the risk involved in performing a liver biopsy in patients with coagulopathy generally advise against routine histologic study in patients with ALF, and nor should the decision to transplant be based on biopsy findings. A liver biopsy could be indicated in cases of diagnostic doubt, especially to rule out neoplastic causes, which contraindicate LT [14]. Other factors, such as age, body mass index, serum bilirubin, creatinine, hypoglycemia, lactate levels, and pH changes, can also be considered determinant.

All these factors help to identify patients with ALF who have a worse prognosis. Recently, the EASL established recommendations for the early transfer to transplant centers of patients with ALF if they fulfill the following criteria [15]:

- ALF due to paracetamol or hyperacute causes:
  - Arterial pH <7.3 or HCO_3 <18
  - INR >3.0 day 2 or >4 thereafter
  - Oliguria and/or elevated creatinine
  - Altered level of consciousness
  - Hypoglycemia
  - Elevated lactate unresponsive to fluid resuscitation
- Non-paracetamol:
  - Arterial pH <7.3 or HCO3 <18
  - INR >1.8
  - Oliguria/renal failure or Na <130 mmol/L
  - Encephalopathy, hypoglycemia, or metabolic acidosis
  - Bilirubin >300 µmol/L (17.6 mg/dL)
  - Shrinking liver size

2.2. Prognostic models

The currently available prognostic models should be applied continuously during the follow-up and clinical management of patients with ALF, even though they are not universally accepted or their recommendations established.

In 1989, the King's College Hospital criteria (KCC) were established (**Table 2**) [16]. These are based on cohort studies and are widely used at the present time. They are based mainly on the etiology, differentiating between ALF secondary to paracetamol and ALF of other causes. They are highly specific, that is, patients who fulfill these criteria have a high likelihood of death if they do not undergo LT. However, their sensitivity is low, as seen from the death of patients who do not meet the criteria, especially in patients with causes other than paracetamol [17]. A meta-analysis found a specificity of 82% for etiologies other than paracetamol and 92–95% for causes related with paracetamol. The sensitivity was about 68%. Both sensitivity and specificity increase if the criteria are applied dynamically [18]. In an attempt to improve the predictive value of the KCC, the measurement of lactate as an indicator of tissue dysfunction and failure of hepatic clearance has been added to the criteria in the UK. This is particularly useful in cases of paracetamol toxicity. An admission arterial lactate >3.5 or >3 mmol/L after fluid resuscitation is a marker of poor prognosis [19, 20].

AFL due to paracetamol

- Arterial pH <7.3 after resuscitation and 24 h since ingestion
- Three following criteria:
  - Hepatic encephalopathy grades 3–4
  - Serum creatinine >300 mol/L (3.4 mg(dl)
  - INR >6.5

ALF not due to paracetamol

- INR >6.5
- Three out of five following criteria:
  - Etiology: indeterminate etiology hepatitis, drug-induced hepatitis
  - Age <10 years or >40 years
  - Interval jaundice encephalopathy >7 days
  - Bilirubin >300 mol/L (17 mg/dl)
  - INR >3.5

Table 2. King's College criteria.

The Clichy criteria, established in 1986, also derive from cohort studies in patients with fulminant hepatitis B (**Table 3**) [21]. Validation studies found less accuracy than for the KCC, with a positive predictive value of 89%, but a negative predictive value of 36%. They are, therefore, very deficient for identifying potential survivors without a LT [22].

The MELD score (**Table 4**), adopted by the United Network for Organ Sharing (UNOS) and The Organ Procurement and Transplantation Network (OPTN), has been validated as a predictor of short-term mortality in patients with hepatic cirrhosis. Retrospective studies have shown that the MELD score has a similar predictive value to the KCC for AFL-associated mortality [23]. In the USA, the prospective data from the Acute Liver Failure Study Group (ALFSG) showed that a MELD >30 in patients with ALF due to paracetamol has a negative predictive value of 82%, such that patients with a MELD <30 have a high likelihood of survival without a LT and with a slightly lower score in cases not related with paracetamol [24].

- Confusion or coma (hepatic encephalopathy 3–4)
- Factor V <20% of normal if age <30 years or factor V <30% if age >30 years

Table 3. Clichy criteria.

$$9.57 \times \log_e^{(creatinine)} + 3.78 \times \log_e^{(bilirubin)} + 11.2 \times \log_e^{(INR)} + 6.43$$

Table 4. MELD (MELD calculator).

In an attempt to improve the prognostic accuracy in ALF patients, other indicators of liver dysfunction have been suggested, such as measures of hepatic metabolism with markers labeled with indocyanine green [25], as well as predictive models of mortality used in other clinical situations. The APACHE II system, designed to predict mortality in intensive care patients, has also been applied in ALF patients, but no cut point has been set demonstrating that it is superior to the KCC and nor can it be applied early on [26].

A prognostic index designed by the ALFSG included variables at the time of presentation of the condition, such as bilirubin, encephalopathy grade, INR, phosphorus, and serum levels of M30 (a direct marker of hepatocyte apoptosis). Although the prognostic value of this index was greater than the KCC and MELD score, measurement of M30 is not generally available [27].

Comparison between these different models, which share some parameters, has found no superiority of one over the others, and no universal recommendations have been established. It is, however, accepted that ALF should be strictly assessed at the reception center and, if the patient meets the criteria for a poor prognosis, they should be referred as soon as possible to a transplant center where the available predictive models can be applied dynamically, mainly the KCC and Clichy criteria, to determine the indication for LT. American and European series show that 50% of patients admitted with ALF receive a LT [28]. Once the indication for a transplant has been made, the patient is included on the active list, in most countries with a higher priority than patients with other indications, thus ensuring an early transplant, usually within days of being placed on the list.

If a donor organ becomes available, the situation of the patient should be reassessed by the transplant team, in order to identify a likely clear improvement after transplant or else an absolute contraindication for transplant, mainly the presence of irreversible brain damage.

3. Outcome of liver transplant in acute liver failure

In Europe LT due to acute or subacute liver failure accounts for some 8% of LT. Patient survival after LT for this reason is 79, 71, 69 and 61%, at 1, 3, 5 and 10 years, respectively [29]. This survival rate is slightly lower during the initial years (first and third) than LT for other reasons but then becomes similar. Most deaths occur between the first and third years posttransplant due, mainly, to neurologic complications and sepsis [30]. Some centers have reported survival rates of up to 86% [31]. Overall survival is probably greatly influenced by patient age, with data from the European Transplant Registry showing 1- and 5-year survival of 51 and 42% in patients older than 60 years [29].

3.1. Factors influencing the results

Multiple factors have been associated with the outcome of patients who receive a LT due to ALF. Three studies [4, 32, 33] have identified a recipient age above 45–50 years as a poor prognostic factor, attributing this to the reduction in physiologic reserve with effect from these ages [4]. A body mass index (BMI) >29 was identified in one study [32]. On the other hand, no specific factor associated with the severity of the ALF, such as coagulopathy, has been found to be associated with a poor prognosis, although the degree of kidney failure, mechanical ventilation, and the use of inotropic drugs were found to be predictive factors in these studies.

Such donor characteristics as age >60 years, ABO incompatibility [34, 35], and the use of a split or small liver have also been related with worse results [18, 36].

Survival has improved greatly over the last decade. This is the result of better management of ALF patients, leading to a lower incidence of pretransplant complications (e.g., renal failure, respiratory problems, sepsis), a lower grade of encephalopathy, and the use of more isogroup grafts. Identification of prognostic factors as well as the creation of transplant indication criteria like the Clichy [37] or King's College [16] criteria has also contributed to this improvement. The earlier indication for transplant, which in turn contributes to the use of more compatible organs and the patient receiving the transplant in better conditions, has been the foundation for the improvement in results over recent years.

The rapid localization of organs for transplant in ALF patients is an important factor that has also contributed greatly to the better results. In countries like Spain, with a high donation rate, it proves relatively easy to find a compatible organ fairly quickly, with 50% of these patients receiving a transplant within 24 h of becoming active on the waiting list, while the mean time to transplant is 40 h. In Spain this has resulted in only around 7% of ALF patients dying while still on the waiting list compared with 30% in the USA [38].

Thus, the optimal selection of candidates for transplant plus the identification of poor prognostic factors and the exclusion of those patients who will not benefit from LT due to their situation have contributed to the improved results. The development of extracorporeal bio-artificial systems, improved organ procurement, and the use of organs from living donors can all contribute to future improvements.

4. Conclusion

Acute liver failure is a potentially severe clinical condition that is associated with a high rate of mortality. Selection of those patients who will benefit from a liver transplant should be based on the early identification of prognostic factors. Survival of patients who receive a transplant due to ALF has improved over recent years, though it is still somewhat lower than that of patients who receive a LT for other reasons.

Conflict of interest

The authors have no conflict of interest to declare.

Author details

Rocío González Grande and Miguel Jiménez Pérez*

*Address all correspondence to: mjimenezp@commalaga.com

Department of Gastroenterology and Hepatology, Liver Transplantation Unit, Regional University Hospital, Málaga, Spain

References

[1] O'Grady JG, Schalm SW, Williams R. Acute liver failure: Redefining the syndromes. Lancet. 1993;**342**:273-275

[2] Polson J, Lee WM. American Association for the Study of Liver Disease. AASLD position paper: The management of acute liver failure. Hepatology. 2005;**41**:1179-1197

[3] Koch DG, Speiser JL, Durkalski V, Fontana RJ, Darven T, McGuire B, et al. The natural history of severe acute liver injury. The American Journal of Gastroenterology. 2017;**112**:1389-1396

[4] Germani G, Theocharidou E, Adam R, Karam V, Wendon J, O'Grady J, et al. Liver transplantation for acute liver failure in Europe: Outcomes over 20 years from the ELTR database. Journal of Hepatology. 2012;**57**:288-296

[5] Lee WM. Etiologies of acute liver failure. Seminars in Liver Disease. 2008;**28**:142-152

[6] Lee WM, Stravitz RT, Larson AM. Introduction to the revised American Association for the Study of the Liver Diseases Position Paper on acute liver failure 2011. Hepatology. 2012;**55**:965-967

[7] Bernuau J, Rueff B, Benhamou JP. Fulminant and subfulminant liver failure: Definitions and causes. Seminars in Liver Disease. 1986;**6**:97-106

[8] Cardoso FS, Marcelino P, Bagulho L, Karvellas CJ. Acute liver failure: An up to date approach. Journal of Critical Care. 2017;**39**:25-30

[9] Castaldo ET, Chari RS. Liver transplantation for acute hepatic failure. HPB Journal. 2006;**8**:29-34

[10] Ostapowicz G, Fontana RJ, Schidodt FV, Larson A, Davern TJ, Han SH, et al. Results of a prospective study of acute liver failure at 17 tertiary care centers in the United States. Annals of Internal Medicine. 2002;**137**(12):947-954

[11] Hoofnagle JH, Carithers RL Jr, Shapiro C, Ascher N. Fulminant hepatic failure: Summary of workshop. Hepatology. 1995;**21**:240-252

[12] Singanayagam A, Bernal W. Update on acute liver failure. Current Opinion in Critical Care. 2015;**21**:134-141

[13] Baker A, Dhawan A, Heaton N. Who needs a liver transplant? (New disease specific indications). Archives of Disease in Childhood. 1998;**79**:460-464

[14] Herrine SK, Moayyedi P, Brown RS, Falck-Ytter YT. American Gastroenterological Association Institute technical review on initial testing and management of acute liver disease. Gastroenterology. 2017;**152**:648-664

[15] European Association for the Study of the Liver. EASL clinical practical guidelines of the management of acute (fulminant) liver failure. Journal of Hepatology. 2017;**66**:1047-1081

[16] O'Grady JG, Alexander GJ, Hayllar KM, Williams R. Early indicators of prognosis in fulminant hepatic failure. Gastroenteroogy. 1989;**97**:439-445

[17] Bailey B, Amre DK, Gaudreault P. Fulminant hepatic failure secondary to acetaminophen poisoning: A systematic review and meta-analysis of prognostic criteria determining the need for liver transplantation. Critical Care Medicine. 2003;**31**:299-305

[18] McPhail MJ, Wendon JA, Bernal W. Meta-analysis of performance of King's College Hospital Criteria in prediction of outcome in non-paracetamol-induced acute liver failure. Journal of Hepatology. 2010;**53**:492-499

[19] Bernal W, Donaldson N, Wyncoll D, Wendon J. Blood lactate as an early predictor of outcome in paracetamol-induced acute liver failure: A cohort study. Lancet. 2002;**359**: 558-563

[20] Gow PJ, Warrilow S, Lontos S, Lubel J, Wongseelashote S, GC MQ, et al. Time to review the selection criteria for transplantation in paracetamol-induced fulminant hepatic failure? Liver Transplantation. 2007;**13**:1762-1763

[21] Bernau J, Godeau A, Poynard T, Dubois F, Lesage G, Yvonnet B, Degott C, et al. Multivariate analysis of prognostic factors in fulminant hepatitis B. Hepatology. 1986;**6**:648-651

[22] Pawles A, Mostefa-Kara N, Florent C, Levy VG. Emergency liver transplantation for acute liver failure: Evaluation of London and Clichy criteria. Journal of Hepatology. 1993;**17**:124-127

[23] Zaman MB, Hoti E, Qasim A, Maguire D, PA MC, Hegarty JE, et al. MELD score as a prognostic model for listing acute liver failure patients for liver transplantation. Transplantation Proceedings. 2006;**38**:2097-2098

[24] Flamm SL, Yu-X Y, Singh S, Falck-Ytter YT, The AGA Institute Clinical Guidelines Committee. American Gastroenterological Association Institute Guidelines for the diagnosis and management of acute liver failure. Gastroenterology. 2017;**152**:644-647

[25] Feng HL, Li Q, Wang GY, Cao WK. Indocyanine green clearance test combined with MELD score in predicting short-term prognosis of patients with acute liver failure. Hepatobiliary & Pancreatic Diseases International. 2014;**13**:271-275

[26] Mitchell I, Bihari D, Chang R, Wendon J, Williams R. Early identification of patient at risk of acetaminophen-induced acute liver failure. Critical Care Medicine. 1998;**26**:279-284

[27] Rutherford A, King LY, Hynan LS, Vedvyas C, Lin W, Lee WM, et al. Development of an accurate index for predicting outcomes of patients with acute liver failure. Gastroenterology. 2012 Nov;**143**(5):1237-1243. DOI: 10.1053/j.gastro.2012.07.113

[28] O'Grady J. Timing and benefit of liver transplantation in acute liver failure. Journal of Hepatology. 2014;**60**:663-670

[29] Disponible. Available from: www.eltr.org [Accessed: October 2017]

[30] Lee WM, Larson AM, Stravitz RT. Introduction to the Revised American Association for the Study of Liver Diseases Position Paper on Acute Liver Failure 2011. Hepatology. 2012;**55**(3):965-967. DOI: 10.1002/hep.25551

[31] Bernal W, Hyyryainen A, Gera A, Audimoolam VK, MJW MP, Auzinger G, et al. Lessons from look-back in acute liver failure? A single centre experience of 3300 patients. Journal of Hepatology. 2013;**59**:74-80

[32] Barshes NR, Lee TC, Balkrishnan R, Karpen SJ, Carter BA, Goss JA, et al. Risk stratification of adult patients undergoing orthotopic liver transplantation for fulminant hepatic failure. Transplantation. 2006;**81**:195-201

[33] Bernal W, Cross TJS, Auzinger G, Sizer E, Heneghan MA, Bowles M, et al. Outcome after wait-listing for emergency liver transplantation in acute liver failure: A single centre experience. Journal of Hepatology. 2009;**50**:306-313

[34] Toso C, Al-Qahtani M, Alsaif FA. ABO-incompatible liver transplantation for critically ill adult patients. Transplant International. 2007;**20**:675-681

[35] Registro Español de Trasplante Hepático. Memoria de resultados 2015. Available from: http://www.ont.es/infesp/ Paginas/RegistroHepatico.aspx [Accessed October 1, 2017]

[36] Neuberger J, Gimson A, Davies M, Akyol M, O'Grady J, Burroughs A, et al. Selection of patients for liver transplantation and allocation of donated livers in the UK. Gut. 2008;**57**:252-257

[37] Bernuau J, Samuel D, Durand R, Saliba M, Bourliere M, Adam R, et al. Criteria for emergency liver transplantation with acute viral hepatitis and factor V level <50% of normal: A prospective study [abstract]. Hepatology. 1991;**14**:49

[38] Escorsell A, Mas A, De la Mata M, the Spanish Group for the Study of acute Liver Failure. Acute liver failure in Spain: Análisis of 267 cases. Liver Transplantation. 2007;**13**:1389-1395

2

Portal Vein Thrombosis in Liver Cirrhosis

Shuai Xue, Peisong Wang, Hui Han and
Guang Chen

Abstract

In liver cirrhosis, portal vein thrombosis (PVT), which is defined as thrombosis that occurs within the main portal vein and intrahepatic portal branches, is one of the most common complications. High incidence of PVT in the setting of liver cirrhosis is mainly due to hypercoagulable state and altered dynamic of blood flow in the portal vein. The clinical manifestations of PVT are variable among different patients, so the diagnosis of PVT is mainly dependent on the imaging examinations, like ultrasound, computed tomography and magnetic resonance imaging. The overall goal of treatment for PVT can be summarized as reducing risk factors of PVT, thus to prevent further expansion of thrombus and maintain portal patency and prevent and treat the symptoms of PVT by anticoagulants, local thrombolysis, transjugular intrahepatic portosystemic shunt and/ or surgery. In future, due to the progress in vascular imaging and innovation in clinical anti-thrombotic drug, PVT could be prevented and cured effectively.

Keywords: portal vein thrombosis, cirrhosis, management, anticoagulant

1. Introduction

Portal vein thrombosis (PVT) is diagnosed when a venous thrombosis occurs within the main portal vein and intrahepatic portal branches [1, 2]. In liver cirrhosis, especially in advanced stages, PVT is one of the most common complications [3–5]. High incidence of PVT in the setting of liver cirrhosis is mainly due to hypercoagulable state and altered dynamics of blood flow in the portal vein [6–8]. Moreover, PVT will deteriorate liver cirrhosis by increasing portal vein pressure and decreasing blood flow into liver. Under severe circumstances, it will worsen symptoms of cirrhosis such as ascites, upper gastrointestinal bleeding, intestinal avascular necrosis and so on [3, 4, 9–11]. However, 30–50% patients with PVT will spontaneously alleviate or recover without any treatment [4, 10, 12, 13]. This highlights the over-diagnosis of PVT in cirrhosis and questions whether PVT treatment will benefit cirrhotic patients, especially when they are diagnosed incidentally on imaging. Right now, there is no guideline or expert consensus on how to manage cirrhotic patients with PVT. A meta-analysis which includes 3735 cirrhotic patients demonstrated that PVT negatively influenced both mortality and hepatic decompensation, despite its limitation of including heterogeneous populations [14]. However, another prospective multicenter study which includes 863 Child-Pugh class A and 380 class B cirrhotic patients found PVT was not a prognostic factor for either mortality or hepatic decompensation [15]. A study that only investigated 42 cirrhotic patients with extrahepatic nonmalignant partial PVT reported that no association was found between progression or regression of partial PVT and clinical outcomes. The model for end-stage liver disease (MELD) score, rather than PVT, was the predictor of worse prognosis in cirrhotic patients [16]. So, at present, the issue of whether PVT does or does not have influence on the natural history of cirrhosis is still controversial [17–19].

2. Prevalence

The prevalence and incidence of PVT in cirrhosis often varies from 1 to 28% among different studies depending on heterogeneity in diagnosis methods, different populations and variable follow-up time [16–22]. In a retrospective study of 150 patients with viral cirrhosis, the cumulative overall incidences of PVT were 12.8% at 1 year, 18.6% at 3 years, 20% at 5 years and 38.7% at 8–10 years, respectively [23]. In another study, which includes 701 cirrhosis patients without hepatocellular carcinoma, the incidence of PVT was 11.2% since they used ultrasound for diagnosis routinely [24]. PVT is more common in advanced cirrhosis and the incidence is positively related with the stage of cirrhosis, which is only 1% in compensated patients but 8.4% in severe cirrhosis waiting for liver transplantation [21, 25–28]. However, there are some limitations in these studies which weaken the magnitude and reliability of these conclusions like different subgroup patients and follow-up times as we previously mentioned. Violi et al. reported a study aimed at evaluating the prevalence of PVT in a broad spectrum of patients with cirrhosis and found 17% of 753 cirrhotic patients had PVT [29]. A multicenter randomized trial that includes 898 well-compensated cirrhosis patients reported that the 5-year cumulative incidence of PVT was 11.9% [30].

3. Pathophysiology

3.1. Hypercoagulable state of blood flow

After liver transplantation, the number of platelets will increase temporarily for a short time, which contributes to the hypercoagulable state of blood [31, 32]. That would be one of the significant reasons for PVT formation in liver transplantation patients. The study showed that surgery not only increased blood platelets but also activated their surface glycoprotein CD62P, reflecting the degree of platelet activation and causing a hypercoagulable state [33, 34]. Postoperative-elevated CD62P is closely related with PVT, which can be used as a sensitive diagnostic biomarker of PVT [9, 35, 36]. Toshiki Matsui also reported that soluble form of glycoprotein VI, as a platelet activation marker, was associated with PVT formation after hepatectomy and splenectomy in patients with liver cirrhosis [37]. Another study from Poland found platelet aggregability was decreased in PVT patients [31]. In another logistic regression model, incidence of PVT was highly related with D-dimer and bilirubin [38, 39]. Additionally, increased whole blood viscosity due to increased number of erythrocytes and ability of aggregation as well as decreased deformability may be reasons for increased PVT formation [34, 40]. Both procoagulant and anticoagulant proteins decreased in liver cirrhosis patients at the same time, owing to decreased synthesis function of the liver, which often largely maintained in a dynamic balance [7, 8, 34, 41]. Therefore, the body is neither to bleed nor to form thrombosis. However, after liver transplantation surgery, venous injury would reduce the flow rate of portal vein; thus, anticoagulant-associated protein S and C decreased as well as anti-thrombin III [21]. Meanwhile, surgery consumes numerous coagulation factors. Factor VIII, VII factor-related antigens and anti-cardiolipin antibody increased, which both resulted in PVT formation. Factor VIII concentration and the ratio of the most powerful procoagulant (factor VIII) and anticoagulant (protein C) were considered as markers to indicate hypercoagulability [25, 38, 42–44]. Studies showed factor VIII was related to PVT in cirrhotic patients independently. Patients with factor VIII level above 129 IU/dl had six times the probability to PVT [45]. Some researchers reported in the literature that procoagulant gene mutations, including coagulation factor V Leiden G1691A, methylenetetrahydrofolate reductase C677T and prothrombin G20210A, may be associated with PVT [46, 47]. Recent studies showed that increased hemagglutinin activated fibrinolysin inhibition gene mutation and blood coagulation factor VII, which were closely related to the occurrence of PVT [1, 2].

3.2. Hemodynamic changes in the portal vein

PVT formation is associated with intrahepatic resistance and poor portal blood flow. Moreover, portal blood flow decreases more if cirrhosis progresses. That's why the incidence of PVT is much higher in advanced-stage cirrhotic patients compared with well-compensated ones [48]. Cirrhotic patients with PVT had low portal flow volumes and high collateral vessel flow velocity. Intraoperative clamp and squeeze will cause vein intimal injury, collagen exposure and activation of the coagulation system. After liver transplantation, blood flow in portal vein is relatively slow, which is easy to form turbulence and thrombosis [9, 25, 49, 50]. Portal vein blood flow velocity and PVT have an important relationship. Studies demonstrated that patients with portal vein blood flow <15 cm/s had higher incidence of PVT [17, 27, 50–52]. So, some researchers often regarded portal vein diameter as an independent risk factor for the formation of PVT. In short, because there are various changes in portal hemodynamics, the incidence of PVT is quite high after liver transplantation.

3.3. Endotoxinemia

Cirrhosis is more likely to damage intestinal mucosal barrier which facilitates bacterial translocation and endotoxinemia [53]. Endotoxinemia not only can increase portal vein pressure but also can activate coagulation cascade. That explains why it can increase the PVT incidence in the portal system [54].

4. Diagnosis

4.1. Clinical manifestations

A study which includes 79 cirrhotic patients has shown that 57% of PVT were symptomatic and among them 39% had gastrointestinal bleeding and 70% had intestinal infarction [24]. Abdominal pain is generally the earliest clinical symptom after the acute formation of PVT. Usually, abdominal pain is limited within a specific region while few are diffuse pain and intermittent colic pain with longer durations. Nausea and vomiting occur in 50% of PVT patients [3, 4, 51, 55–57]. A few patients will have diarrhea or bloody stool. If complete intestinal obstruction occurs suddenly, abdominal pain is paroxysmal accompanied by significant nausea, vomiting without fart and defecation. Under this circumstance, there are no obvious physical examination signs, that the degree of pain is not consistent with the signs of the abdomen [19, 58, 59]. Increased anterior hepatic obstructive factors will cause decreased portal vein blood flow which aggravates liver damage, increases portal pressure, causes repeated upper gastrointestinal bleeding and refractory ascites and so on. In some severe cases, clinical manifestations of intestinal necrosis such as persistent abdominal pain, bloating, hemafecia, hematemesis, shock and peritoneal irritation will occur [18, 24, 26]. Abdominal puncture can be bloody ascites. In the event of intestinal necrosis, disease mortality rate can rise to 20–60%. Patients often suffer from persistent abdominal pain, hemafecia, abdominal cramps, ascites, multiple organ failure and so on. For chronic PVT, patients will have refractory bloating, diarrhea, upper abdominal pain and ascites due to gastrointestinal congestion and insufficient perfusion of liver portal vein [24]. The clinical manifestations of PVT are variable among different patients, so the clinical diagnosis of PVT is mainly dependent on the imaging examination.

4.2. Imaging

Ultrasound, the most common imaging way, is simple and easy to accurately evaluate PVT [60]. Thus, it is the preferred imaging method for diagnosis. Ultrasound diagnosis of PVT is characterized by abnormal echo in the portal vein, unclear boundary with the wall, CDFI: no blood flow signal, portal venous cavernous hemangioma; portal vein expansion before thrombosis site; and no display of portal vein if PVT is formed within a wide range [11, 17, 18, 60, 61]. The sensitivity and specificity of ultrasonography to diagnose PVT are up to 60 and 100% [60, 62]. Ultrasound can clearly demonstrate the blood flow, vascular diameter and the changes and the presence of thrombi. Ultrasound can also determine the formation of collateral circulation simultaneously through CDFI. But the ultrasound cannot reflect directly the situation of the portal vein and its branches, and the experience of the operator affects the accuracy of the diagnosis. Ultrasound angiography or ultrasound endoscopy can diagnose PVT more accurately that even raises the diagnostic sensitivity to 81% [24]. Some authors recommended contrasting enhanced ultrasound as the first-line imaging and "gold standard method" for the diagnosis of PVT [63, 64]. But ultrasound angiography and endoscopy also have some limitations. Firstly, they cannot evaluate the portal vein within the part of the liver and superior mesenteric vein end accurately. Moreover, they cannot assess the surrounding organs which may be affected by PVT [50, 63, 64].

Enhanced computer tomography (CT) or enhanced magnetic resonance imaging (MRI) examination by intravenous injection contrast can effectively solve the above deficiencies. By comparison with contrast, we can discover intraluminal filling defects and perfusion conditions for nearby organs at different times of the imaging process. CT angiography (CTA) and magnetic resonance angiography (MRA) greatly increase the accuracy of diagnosis. Some studies have showed that the sensitivity and the specificity for CTA were 86 and 95%. For MRA, the sensitivity was 100% and specificity was 98% [60, 65–67]. Typical CT signs of PVT are very intuitive: no-enhanced low-density intraluminal stripe or massive lesions within portal static. Occasionally, CT can also find an enhanced ring around thrombus due to nourishing small blood vessels. Moreover, CT can also help to diagnose primary liver cancer, cirrhosis and evaluate intestinal ischemia and necrosis. CTA has several advantages including short scan time, fast imaging speed and reduced motion artifact [67]. However, its main drawbacks can be related to some complications like contrast agent allergy, contrast agent nephropathy and other adverse reactions. The safety of MRA contrast is significantly better than that of CTA. But MRA has the same disadvantages like motion artifacts, long-signal acquisition time and limited imaging range [66]. Therefore, patients with suspicious PVT should be enrolled in contract CT or MRI imaging, which can be more accurate for clinical diagnosis.

Angiography is the traditional method for diagnosis of PVT. It is not the routine examination of PVT because of its invasive feature. Angiography includes two categories: indirect and direct. Indirect angiography is through splenic artery and superior mesenteric artery to image [2, 65]. In this way, we can see the portal vein filling defect as well as the collateral circulation. The most important thing is we can put the catheter into the superior mesenteric artery and/or splenic artery branch to infuse thrombolytic drugs after indirect angiography. It means we can finish diagnosis and follow treatment after invasive process at one time. Direct angiography is divided into: percutaneous transhepatic portal angiography, which can display directly portal vein system and evaluate portal hemodynamics, and umbilical portal vein angiography, which is indicated for splenic vein thrombosis, spleen resection and failure of arterial portal angiography [50].

4.3. Laboratory tests

Usually, prothrombin time (PT) and activated partial thromboplastin time (APTT) were used as predictors for the coagulation state with cirrhosis, and even the predictive ability was poor [7, 34, 68]. Because they could not explain and represent natural anticoagulants such as antithrombin and protein C in vivo, the thrombin generation test, which used tissue factor as trigger and phospholipids as platelet substitutes, was considered more appropriate for evaluating thrombin generation. The test was regarded as representation of the balance between the pro- and anticoagulant proteins in plasma [33, 44]. Another test named thromboelastography (TEG) can monitor all kinds of hemostatic functions (coagulation, anticoagulation, fibrinolysis) continuously to predict thrombosis formation and dissolution dynamically. This test also emphasized the dynamic assessment of balanced status in blood coagulation and anticoagulation process [17, 18]. This is a new laboratory test to evaluate whether the blood is hypercoagulable, whether there is the formation of thrombus and whether the thrombus is stable. The effectiveness of clinical application needs to be further studied. Additionally, we can exclude PVT patients with a 90% negative predictive value when the D-dimer level is less than 1.82 mg/l [38, 39, 69, 70]. Systemic evaluation of coagulation tests, including PT, international standardization ratio, partial thromboplastin time, and so on, could not fully assess the patient's coagulation abnormalities. Dynamic monitoring of vitamin K-related coagulation factors, fibrinogen, platelet function, fibrinolysis status as well as other coagulation factors simultaneously is essential.

5. Classification

According to PVT imaging findings preoperatively, Yerdel found a classification system as the following: grade I, <50% portal vein obstruction with or without micro-thrombus of the superior mesenteric vein; grade II, >50% portal vein obstruction with or without micro-thrombus of the superior mesenteric vein; grade III, complete portal vein and proximal superior mesenteric vein obstruction; and grade IV, complete portal vein and entire superior mesenteric vein obstruction [71].

6. PVT treatment

The overall goal of treatment for PVT can be summarized as reducing risk factors of PVT, thus to prevent further expansion of thrombus and maintain portal patency, prevent and treat the symptoms of PVT. For acute PVT, the aim is to prevent thrombus extension and intestinal infarction, whereas for chronic PVT, it is to prevent recurrent thrombosis, gastrointestinal bleeding and portal cholangiopathy [20, 35, 51].

6.1. Non-surgical treatment

The incidence of PVT is high in cirrhotic patients, but clinical studies found that 30–50% of patients with PVT could alleviate without any treatment. Longest diameter of portal vein and blood flow of the largest collateral circulation vein were closely related with the incidence of spontaneous alleviation in PVT patients [1, 21]. But another study demonstrated that untreated PVT was associated with increased mortality, especially in patients with low Child-Pugh scores. And there were strong correlations between anticoagulation therapy and lower thrombus progress rate as well as higher recanalization rate [11, 72, 73]. Furthermore, PVT has been reported as an independent risk factor for recurrent and refractory acute variceal bleeding [23, 74]. There is inconsistent guidance on the anticoagulant management of PVT. However, once the PVT is diagnosed, the optimal time of prevention and treatment often has been missed. Serious complications would increase mortality greatly for PVT patients. So, it is recommended for cirrhotic patients that routine color Doppler ultrasound assessment should be performed. Early diagnosis, early anticoagulant and thrombolytic therapy can effectively improve the prognosis of patients. A meta-analysis from Italy, which includes 8 studies comprising 353 patients with cirrhosis and PVT, demonstrated anticoagulant therapy (low-weight heparin or warfarin) could increase recanalization and reduce progression of thrombosis effectively [75]. Meanwhile, these anticoagulants will not increase the incidence of any kinds of bleedings [75]. Another study from Italy found the benefits patients got overweighed the potential minor bleeding risk [76]. And they also concluded that portal hypertension, rather than anticoagulants, would be the real reason for the risk of major bleeding among cirrhotic patients with PVT. A prospective study from China which focused on patients with cirrhosis undergoing elective transjugular intrahepatic portosystemic shunt (TIPS) found that warfarin treatment within 12 months achieved a much higher rate of complete recanalization [77]. The commonly used drugs include warfarin, low molecular weight heparin and urokinase[78–81]. Most patients with acute PVT were recommended early anticoagulant therapy at least for 6 months. A systematic review and meta-analysis that summarized different regiments of anticoagulation has been reported [82]. In this study, the overall rate of portal vein recanalization was 37–93% and the anti-coagulation related bleeding was 0–18% [82]. In this way, we can not only reduce the incidence of PVT greatly but also increase PVT recanalization rate up to 39.3–100.0%.

In recent years, inhibitors of activated factor Xa (e.g., rivaroxaban) have been used in the prevention of clinical PVT. The advantages are convenient oral administration, no effect on the international standardization ratio and no need to monitor blood coagulation indicators. Hyeyoung Yang et al. reported a 63-year-old female who experienced complete resolution of recurrent acute PVT in liver cirrhosis after rivaroxaban treatment [83]. The disadvantage is there is no effective antagonist. When bleeding happens during anticoagulant therapy, the consequence is serious. However, some new oral anticoagulants' antidotes have been under investigation like andexanet alfa, P-glycoprotein substrates and drugs inducing CYP3A4. They all could inhibit the concentration or absorption of new oral anticoagulants and attenuate their effects remarkably [83, 84].

In short, clinical non-surgical methods are still mainly treatments of PVT in cirrhotic patients.

6.2. Local thrombolytic treatment

Local thrombolysis is divided into indirect way (femoral artery-superior mesenteric artery indwelling catheter thrombolysis) and direct way (percutaneous transhepatic portal vein thrombolysis) [13, 17, 18, 27, 35, 56, 85].

The advantages of the femoral artery-superior mesenteric artery catheter thrombolysis are simple and relative small trauma. It is just suitable for mild PVT without vascular occlusion. Because when PVT is found by this method, portal vein branches are usually in the stenosis or occlusion state by obstruction of thrombosis. Most of the drugs we injected for thrombolysis cannot reach the site of thrombus effectively. So, indications of this method are limited.

The advantages of the percutaneous transhepatic portal vein thrombolysis method are simple and show high success rates. However, we must stop this treatment when the patient has: (1) APTT significantly longer; (2) the international standardization ratio > 2; and (3) obvious abdominal pain, bloating, vomiting, hemafecia, increased puncture-point bleeding, more subcutaneous ecchymosis, hemoglobin continuing to decrease, faster heart rate, lower blood pressure and other signs of active bleeding.

6.3. TIPS

When severe PVT happened, thrombus blocked more than 50% lumen or completely blocked, anticoagulant therapy was unlikely to recanalization. Under this condition, we can choose TIPS. This method has the advantages as the following: the risk of thrombolysis is relatively small, and punctures can often reach directly to the thrombus site; at the same time intravascular technology (balloon plasty, stent replacement, thrombectomy and thrombolytic therapy surgery) can be applied to achieve the goal of treatment of PVT. A study from China which compared transcatheter selective superior mesenteric artery urokinase infusion and TIPS has found they were safe and effective for acute symptomatic PVT in cirrhosis [86]. But the operation was a relative difficult and lethal event as well as severe complications were still possible, so it is particularly important to assess the risk-benefit ratio of TIPS preoperatively. At present, the TIPS therapy methods for PVT are the following [87–89]:

A. TIPS placement → portosystemic shunt → portal vein recanalization;

B. TIPS placement through percutaneous ways portal vein recanalization;

C. TIPS placement between hepatic vein and collateral vessel → no portal vein recanalization

For cirrhotic patients with refractory variceal bleeding and ascites, TIPS was considered as one of the major treatment strategies if the patient did not have PVT. PVT has changed natural history of liver cirrhosis and affected outcomes. So, in this circumstance, TIPS should be recommended with caution. No convincing evidence has been published to verify the superiority of TIPS over traditional anticoagulants. TIPS should only be recommended for severe PVT patients although technical difficulty rose sharply when severe PVT was diagnosed [89]. That means reliable predictors for PVT progression should be further investigated in future.

6.4. Surgical treatment of PVT

Surgery is relatively high risk. The commonly used methods are (1) PVT excision; (2) portal vein stent implantation, mainly aimed to relieve portal vein obstruction; (3) liver transplantation. During treatment, if the patient has the sustained abdominal pain, abdominal distension and other signs of peritonitis, laparotomy exploration should be performed early to prevent the occurrence of intestinal necrosis. When intestinal necrosis is diagnosed, intestinal and mesangial resections should be performed. At the same time, the intestinal end-to-end anastomosis should be done. Anticoagulation was continued after surgery to prevent thrombus reformation.

7. PVT prevention

Kawanaka et al. have shown that anti-thrombin III (AT III) activity and splenic vein diameter were the risk factors of PVT after surgery. Moreover, they used those risk factors to formulate risk stratification system [90]. According to the risk stratification, doctors can decide whether to give prevention or not: low risk: AT III activity ≥70% and splenic vein straight diameter <10 mm, no preventive treatment; intermediate risk: AT III activity <70% or splenic

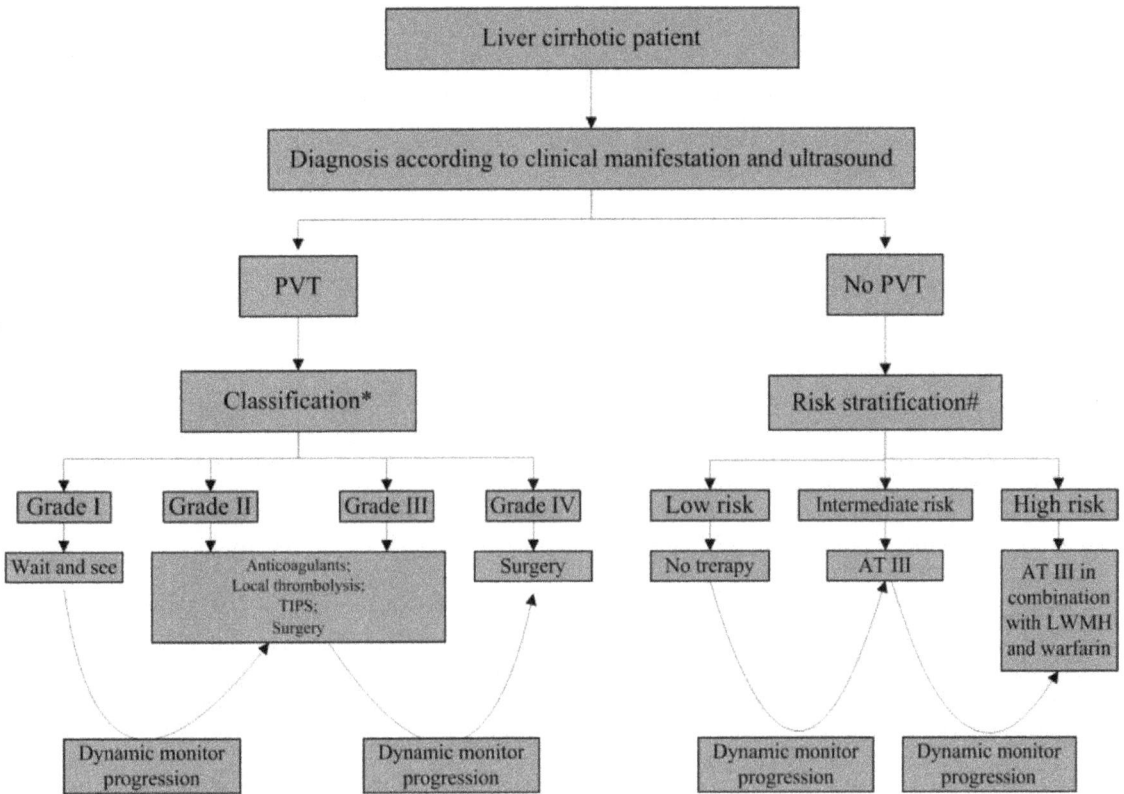

Figure 1. Algorithm for the treatment of portal vein thrombosis in liver cirrhosis. *Abbreviations*: PVT, portal vein thrombosis; TIPS, transjugular intrahepatic portosystemic shunt; AT III, anti-thrombin III therapy; LWMH, low-weight molecular heparin; *according to Yerdel's study [68]; # according to Kawanaka's study [90].

vein diameter ≥10 mm, simple AT III prevention treatment; and high risk: splenic vein diameter ≥15 mm or from the liver collateral circulation vein diameter ≥10 mm, AT III, low molecular weight heparin in conjunction with warfarin [90].

Enoxaparin was found to prevent PVT in advanced cirrhotic patients. Daily subcutaneous enoxaparin (4000 IU/day) could significantly reduce incidence of PVT in the short and long term [91, 92]. And enoxaparin can also decrease the liver decompensation rate and improve survival of patients who received liver transplantation [52, 91, 92].

Surgery on the portal vein system should be gentle and accurate. We should prevent unnecessary damage to the vascular endothelium and avoid ligation of chunk tissue. If there is no obvious bleeding tendency, surgeons should not use hemostatic after surgery which may result in thrombosis (**Figure 1**).

8. Conclusion

PVT was a clinical rare deep venous thrombosis but highly occurred in liver cirrhotic patients. Local or systemic factors alone or in combination make contribution to the formation of PVT. In clinical, PVT should be given enough attention due to its severe threat to the patient's life and health. The overall treatment principles are early diagnosis, early treatment and pre-vention combined with treatment. In the future, due to the progress in vascular imaging and innovation in clinical anti-thrombotic drug, PVT could be prevented and cured effectively.

Author details

Shuai Xue, Peisong Wang, Hui Han and Guang Chen*

*Address all correspondence to: cg9293@sina.com

The General Surgery Center, The First Hospital of Jilin University, Changchun, Jilin, China

References

[1] Chawla YK, Bodh V. Portal vein thrombosis. Journal of Clinical and Experimental Hepatology. 2015;**5**(1):22-40

[2] Basit SA, Stone CD, Gish R. Portal vein thrombosis. Clinics in Liver Disease. 2015;**19**(1):199-221

[3] Yang ZNJ, Costa KA, Novelli EM, Smith RE. Venous thromboembolism in cirrhosis. Clinical and Applied Thrombosis-Hemostasis. 2014;**20**(2):169-178

[4] Handa P, Crowther M, Douketis JD. Portal vein thrombosis: A clinician-oriented and practical review. Clinical and Applied Thrombosis-Hemostasis. 2014;**20**(5):498-506

[5] Tsochatzis EA, Bosch J, Burroughs AK. Liver cirrhosis. Lancet. 2014;**383**(9930):1749-1761

[6] Cai CC, Liu SY. A meta-analysis of portal vein thrombosis in patients with liver cirrhosis. Journal of Gastroenterology and Hepatology. 2013;**28**:847

[7] Schaden E, Saner FH, Goerlinger K. Coagulation pattern in critical liver dysfunction. Current Opinion in Critical Care. 2013;**19**(2):142-148

[8] Mucino-Bermejo J, Carrillo-Esper R, Uribe M, Mendez-Sanchez N. Coagulation abnor-malities in the cirrhotic patient. Annals of Hepatology. 2013;**12**(5):713-724

[9] Ghabril M, Agarwal S, Lacerda M, Chalasani N, Kwo P, Tector AJ. Portal vein throm-bosis is a risk factor for poor early outcomes after liver transplantation: Analysis of risk factors and outcomes for portal vein thrombosis in waitlisted patients. Transplantation. 2016;**100**(1):126-133

[10] Girleanu I, Stanciu C, Cojocariu C, Boiculese L, Singeap AM, Trifan A. Natural course of nonmalignant partial portal vein thrombosis in cirrhotic patients. Saudi Journal of Gastroenterology. 2014;**20**(5):288-292

[11] Borjas-Almaguer OD, Cortez-Hernandez CA, Gonzalez-Moreno EI, Bosques-Padilla FJ, Gonzalez-Gonzalez JA, Garza AA, et al. Portal vein thrombosis in patients with cirrhosis: Just a common finding or a predictor of poor outcome? Annals of Hepatology. 2016;**15**(6):902-906

[12] Berry K, Taylor J, Liou IW, Ioannou GN. Portal vein thrombosis is not associated with increased mortality among patients with cirrhosis. Clinical Gastroenterology and Hepatology. 2015;**13**(3):585-593

[13] Qi XS, Han GH, Fan DM. Management of portal vein thrombosis in liver cirrhosis. Nature Reviews Gastroenterology & Hepatology. 2014;**11**(7):435-446

[14] Stine JG, Shah PM, Cornella SL, Rudnick SR, Stukenborg GR, Northup P. Portal vein thrombosis, mortality and hepatic decompensation in patients with cirrhosis: A meta-analysis. Hepatology. 2015;**62**:943A-A

[15] Nery F, Chevret S, Condat B, de Raucourt E, Boudaoud L, Rautou PE, et al. Causes and consequences of portal vein thrombosis in 1,243 patients with cirrhosis: Results of a longitudinal study. Hepatology. 2015;**61**(2):660-667

[16] Luca A, Caruso S, Milazzo M, Marrone G, Mamone G, Crino F, et al. Natural course of extrahepatic nonmalignant partial portal vein thrombosis in patients with cirrhosis. Radiology. 2012;**265**(1):124-132

[17] von Kockritz L, De Gottardi A, Trebicka J, Praktiknjo M. Portal vein thrombosis in patients with cirrhosis. Gastroenterology Report. 2017;**5**(2):148-156

[18] Fujiyama S, Saitoh S, Kawamura Y, Sezaki H, Hosaka T, Akuta N, et al. Portal vein thrombosis in liver cirrhosis: Incidence, management, and outcome. BMC Gastroenterology. 2017;**17**(1):112

[19] Loudin M, Ahn J. Portal vein thrombosis in cirrhosis. Journal of Clinical Gastroenterology. 2017;**51**(7):579-585

[20] Haris M, Thachil J. The problem with incidental and chronic portal vein thrombosis. European Journal of Internal Medicine. 2017;**39**:E29-E30

[21] Chen H, Turon F, Hernandez-Gea V, Fuster J, Garcia-Criado A, Barrufet M, et al. Nontumoral portal vein thrombosis in patients awaiting liver transplantation. Liver Transplantation. 2016;**22**(3):352-365

[22] Cruz-Ramon V, Chinchilla-Lopez P, Ramirez-Perez O, Mendez-Sanchez N. Effects of portal vein thrombosis on the outcomes of liver cirrhosis: A Mexican perspective. Journal of Translational Internal Medicine. 2017;**5**(4):189-191

[23] Maruyama H, Okugawa H, Takahashi M, Yokosuka O. De novo portal vein thrombosis in virus-related cirrhosis: Predictive factors and long-term outcomes. American Journal of Gastroenterology. 2013;**108**(4):568-574

[24] Amitrano L, Guardascione MA, Brancaccio V, Margaglione M, Manguso F, Iannaccone L, et al. Risk factors and clinical presentation of portal vein thrombosis in patients with liver cirrhosis. Journal of Hepatology. 2004;**40**(5):736-741

[25] Lankarani KB, Homayon K, Motevalli D, Heidari ST, Alavian SM, Malek-Hosseini SA. Risk factors for portal vein thrombosis in patients with cirrhosis awaiting liver transplantation in shiraz, Iran. Hepatitis Monthly. 2015;**15**(12):e26407

[26] Eshraghian A, Nikeghbalian S, Kazemi K, Shamsaeefar A, SAM H. Prevalence and risk factors of portal vein thrombosis in patients with liver cirrhosis and its impact on outcomes after liver transplantation. Transplant International. 2017;**30**:146

[27] Qi XS, Li HY, Liu X, Yao H, Han GH, Hu FR, et al. Novel insights into the development of portal vein thrombosis in cirrhosis patients. Expert Review of Gastroenterology & Hepatology. 2015;**9**(11):1421-1432

[28] Francoz C, Belghiti J, Vilgrain V, Sommacale D, Paradis V, Condat B, et al. Splanchnic vein thrombosis in candidates for liver transplantation: Usefulness of screening and anticoagulation. Gut. 2005;**54**(5):691-697

[29] Violi F, Corazza RG, Caldwell SH, Perticone F, Gatta A, Angelico M, et al. Portal vein thrombosis relevance on liver cirrhosis: Italian venous thrombotic events registry. Internal and Emergency Medicine. 2016;**11**(8):1059-1066

[30] Nery FG, Chaffaut C, Condat B, de Raucourt E, Boudaoud L, Rautou PE, et al. Portal vein thrombosis (PVT) in compensated cirrhosis: A prospective cohort study on 898 patients. Hepatology. 2013;**58**:271A-272A

[31] Wosiewicz P, Zorniak M, Hartleb M, Baranski K, Onyszczuk M, Pilch-Kowalczyk J, et al. Portal vein thrombosis in cirrhosis is not associated with intestinal barrier disruption or increased platelet aggregability. Clinics and Research in Hepatology and Gastroenterology. 2016;**40**(6):722-729

[32] Colli A, Gana JC, Yap J, Adams-Webber T, Rashkovan N, Ling SC, et al. Platelet count, spleen length, and platelet count-to-spleen length ratio for the diagnosis of oesophageal varices in people with chronic liver disease or portal vein thrombosis. Cochrane Database of Systematic Reviews. 2017;**4**:CD008759

[33] Khoury T, Ayman A, Cohen J, Daher S, Shmuel C, Mizrahi M. The complex role of anticoagulation in cirrhosis: An updated review of where we are and where we are going. Digestion. 2016;**93**(2):149-159

[34] Tripodi A, Primignani M, Braham S, Chantarangkul V, Clerici M, Moia M, et al. Coagulation parameters in patients with cirrhosis and portal vein thrombosis treated sequentially with low molecular weight heparin and vitamin K antagonists. Digestive and Liver Disease. 2016;**48**(10):1208-1213

[35] Sharma AM, Zhu D, Henry Z. Portal vein thrombosis: When to treat and how? Vascular Medicine. 2016;**21**(1):61-69

[36] Dell'Era A, Seijo S. Portal vein thrombosis in cirrhotic and non cirrhotic patients: From diagnosis to treatment. Expert Opinion on Orphan Drugs. 2016;4(9):927-940

[37] Matsui T, Usui M, Wada H, Iizawa Y, Kato H, Tanemura A, et al. Platelet activation assessed by glycoprotein VI/platelet ratio is associated with portal vein thrombosis after hepatectomy and splenectomy in patients with liver cirrhosis. Clinical and Applied Thrombosis/Hemostasis. 2017;24(2):254-262. DOI: 10.1177/1076029617725600

[38] Zhang DL, Hao JY, Yang N. Value of D-dimer and protein S for diagnosis of portal vein thrombosis in patients with liver cirrhosis. Journal of International Medical Research. 2013;41(3):664-672

[39] Dai JN, Qi XS, Li HY, Guo XZ. Role of D-dimer in the development of portal vein thrombosis in liver cirrhosis: A meta-analysis. Saudi Journal of Gastroenterology. 2015;21(3):165-174

[40] Wu XM, Yao ZP, Zhao L, Zhang Y, Cao MH, Li T, et al. Phosphatidylserine on blood cells and endothelial cells contributes to the hypercoagulable state in cirrhosis. Liver International. 2016;36(12):1800-1810

[41] Cui SB, Fu ZM, Feng YM, Xie XY, Ma XW, Liu TT, et al. The disseminated intravascular coagulation score is a novel predictor for portal vein thrombosis in cirrhotic patients with hepatitis B. Thrombosis Research. 2018;161:7-11

[42] Singhal A, Karachristos A, Bromberg M, Daly E, Maloo M, Jain AK. Hypercoagulability in end-stage liver disease: Prevalence and its correlation with severity of liver disease and portal vein thrombosis. Clinical and Applied Thrombosis-Hemostasis. 2012;18(6):594-598

[43] Girolami A, Cosi E, Ferrari S, Girolami B. Heparin, coumarin, protein C, antithrombin, fibrinolysis and other clotting related resistances: Old and new concepts in blood coagulation. Journal of Thrombosis and Thrombolysis. 2018;45(1):135-141

[44] Qi XS, Chen H, Han GH. Effect of antithrombin, protein C and protein S on portal vein thrombosis in liver cirrhosis: A meta-analysis. American Journal of the Medical Sciences. 2013;346(1):38-44

[45] Martinelli I, Primignani M, Aghemo A, Reati R, Bucciarelli P, Fabris F, et al. High levels of factor VIII and risk of extra-hepatic portal vein obstruction. Journal of Hepatology. 2009;50(5):916-922

[46] Pasta L, Pasta F, D'Amico M. PAI-1 4G-4G, MTHFR 677TT, V Leiden 506Q, and Prothrombin 20210A in splanchnic vein thrombosis: Analysis of individual patient data from three prospective studies. Journal of Clinical and Experimental Hepatology. 2016;6(1):10-14

[47] Ventura P, Venturelli G, Marcacci M, Fiorini M, Marchini S, Cuoghi C, et al. Hyperhomocysteinemia and MTHFR C677T polymorphism in patients with portal vein thrombosis complicating liver cirrhosis. Thrombosis Research. 2016;141:189-195

[48] Werner KT, Sando S, Carey EJ, Vargas HE, Byrne TJ, Douglas DD, et al. Portal vein thrombosis in patients with end stage liver disease awaiting liver transplantation: Outcome of anticoagulation. Digestive Diseases and Sciences. 2013;**58**(6):1776-1780

[49] Nazzal M, Sun YF, Okoye O, Diggs L, Evans N, Osborn T, et al. Reno-portal shunt for liver transplant, an alternative inflow for recipients with grade III-IV portal vein thrombosis: Tips for a better outcome. International Journal of Surgery Case Reports. 2017;**41**:251-254

[50] Seijo S, Garcia-Criado A, Darnell A, Garcia-Pagan JC. Diagnosis and treatment of portal thrombosis in liver cirrhosis. Gastroenterologia Y Hepatologia. 2012;**35**(9):660-666

[51] Manzano-Robleda MD, Barranco-Fragoso B, Uribe M, Mendez-Sanchez N. Portal vein thrombosis: What is new? Annals of Hepatology. 2015;**14**(1):20-27

[52] Mancuso A. Management of portal vein thrombosis in cirrhosis: An update. European Journal of Gastroenterology & Hepatology. 2016;**28**(7):739-743

[53] Lin RS, Lee FY, Lee SD, Tsai YT, Lin HC, Lu RH, et al. Endotoxemia in patients with chronic liver-diseases—Relationship to severity of liver-diseases, presence of esophageal-varices, and hyperdynamic circulation. Journal of Hepatology. 1995;**22**(2):165-172

[54] Rosenqvist K, Eriksson LG, Rorsman F, Sangfelt P, Nyman R. Endovascular treatment of acute and chronic portal vein thrombosis in patients with cirrhotic and non-cirrhotic liver. Acta Radiologica. 2016;**57**(5):572-579

[55] Buresi M, Hull R, Coffin CS. Venous thromboembolism in cirrhosis: A review of the literature. Canadian Journal of Gastroenterology. 2012;**26**(12):905-908

[56] Llop E, Seijo S. Treatment of non-cirrhotic, non-tumoural portal vein thrombosis. Gastroenterologia Y Hepatologia. 2016;**39**(6):403-410

[57] Ambrosino P, Tarantino L, Di Minno G, Paternoster M, Graziano V, Petitto M, et al. The risk of venous thromboembolism in patients with cirrhosis a systematic review and meta-analysis. Thrombosis and Haemostasis. 2017;**117**(1):139-148

[58] Harding DJ, Perera M, Chen F, Olliff S, Tripathi D. Portal vein thrombosis in cirrhosis: Controversies and latest developments. World Journal of Gastroenterology. 2015;**21**(22):6769-6784

[59] Cagin YF, Atayan Y, Erdogan MA, Dagtekin F, Colak C. Incidence and clinical presentation of portal vein thrombosis in cirrhotic patients. Hepatobiliary & Pancreatic Diseases International. 2016;**15**(5):499-503

[60] Margini C, Berzigotti A. Portal vein thrombosis: The role of imaging in the clinical setting. Digestive and Liver Disease. 2017;**49**(2):113-120

[61] Stine JG, Wang J, Shah PM, Argo CK, Intagliata N, Uflacker A, et al. Decreased portal vein velocity is predictive of the development of portal vein thrombosis: A matched case-control study. Liver International. 2018;**38**(1):94-101

[62] Alam S, Pervez R. Validity of colour doppler sonography for evaluation of portal venous system in hepatocellular carcinoma. Journal of the Pakistan Medical Association. 2013;**63**(3):365-368

[63] Danila M, Sporea I, Popescu A, Sirli R. Portal vein thrombosis in liver cirrhosis— The added value of contrast enhanced ultrasonography. Medical Ultrasonography. 2016;**18**(2):218-223

[64] Tarantino L, Ambrosino P, Di Minno MND. Contrast-enhanced ultrasound in differentiating malignant from benign portal vein thrombosis in hepatocellular carcinoma. World Journal of Gastroenterology. 2015;**21**(32):9457-9460

[65] Berzigotti A, Garcia-Criado A, Darnell A, Garcia-Pagan JC. Imaging in clinical decision-making for portal vein thrombosis. Nature Reviews Gastroenterology & Hepatology. 2014;**11**(5):308-316

[66] Ahn JH, Yu JS, Cho ES, Chung JJ, Kim JH, Kim KW. Diffusion-weighted MRI of malignant versus benign portal vein thrombosis. Korean Journal of Radiology. 2016;**17**(4):533-540

[67] Qi XS, Han GH, He CY, Yin ZX, Guo WG, Niu J, et al. CT features of non-malignant portal vein thrombosis: A pictorial review. Clinics and Research in Hepatology and Gastroenterology. 2012;**36**(6):561-568

[68] Qi XS, Su CP, Ren WR, Yang M, Jia J, Dai JN, et al. Association between portal vein thrombosis and risk of bleeding in liver cirrhosis: A systematic review of the literature. Clinics and Research in Hepatology and Gastroenterology. 2015;**39**(6):683-691

[69] Zhang DL, Hao JY. Evaluation of D-dimer and protein S in cirrhotic patients with portal vein thrombosis. Journal of Gastroenterology and Hepatology. 2013;**28**:909-910

[70] Dai JN, Qi XS, Peng Y, Hou Y, Chen J, Li HY, et al. Association between D-dimer level and portal venous system thrombosis in liver cirrhosis: A retrospective observational study. International Journal of Clinical and Experimental Medicine. 2015;**8**(9):15296-15301

[71] Yerdel MA, Gunson B, Mirza D, Karayalcin K, Olliff S, Buckels J, et al. Portal vein thrombosis in adults undergoing liver transplantation—Risk factors, screening, management, and outcome. Transplantation. 2000;**69**(9):1873-1881

[72] Giannini EG, Stravitz RT, Caldwell SH. Portal vein thrombosis and chronic liver disease progression: The closer you look the more you see. Hepatology. 2016;**63**(1):342-343

[73] Wang Z, Jiang MS, Zhang HL, Weng NN, Luo XF, Li X, et al. Is post-TIPS anticoagulation therapy necessary in patients with cirrhosis and portal vein thrombosis? A randomized controlled trial. Radiology. 2016;**279**(3):943-951

[74] Abdel-Razik A, Mousa N, Elhelaly R, Tawfik A. De-novo portal vein thrombosis in liver cirrhosis: Risk factors and correlation with the model for end-stage liver disease scoring system. European Journal of Gastroenterology & Hepatology. 2015;**27**(5):585-592

[75] Loffredo L, Pastori D, Farcomeni A, Violi F. Effects of anticoagulants in patients with cirrhosis and portal vein thrombosis: A systematic review and meta-analysis. Gastroenterology. 2017;**153**(2):480

[76] Naeshiro N, Aikata H, Hyogo H, Kan H, Fujino H, Kobayashi T, et al. Efficacy and safety of the anticoagulant drug, danaparoid sodium, in the treatment of portal vein thrombosis in patients with liver cirrhosis. Hepatology Research. 2015;**45**(6):656-662

[77] Qi XS, He CY, Guo WG, Yin ZX, Wang JH, Wang ZY, et al. Transjugular intrahepatic portosystemic shunt for portal vein thrombosis with variceal bleeding in liver cirrhosis: Outcomes and predictors in a prospective cohort study. Liver International. 2016;**36**(5):667-676

[78] De Gottardi A, Trebicka J, Klinger C, Plessier A, Seijo S, Terziroli B, et al. Antithrombotic treatment with direct-acting oral anticoagulants in patients with splanchnic vein thrombosis and cirrhosis. Liver International. 2017;**37**(5):694-699

[79] Jairath V, Burroughs AK. Anticoagulation in patients with liver cirrhosis: Complication or therapeutic opportunity? Gut. 2013;**62**(4):479-482

[80] Leonardi F, De Maria N, Villa E. Anticoagulation in cirrhosis: A new paradigm? Clinical and Molecular Hepatology. 2017;**23**(1):13-21

[81] Dhar A, Mullish BH, Thursz MR. Anticoagulation in chronic liver disease. Journal of Hepatology. 2017;**66**(6):1313-1326

[82] Qi XS, De Stefano V, Li HY, Dai J, Guo XX, Fan DM. Anticoagulation for the treatment of portal vein thrombosis in liver cirrhosis: A systematic review and meta-analysis of observational studies. European Journal of Internal Medicine. 2015;**26**(1):23-29

[83] Lenz K, Dieplinger B, Buder R, Piringer P, Rauch M, Voglmayr M. Successful treatment of partial portal vein thrombosis (PVT) with low dose rivaroxaban. Zeitschrift Fur Gastroenterologie. 2014;**52**(10):1175-1177

[84] Yang H, Kim SR, Song MJ. Recurrent acute portal vein thrombosis in liver cirrhosis treated by rivaroxaban. Clinical and Molecular Hepatology. 2016;**22**(4):499-502

[85] Qi XS, Wang J, Chen H, Han GH, Fan DM. Nonmalignant partial portal vein thrombosis in liver cirrhosis: To treat or not to treat? Radiology. 2013;**266**(3):994-995

[86] Jiang TT, Luo XP, Sun JM, Gao J. Clinical outcomes of transcatheter selective superior mesenteric artery urokinase infusion therapy vs transjugular intrahepatic portosystemic shunt in patients with cirrhosis and acute portal vein thrombosis. World Journal of Gastroenterology. 2017;**23**(41):7470-7477

[87] Zhao MF, Yue ZD, Zhao HW, Wang L, Fan ZH, He FL, et al. Techniques of TIPS in the treatment of liver cirrhosis combined with incompletely occlusive main portal vein thrombosis. Scientific Reports. 2016;**6**:33069

[88] Wang L, He FL, Yue ZD, Zhao HW, Fan ZH, Zhao MF, et al. Techniques and long-term effects of transjugular intrahepatic portosystemic shunt on liver cirrhosis-related thrombotic total occlusion of main portal vein. Scientific Reports. 2017;**7**(1):10868

[89] Fagiuoli S, Bruno R, Venon WD, Schepis F, Vizzutti F, Toniutto P, et al. Consensus con-
      ference on TIPS management: Techniques, indications, contraindications. Digestive and
      Liver Disease. 2017;**49**(2):121-137

[90] Kawanaka H, Akahoshi T, Itoh S, Iguchi T, Harimoto N, Uchiyama H, et al. Optimizing
      risk stratification in portal vein thrombosis after splenectomy and its primary prophy-
      laxis with antithrombin III concentrates and danaparoid sodium in liver cirrhosis with
      portal hypertension. Journal of the American College of Surgeons. 2014;**219**(5):865-874

[91] Villa E, Camma C, Marietta M, Luongo M, Critelli R, Colopi S, et al. Enoxaparin prevents
      portal vein thrombosis and liver decompensation in patients with advanced cirrhosis.
      Gastroenterology. 2012;**143**(5):1253

[92] Fortea JI, Zipprich A, Fernandez-Mena C, Puerto M, Bosoi CR, Almagro J, et al. Enoxaparin
      does not ameliorate liver fibrosis or portal hypertension in rats with advanced cirrhosis.
      Liver International. 2018;**38**(1):102-112

3

Caffeine with Links to NAFLD and Accelerated Brain Aging

Ian James Martins

Abstract

Nutritional diets are essential to prevent nonalcoholic fatty liver disease (NAFLD) in the global obesity and diabetes epidemic. The ingestion of palmitic acid-rich diets induces NAFLD in animal and human studies. The beneficial properties of olive oil (oleic acid) may be superseded by ingestion of palmitic acid-rich diets. Hepatic caffeine metabolism is regulated by palmitic and oleic acid with effects of these fats on amyloid beta metabolism. Healthy fats such as olive oil may facilitate rapid amyloid beta clearance in the periphery to maintain drug therapy in diabetes and various neurological diseases. Repression of the anti-aging gene sirtuin 1 (Sirt 1) prevents the beneficial properties of olive oil. Brain disorders induce NAFLD and supersede caffeine's therapeutic effects in the prevention of NAFLD. Delayed hepatic caffeine metabolism in NAFLD and increased caffeine transport to the brain with aging-induced mitophagy in neurons with induction of type 3 diabetes and neurodegenerative disease.

Keywords: caffeine, nonalcoholic fatty liver disease, brain aging, palmitic acid, mitochondria

1. Introduction

The global increase in nonalcoholic fatty liver disease (NAFLD) is linked to various induction factors such as excessive caloric intake, genetic, environmental inducing factors and psychosocial factors that override the liver's ability to metabolize lipids and determine excess body fat (adipose tissue size) with the risk of dyslipidemia, obesity, cardiovascular disease, hypertension, and insulin resistance that lead to population mortality in developed countries. In developed countries, the Western diet is known to be high in fat and glucose and closely involved in early liver disease associated with excess transfer of fat to the adipose tissue (visceral fat) and the induction of the metabolic syndrome and obesity. Increased susceptibility to obesity in man compared with other species now indicates NAFLD to be the clinical condition involved in the induction of obesity in man [1–3]. In North America, the rate of childhood obesity has doubled in the last 20 years and similar statistics are reported in countries like Thailand, China, Brazil, and South Africa. The prevalence of childhood and adolescent obesity has increased since 1980 with concerns for NAFLD to exceed 50% of the childhood population [4–6]. Early dietary intervention in genetic and obese/diabetic mice models has indicated reversal and stabilization of NAFLD with relevance to the global NAFLD and neurodegeneration. Education programs such as food restriction programs (**Figure 1**) have been performed but induction of global NAFLD has not decreased in the world [7, 8]. The projected health care costs by the year 2018 in relation to obesity/diabetes-related medical expenses in the United States have been reported to be 344 billion dollars accounting for 21% of total health care costs. Excessive caloric intake, genetic, environmental inducing agents, and psychosocial factors all contribute to the cause of NAFLD (**Figure 1**) with the reduced metabolism of lipids involved in the development of obesity in middle adult life. In the global population, the prevalence of NAFLD has increased from 15% in 1980 to 25% in 2010 with NAFLD to increase to 40% of the global population by the year 2050. In the developing world, the increased obesity/diabetes epidemic is now associated with diet and the presence of specific chemicals such as xenobiotics [9]. The interactions between the brain, liver, and adipose tissue are defective [10] with reduced adipose tissue-liver crosstalk [10–12] responsible for the defective hepatic metabolism of dietary fat, xenobiotics, and drugs and related to the induction of global NAFLD epidemic. Major interests in caffeine intake have accelerated with relevance to global mitophagy, amyloid beta aggregation, NAFLD, and neurodegenerative

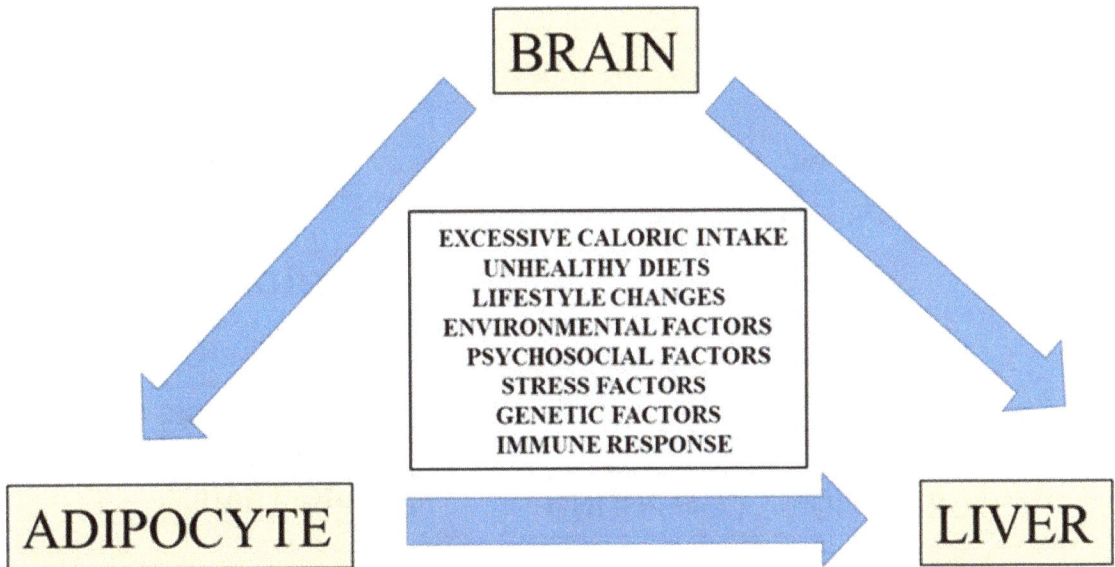

Figure 1. Inducing factors for NAFLD override the brain regulation of the adipose tissue-liver crosstalk. The dose of caffeine used in healthy diets has become important with relevance to the brain control of liver function. Palmitic acid-rich diets induce NAFLD and delay caffeine metabolism with increased caffeine transport to the brain. Other factors such as stress and psychosocial factors disturb brain function with altered cellular lipid metabolism which is now linked to obesity and the NAFLD epidemic.

disease [13]. Caffeine is an appetite suppressant with effects on improving liver fat metabolism and adipogenesis [14] and important to the adipose tissue-liver crosstalk. Brain regulation of the adipose tissue-liver crosstalk is impaired by various inducing factors with excess transport of caffeine to the brain that interferes with the circadian rhythm with relevance to accelerated aging [14–17]. Inducing factors for NAFLD (**Figure 1**) override the beneficial effects of caffeine on adipocyte/liver fat metabolism [18, 19] and the dose of caffeine used in diets has become important with relevance to the NAFLD epidemic since the pharmacokinetics of caffeine may be completely impaired in the liver (NAFLD) in overweight/obese individuals [2, 20–27].

Unhealthy diets (**Figure 1**) that contain palmitic acid (cream, butter, and cheese) increase cholesterol levels and induce NAFLD [28–32] and neurodegeneration with complete impairment of caffeine actions with relevance to its role as a modulator of receptors relevant to the adipose tissue and liver fat metabolism. Palmitic acid diets alter cell cholesterol and phospholipid dynamics with increased contents of phospholipids such as dipalmitoylphosphatidylcholine (DPPC) that are relevant to increased membrane cholesterol content [33, 34] with relevance to delayed hepatic caffeine and amyloid beta transport and metabolism. Palmitic acid and DPPC have major effects on membrane cholesterol formation that stimulate amyloid beta formation [35, 36]. Amyloid beta is a 4-kDa hydrophobic peptide (**Figure 2**) released from neurons in the brain for metabolism by the liver [37] with recent research that caffeine (hydrophobic

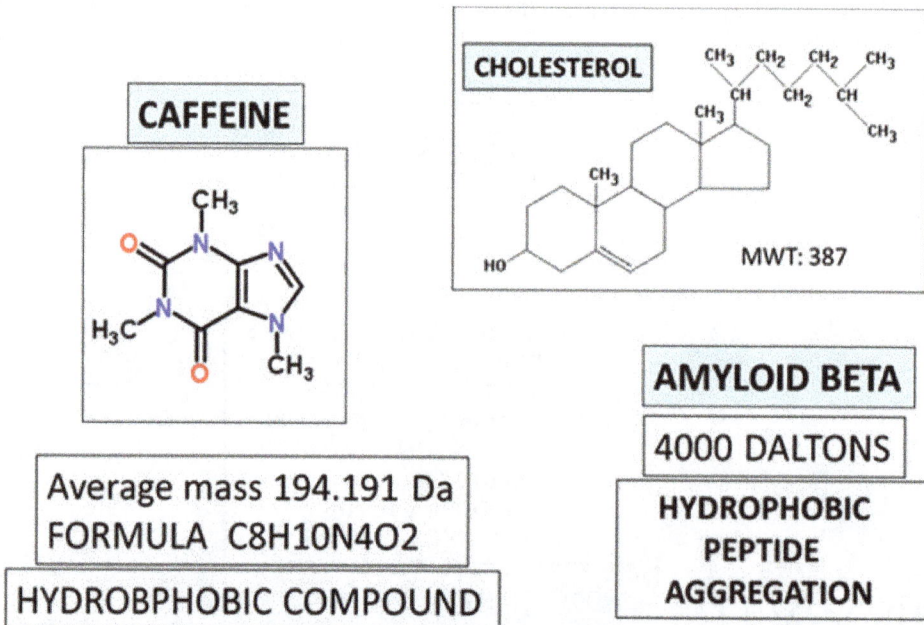

Figure 2. Increased cholesterol levels have been associated with toxic amyloid beta formation. Diets with increased palmitic acid increase cell cholesterol and the phospholipid dipalmitoylphosphatidylcholine (DPPC) with relevance to delayed cell amyloid beta transport and caffeine metabolism. Caffeine is a hydrophobic compound and its increased insertion into the cell membrane with aging is related to abnormal cholesterol and amyloid beta metabolism with the induction of mitophagy. The consumption of olive oil (oleic acid) is associated with the phospholipid 1-palmitoyl-2-oleolylphosphatidylcholine (POPC) and is related to rapid amyloid beta and caffeine metabolism.

compound, **Figure 2**) improves brain-liver amyloid beta transport and metabolism with the prevention of neurodegeneration [38, 39]. DPPC/cholesterol interactions accumulate cellular caffeine with corruption of the brain-liver amyloid beta metabolism with accelerated brain aging associated with toxic amyloid beta aggregation (**Figure 2**). Increased cell phospholipid dynamics with consumption of olive oil (oleic acid) are associated with phospholipids such as 1-palmitoyl-2-oleolylphosphatidylcholine (POPC) that is a common pattern of naturally occurring phospholipids in cells and relevant to cell phospholipid dynamics [40] and rapid caffeine metabolism. Palmitic acid and DPPC are sensitive to cholesterol with toxic effects involved in the interference with brain-liver amyloid beta and caffeine metabolism with relevance to caffeine-induced mitophagy [41, 42] and the induction of NAFLD and neurodegeneration in global communities.

2. Defective adipose tissue-liver crosstalk in the induction of the global NAFLD epidemic

New quantitative genetic methods such as the use of DNA and RNA microarrays have been used to examine novel genetic pathways and now identify a single gene to be involved in the NAFLD and obesity epidemic. The anti-aging gene sirtuin 1 (Sirt 1) has now been implicated as a NAD(+)-dependent class III histone deacetylase (HDAC) protein that targets transcription factors to adapt gene expression to metabolic activity, insulin resistance, and inflammation in chronic diseases [43–46]. Sirt 1 is involved in food intake regulation [47, 48], gluconeogenesis in the liver [49], fat mobilization from white adipose tissue, cholesterol metabolism, and energy metabolism [50, 51]. In adipose tissue, Sirt 1 activates fat mobilization by inhibiting peroxisome proliferator-activated receptor gamma (PPAR-gamma) [52, 53] and in the pancreas Sirt 1 repression decreases insulin secretion with effects on beta cell uncoupling protein 2 levels [54]. Sirt 1 influences mitochondrial biogenesis in the adipose tissue and liver with relevance to NAFLD [10]. Furthermore, diet and nutrigenomics are involved in Sirt 1 regulation of DNA repair with transcription factors regulated by Sirt 1 connected to the nuclear receptors such as peroxisome proliferator-activated receptor (PPARalpha, PPARgamma), liver X receptor, pregnane X receptor, and farnesoid X receptor involved in liver metabolic homeostasis with roles in lipid metabolism in adipose tissue [9].

The effects of dysregulated Sirt 1 on adipocyte differentiation [55–59] and regulation of gene expression involves the secretion of adiponectin [60–62] with adipocyte size negatively correlated with adiponectin levels, adipose tissue ceramide metabolism, and HDL levels [63–67]. Adiponectin is mainly secreted from the adipose tissue into the bloodstream and inversely correlated with body fat in adults. Adiponectin self-associates into larger structures from trimers to form hexamers or dodecamers with the high-molecular weight form, biologically more active with regard to glucose homeostasis. High fat intake is associated with decreased adiponectin levels [68] and downregulation of Sirt 1 [10] with low adiponectin levels associated with the metabolic syndrome, NAFLD [69–71] with effects on hypercholesterolemia (low high-density lipoproteins, apolipoprotein AI levels and high low-density lipoprotein, apolipoprotein B levels) associated with insulin resistance and NAFLD (**Figure 3**). Adiponectin

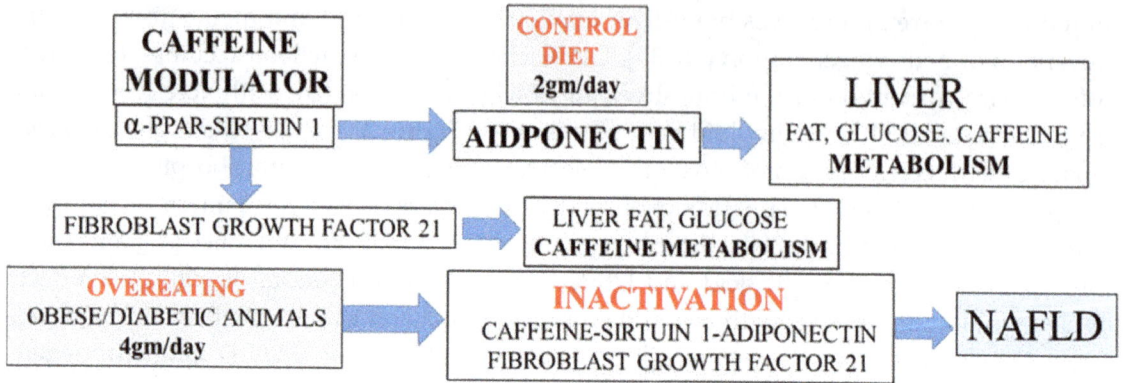

Figure 3. Dietary fat consumption in man needs to be carefully controlled to allow caffeine to modulate cell Sirtuin 1 activity that is involved in mitochondrial biogenesis and the metabolism of cellular fatty acids. Diets that are low in calories activate Sirtuin 1 and allow caffeine-induced modulation of adiponectin levels essential for the adipose tissue-liver crosstalk and the hepatic metabolism of glucose and fatty acids. In rodents, feeding mice 2 g/day instead of 4 g/day increases hepatic fatty acid metabolism and activates hepatic Sirtuin 1 involved in glucose and fatty acid metabolism. Sirtuin 1 is involved in adipose tissue-liver FGF21 production essential for mitochondrial function in the brain and the metabolism of fatty acids, glucose, and caffeine in the liver. The calculated fat content by (Martins IJ, author) in man is related to between 20 and 30 g/day and fat intake at this consumption rate is essential for the prevention of NAFLD.

deficiency has been shown to reduce hepatic ATP-binding cassette transporter ABCA1 (ABCA1) and apo AI synthesis with relevance to the reverse cholesterol transport [72]. FGF21 is now associated with NAFLD [73–76] with hepatic FGF21 shown to regulate lipolysis (fatty acid release) with FGF21 critical in the reduction of adipose tissue ceramides. In insulin resistance and AD, FGF21 and adiponectin levels are implicated in increased cellular ceramide levels and NAFLD [77–81] associated with cholesterol displacement in membranes [82–84] with relevance to amyloid beta aggregation [85]. Sirt 1/adiponectin/FGF21 dysregulation determine hepatic cholesterol metabolism with effects on plasma apo B levels mediated via Sirt 1 and transcription factor C/EBPalpha, which regulates the transcription of the apo B gene [85]. Adipocytes from obese and diabetic individuals are associated with increased adipocyte APP gene expression and plasma amyloid beta levels that implicate adiponectin and Sirt 1 dysregulation with cholesterol and amyloid beta metabolism [86–90]. High-calorie diets downregulate Sirt 1 with reduced adiponectin expression in obesity and diabetes [91] associated with adipose tissue transformation and liver development [60, 86]. Fasting and feeding regulate PPAR alpha-Sirt 1 expression related to hepatic FGF21 production and have become important to NAFLD and the metabolic syndrome [85]. FGF21 is an important activator of Sirt 1-mediated release of adiponectin [85]. FGF21 binds to FGF receptor and beta klotho receptor complex [85] and activates adipose tissue Sirt 1 by increase in NAD+ and activation of peroxisome proliferator-activated receptor gamma coactivator 1-alpha (PGC1-alpha) and AMP-activated protein kinase (AMPK). Unhealthy diets and Sirt 1 repression effect the release of adipose tissue adipokines (adiponectin and leptin) and cytokines (tumor necrosis factor alpha, interleukin-6 and C-reactive protein levels, and Ang II) [92] with FGF21 [73–76] implicated in NAFLD and other chronic diseases associated with accelerated brain aging. In man, caffeine has been associated with increased adiponectin levels with relevance to beneficial effects on liver function [93, 94]. Caffeine and its effects on the adipose tissue-liver crosstalk involve caffeine related to adipose tissue adiponectin release essential for liver function. Caffeine is a modulator of histone deacetylase and its effects as a histone deacetylase modulator [27, 95] in the adipose tissue-liver crosstalk involve the dose of caffeine that is of critical importance to Sirt 1/adiponectin release [85, 96, 97] essential to maintain hepatic metabolism of fatty acids and glucose [18, 98]. Caffeine is important to reduce inflammatory processes [99, 100] with adipose tissue transformation and release of inflammatory cytokines that induce NAFLD [100]. Sirt 1 is involved in autoimmunity [101, 102] with relevance to regulation of various immune cell events in the adipose tissue and liver.

Assessment of hepatic lipid metabolism has been extensively conducted in obese and diabetic rodents with relevance to NAFLD in man [103–107]. In rodents with diets (5% fat), the intake of food per day was approximately 2 g/day and the hepatic metabolism of injected labeled lipoproteins was rapid and cleared and metabolized from the blood plasma within 30 min. In obese and diabetic rodents that had appetite dysregulation consumed approximately 4 g/day (**Figure 3**), the hepatic clearance and metabolism of fats were defective. The excess and ingested fat in obese/diabetic rodents completely downregulated hepatic Sirt 1 with relevance to the NAFLD that develops in these mice with the aging process. In Sirt 1 knockout mice [108, 109], NAFLD develops with relevance to the importance of Sirt 1 in liver fat and cholesterol metabolism [110]. The primary role of fat intake was assessed in obese/diabetic mice that were only allowed to consume 2 g/day (**Figure 3**) instead of 4 g/day and hepatic lipid metabolism was improved in these obese/diabetic rodent experiments with relevance to calorie-sensitive regulation of hepatic Sirt 1 (**Figure 3**). Dietary fat consumption in man needs to be carefully controlled to allow caffeine/adiponectin effects to prevent the induction of NAFLD. The calculated fat content in man has now been determined by author's calculations to be approximately 20–30 g/day [13] and differs from other international researchers [111]. In several laboratories, cellular cholesterol levels are associated with increased amyloid beta formation in the brain and periphery [37], and Sirt 1 downregulation is associated with defective caffeine and cholesterol metabolism (**Figure 4**) with relevance to hepatic amyloid beta clearance and induction of NAFLD [112]. Increased plasma caffeine levels displace amyloid beta and fatty acids from albumin by competition for albumin binding sites [113] with relevance to amyloid beta aggregation [114]. Increased caffeine membrane levels in the liver and brain may affect cholesterol efflux with toxic amyloid beta aggregation (**Figure 4**) relevant to cell apoptosis. Sirt 1 is essential for neuron proliferation with effects of excess cell caffeine that interferes with cell magnesium levels (**Figure 4**) and supersedes the anti-amyloid beta aggregation properties of caffeine [115]. Magnesium deficiency has been associated with hypercholesterolemia and induction of NAFLD [116]. Magnesium is now relevant to maintenance of peripheral hepatic amyloid beta metabolism with magnesium levels critical to the prevention of high-cell cholesterol-induced amyloid beta formation. In NAFLD (**Figure 4**), caffeine consumption should be carefully controlled to prevent magnesium deficiency [117] and to assist with the reduction in hepatic fibrosis in NAFLD [118].

Palmitic acid-rich diets (20–30 g fat/day) should carefully calculate palmitic acid consumption per day to prevent interference of the adipose tissue-crosstalk and induction of NAFLD [13]. Palmitic acid is an Sirt 1 inhibitor [119, 120] with induction of cell cholesterol efflux disturbances

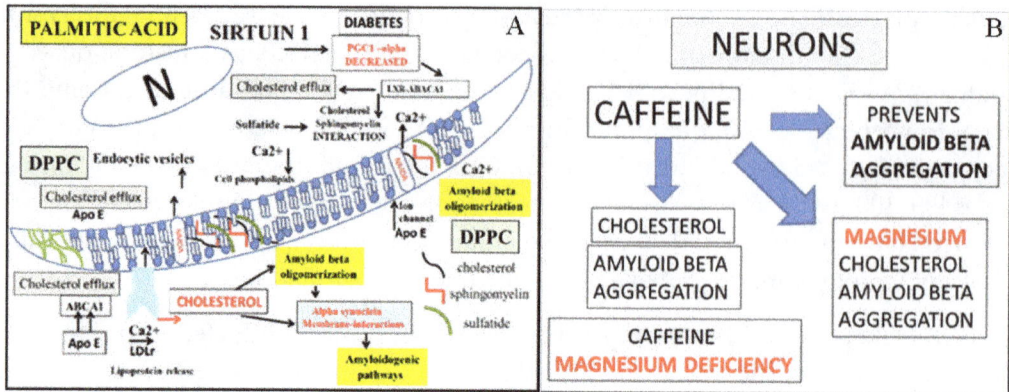

Figure 4. In panel A, palmitic acid as an inhibitor of Sirt 1 is associated with defective caffeine and cholesterol metabolism with relevance to hepatic amyloid beta clearance and induction of NAFLD. Cell caffeine levels are associated with calcium-induced amyloid beta oligomer formation with mitophagy in the liver and brain. In panel B, irreversible effects with aging of palmitic acid induce cell DPPC/cholesterol formation and interfere with caffeine's anti-amyloid beta oligomer properties with increased cell caffeine levels related to magnesium deficiency (NAFLD) and increased cholesterol associated amyloid beta aggregation.

relevant to cell amyloid beta-induced mitophagy [121] with liver inflammation. Palmitic acid induces DPPC phospholipid/cholesterol membrane changes that delay caffeine metabolism with increased cell caffeine levels associated with calcium-induced amyloid beta oligomer formation in the liver and brain [27]. Palmitic acid converts to glucose in cells and with increased palmitic acid levels that are not controlled with aging may inactivate cell Sirt 1 glucose regulation (gluconeogenesis) and nullify the brain to liver amyloid beta clearance pathway with defective adipose tissue-liver crosstalk [10] relevant to induction of chronic diseases.

The gene-environment interaction identifies Sirt 1 in many global populations as the defective gene involved in the defective nuclear-mitochondria interactions in the adipose tissue and the liver relevant to the mitochondrial theory of aging [10]. Sirt 1 targets transcription factors such as peroxisome proliferator-activated receptor gamma coactivator 1-alpha (PGC1-alpha) and p53 to adapt gene expression to mitochondrial function by deacetylation of PGC1-alpha and p53 transcription factors [10], which are important to mitochondrial DNA homeostasis and mitochondrial biogenesis [122–126]. Inhibitors and activators of Sirt 1 [112] have been identified that may override caffeine and its role as a Sirt 1 modulator [27, 95, 112]. Inhibitors include alcohol, sirtinol, suramin and activators include leucine, pyruvic acid, and alpha-lipoic acid. These inhibitors may induce mitochondrial apoptosis and may override the adipose tissue-liver interaction with the induction of NAFLD. Sirt 1 is now referred to as the heat-shock gene with its critical role in heat-shock protein (HSP) metabolism [127, 128]. HSP is a chaperone for amyloid beta and with Sirt 1 repression is important to HSP-amyloid beta-induced endoplasmic reticulum stress relevant to mitophagy and induction of NAFLD [129, 130]. *Caenorhabditis elegans* sirtuins have similar homology to human Sirt 1 with relevance to effects of caffeine on Sirt 1 circadian dysregulation [129]. Induction of HSP from cells in the nematode *C. elegans* has been used for toxicological studies and indicates caffeine doses that induce HSP release with relevance to programmed cell death [129].

3. Accelerated brain aging and type 3 diabetes-induced NAFLD and chronic diseases

In the developed and developing world, the induction of NAFLD has become one of the major interests with its primary or secondary role in the induction of various chronic diseases. Accelerated brain aging with appetite dysregulation indicates that NAFLD may play a secondary role in the induction of various chronic diseases (**Figure 5**). Mitophagy and the induction of neurodegeneration with ****type 3 diabetes are now the primary defects with accelerated NAFLD connected to various chronic diseases (**Figure 5**). Major concerns for suprachiasmatic nucleus (SCN) defects in the hypothalamus may involve appetite dysregulation [11], core-body temperature defects [131], and whole-body glucose disorders (type 3 diabetes) may induce toxicity to the liver and various other organs. Factors such as stress, psychosocial, environmental factors [9], and sleep disorders [132] disturb SCN regulation of the circadian rhythm with toxic effects of glucose, cholesterol, caffeine, and amyloid beta levels to the brain and various tissues (**Figure 5**). Higher brain dysregulation corrupts the hypothalamus-pituitary axis, sympathetic and nonsympathetic pathways that have direct neural innervation to organs such as the liver. Defective hepatic caffeine metabolism may induce magnesium deficiency, apelinergic system imbalances [133, 134], interference with sympathetic pathways [26] connected to mitophagy, and various chronic diseases.

The ingestion of the amount of fat is critical to the adipose tissue-liver cross with immune reactivity [10, 135] connected to mitophagy and induction of NAFLD. Multiple theories of aging have been proposed and the immune theory of aging may involve adipose tissue transformation with activation of immune responses that involve macrophages and immune cells that lead to liver inflammation [10, 99] and the induction of NAFLD. The defect in the neural loop (autonomic nervous system) between the brain and adipose tissue [136] now may be

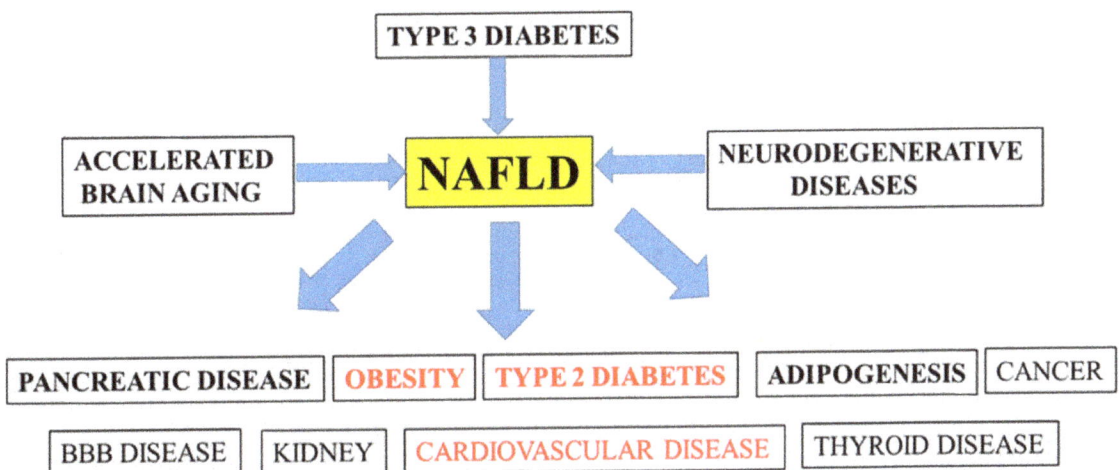

Figure 5. Defects in the suprachiasmatic nucleus (SCN) that involve appetite dysregulation, core-body temperature defects, and whole-body glucose disorders (type 3 diabetes) may induce NAFLD and various other chronic diseases. The primary role in the induction of NAFLD may be related to mitophagy-induced neurodegeneration with relevance to circadian rhythm disorders and complete nullification of hepatic caffeine metabolism by interference with the adipose tissue-liver crosstalk.

related to immunometabolism disorders with adipose tissue transformation. The nature of dietary fat with relevance to adipose tissue as the organ most susceptible to programmed cell death pathways involves transformation that is now important to determine the release of adipocyte inflammatory cytokines, hormones, and heat-shock proteins (HSP) that trigger liver inflammation and NAFLD in global communities [135]. Immunometabolism and accelerated aging are now connected to the adipose tissue and liver crosstalk with the mitochondria theory of aging important to both immune function [10] and metabolism of fats in the adipose tissue and liver. The transcription factor p53 is involved in immune responses, metabolism, and mitochondrial apoptosis [10, 123, 125] with diet, drugs, and environment [9] critical to the regulation of Sirt 1/p53 immunometabolism and induction of NAFLD in the developed world.

Rapid urbanization from 20 to 60% has occurred in Africa, India, China, and Asia and possibly involved with the large global diabetic population in these developing countries. The number of people with diabetes is projected to be double in Africa, Asia, and India. In Asia, the diabetic epidemic has escalated and accounts for 60% of the world diabetic population [137]. The diabetic epidemic has been associated with NAFLD in developing countries of Latin America, Asia [138], India, and Africa with prevalence (20–40%) [9] similar to developed countries [138–141]. Evidence from various studies [9] indicates that environmental factors (xenobiotics) are the major determinants of the increasing rate of diabetes (**Figure 6**). Major threats of xenobiotics such as environmental pollutants may increase with age in individuals

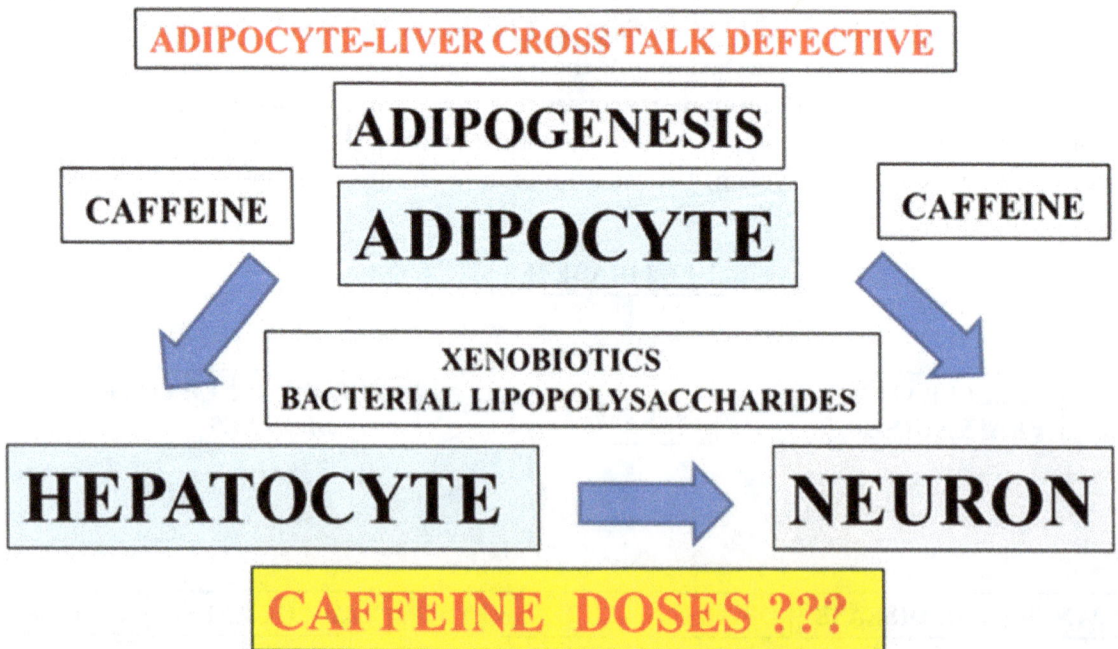

Figure 6. Caffeine is essential for the release of adiponectin from adipose tissue in obesity but the therapeutic effects of caffeine may be superseded with relevance to adipogenesis disorders. In the developing world, xenobiotics induce mitophagy in the adipose tissue and liver and supersede caffeine's protective effects on the mitochondria. In the developing world, plasma LPS levels have increased with effects on the induction of NAFLD and interference with neuron function. Caffeine doses should be carefully controlled with relevance to LPS cell membrane transformations that override caffeine and cell membrane interactions and promote caffeine effects on albumin involved in amyloid beta and fatty acid transport between the brain and the liver.

from developing countries. The NAFLD epidemic is connected to unhealthy diets and reduced hepatic xenobiotic metabolism with blood-brain barrier disorders [9] involved with interference of brain Sirt 1's role in DNA repair [10] with the induction of neuronal apoptosis and type 3 diabetes. The association between xenobiotics in food and the beneficial effects of caffeine (Sirt 1 modulation) on insulin resistance [142, 143] may be superseded with caffeine consumption in these individuals to be revised with relevance to toxic xenobiotic effects associated with delayed caffeine metabolism relevant to NAFLD and neurodegenerative diseases.

The interests in bacterial lipopolysaccharides (LPS) and their influence on cell membrane fluidity in the brain has accelerated with the increase in plasma LPS levels in individuals (30%) of the developing world [144, 145]. LPS is a critical repressor of Sirt 1 actions with the induction of dyslipidemia, mitophagy, and NAFLD [145]. LPS from Gram-negative bacteria is an amphiphile (covalently linked segments, surface carbohydrate polymer O-specific chain, core oligosaccharide, Lipid A) that can rapidly insert into cell membranes and transform mammalian cells. LPS may supersede POPC properties of the cell membrane and induce amyloid beta oligomerization [144].

4. Nutritional diets maintain brain and adipose tissue-liver crosstalk with prevention of NAFLD

In developed world, the consumption of fat consumed in man is between 44 and 78 g/day [111, 146]. The amount of fat consumed (20–30 g/day) is critical to maintain the brain regulation of the adipose tissue-liver crosstalk and connected to the maintenance of the circadian rhythm (12 h light/12 h dark cycle) that is critical to hepatic amyloid beta and glucose metabolism [147, 148]. The SCN is controlled by Sirt 1 with its dysfunction connected to brain circuitry disorders (**Figure 7**) and disconnections between the autonomic nervous system and the liver [148]. The amount of fat consumed with the aging process inactivates the effects of caffeine by interfering with hepatic caffeine metabolism with increased transport to the brain (**Figure 7**). In the brain, SCN neurons are sensitive to caffeine [149] with complete inactivation of the brain to adipose tissue-liver crosstalk and interfere with caffeine's beneficial effects on the sympathetic nervous system and reversal of NAFLD. Caffeine and its role in thermogenesis by modulation of mitochondrial function versus mitochondrial apoptosis are relevant to the consumption of various fats and diets in the developed and developing world. Sirt 1 is now referred as the gene involved in mitochondrial biogenesis that is critical to maintain cell function with the prevention of cell apoptosis [9–12, 122–125]. Sirt 1 is critical to SCN function and the maintenance of core-body temperature with essential control of the adipose tissue-liver crosstalk [131, 150]. The consumption of coconut oil (saturated fat) and palm oil (palmitic acid) should be carefully evaluated in individuals with core-body temperature disorders. These fats are solid at temperatures between 20 and 24°C and with abnormal body temperature dysregulation may be involved in the induction of NAFLD when compared with the consumption of olive oil (monounsaturated) that is liquid at a temperature (4°C) [130, 150]. Fish contains high levels of omega-3 fatty acids, docosahexaenoic acid (DHA 22:6n-3), and eicosapentaenoic acid (EPA 20:5n-3). These fatty acids are essential for liver fat metabolism with prevention of NAFLD [151, 152] and brain function but with changes in core body temperature (**Figure** 7), therapeutic lipids essential for the prevention of NAFLD may be completely inactivated [130, 131, 150]. Palmitic acid content in milk should be carefully controlled to allow the therapeutic effects of caffeine with relevance to mitochondrial thermogenesis and SCN regulation (**Figure** 7). Nutritional diets with timed meals are important for the prevention of NAFLD and with consumption of essential foods which include protein, eggs, cottage cheese, dairy, red meat, poultry, legumes, nuts, and seeds. These foods may contain minerals such as magnesium and zinc that are needed by many enzymes involved with DNA replication and repair with total magnesium intake that should be between 400 mg and 800 mg/day. Zinc deficiency has been reported in global communities with both minerals important to prevent liver and brain diseases and to allow effective vitamin and caffeine therapy. Vitamins such as vitamin B12, folic acid, vitamin B6, vitamins C, D, and E are essential to maintain liver and brain function. The consumption of phosphatidylinositol (PI) (g/day) is essential and lack of PI may not allow the maintenance of SCN function and whole body glucose homeostasis. In individuals with strenuous exercise, the PI half-life is rapid and may require PI ingestion of (g/day) to prevent amyloid beta aggregation and induction of NAFLD [153, 154]. Strenuous exercise may induce magnesium deficiency [116] and magnesium consumption needs revision to prevent SCN disturbances with type 3 diabetes and NAFLD.

The major defects with relevance to the global NAFLD epidemic involve the defective brain circadian circuitry and the adipose tissue-liver crosstalk [136, 155]. The SCN control of the

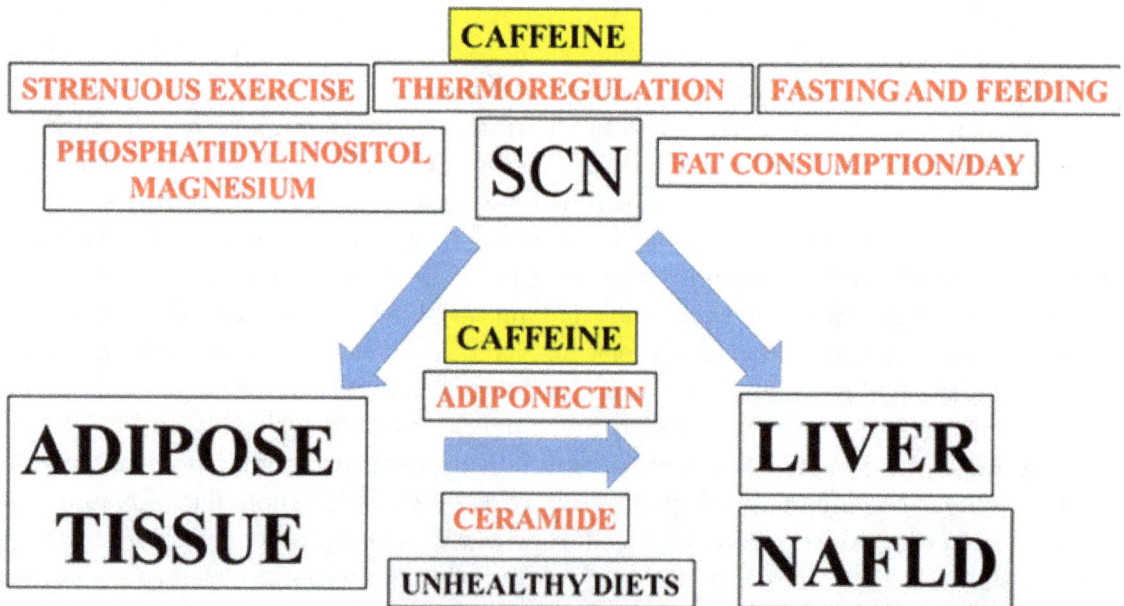

Figure 7. In the current global NAFLD epidemic, plasma ceramides indicate that the adipose tissue-liver crosstalk is completely defective with the release of toxic ceramides into the blood plasma. Sirt 1 downregulation is possibly connected to cell ceramide formation with adipose tissue disorders, liver steatosis development, and complete inactivation of caffeine's involvement in the prevention of NAFLD [94]. Integration of factors such as stress, sleep disorders, and environmental factors (strenuous exercise) inactivate the SCN regulation of the circadian rhythm with toxic effects of glucose, cholesterol, caffeine, and amyloid beta levels to mitochondria in various peripheral tissues.

adipose tissue metabolism allows adipocyte adiponectin release with essential effects on liver glucose and lipid homeostasis [155]. Sirt 1 and its modulation by caffeine have become important with caffeine involved in increased adiponectin levels in man. Apart from caffeine, other foods have been assessed to increase adiponectin levels such as omega-3 supplementation, fruit intake, green tea, magnesium, and hypolipidemic drugs are all involved in the modification of adiponectin levels [156–159]. In individuals with NAFLD, long-term dietary salt restriction is essential to increase adiponectin levels. Fasting and feeding is essential to maintain SCN circadian regulation of liver function that involves peripheral glucose homeostasis with adiponectin release critical to maintain insulin sensitivity and prevent NAFLD [85]. Gamma PPAR-Sirt 1 function in adipocytes is critical to adiponectin release with low adiponectin levels unsuitable to the maintenance of liver ceramide levels that are toxic to the liver and involved in insulin resistance. Ceramide levels and NAFLD [81–84] are now closely linked with programmed cell death. Alcohol consumption should be carefully controlled (Sirt 1 inhibition) with relevance to adiponectin levels in man [160]. Pyruvic acid, leucine, quercetin, green tea catechins, grape seed extract, curcumin, alpha lipoic acid, and resveratrol are Sirt 1 activators essential for SCN maintenance and the adipose tissue-liver cross talk. High-protein diets should be avoided to reduce amyloid beta formation by cells and to reduce the arginine content of the diet that switches leucine (Sirt 1 activator) for arginine in cells and tissues [132].

High-fiber diets [37] in various foods have become important with the consumption of phytosterols [37] involved in reducing intestinal cholesterol absorption and increased hepatic cholesterol metabolism relevant to the prevention of NAFLD in man. Phytosterols should be consumed (1–2 g/day) and excessive intake of phytosterols leads to neurotoxicity with neurodegeneration [37]. Phytosterols cross the blood–brain barrier in neurons to maintain neuron amyloid beta homeostasis [161]. Consumption of plant-based foods essential for phytosterol ingestion should be assessed for caffeine content since approximately 40 caffeine containing plants have been reported. Other caffeine containing foods such as coca cola, energy drinks, caffeine tablets, dark chocolate, chocolate chips, and energy mints should be assessed for caffeine content (mg). Vegetarians should carefully regulate phytosterol consumption over their lifespan to prevent interference with the beneficial effects of caffeine on cholesterol metabolism with relevance to NAFLD [37]. Excessive fructose consumption (fruit, fruit juices) should be avoided with fructose reported as a Sirt 1 inhibitor [162, 163] with the induction of NAFLD. In the developing world, very low carbohydrate diets should be consumed to prevent the absorption of LPS into the blood stream with beneficial effects on magnesium deficiency and the induction of NAFLD [164]. Diets with low-fat contents and without alcohol are essential to prevent the transport of LPS into lipoproteins and proteins in the blood plasma. LPS interferes with the SCN and adipose tissue-liver crosstalk [10, 85, 135, 136] and delays hepatic drug metabolism [165, 166] with premature brain aging and chronic disease progression (**Figure 6**). LPS induces changes in plasma albumin contents [112] in individuals in the developing world with relevance to interference with caffeine and its therapeutic properties with relevance to SCN regulation of adipose tissue-liver crosstalk. In recent studies, caffeine intake and glucose dyshomeostasis that supersede insulin therapy [142, 143] has raised concerns with relevance to glucose/amyloid beta-induced mitochondrial apoptosis and the induction of NAFLD. In the global chronic disease, adiponectin levels are low and to prevent mitochondrial apoptosis, a number of agents are required to maintain mitochondrial function and to prevent cell apoptosis. Diets that contain magnesium, pyrroloquinoline, quinone, resveratrol, and rutin stimulate mitochondrial biogenesis essential to stimulate SCN neuron mitochondrial function [167] with relevance to the global NAFLD epidemic and chronic diseases.

5. Conclusion

In global world, diabetes and mitochondrial disease are expected to cost the developing world US $400 million in the next 30 years. The quality of food consumed has raised major concerns with mitochondrial apoptosis linked to programmed cell death and nonalcoholic fatty liver disease (NAFLD). The amount, nature, and time of day of fat consumption are essential to maintain mitochondrial biogenesis. In the developed and developing world, nutritional interventions are essential to prevent NAFLD and ingestion of caffeine (appetite suppressant) that is associated with the prevention of adipocyte dysfunction and linked to liver function may be completely inactivated by unhealthy diets. In the developing world, bacterial lipopolysaccharides (LPS) may override healthy fat consumption and induce NAFLD. In the developing world, diets that contain LPS, mycotoxins, and xenobiotics interfere with caffeine metabolism with relevance to mitophagy and induction of NAFLD relevant to the survival of various species and man.

Acknowledgements

This work was supported by grants from Edith Cowan University, the McCusker Alzheimer's Research Foundation, and the National Health and Medical Research Council.

Author details

Ian James Martins[1,2,3]

Address all correspondence to: i.martins@ecu.edu.au

1 Centre of Excellence in Alzheimer's Disease Research and Care, School of Medical and Health Sciences, Edith Cowan University, Joondalup, Australia

2 School of Psychiatry and Clinical Neurosciences, The University of Western Australia, Nedlands, Australia

3 McCusker Alzheimer's Research Foundation, Hollywood Medical Centre, Nedlands, Australia

References

[1] de la Monte SM, Longato L, Tong M, Wands JR. Insulin resistance and neurodegeneration: Roles of obesity, type 2 diabetes mellitus and non-alcoholic steatohepatitis. Current Opinion in Investigational Drugs. 2009;**10**:1049-1060

[2] Fabbrini E, Sullivan S, Klein S. Obesity and non-alcoholic fatty liver disease: Biochemical, metabolic, and clinical implications. Hepatology. 2010;**51**:679-689

[3] Bleich SN, Cutler D, Murray C, Adams A. Why is the developed world obese? Annual Review of Public Health. 2008;**29**:273-295

[4] Brody J. The global epidemic of childhood obesity: Poverty, urbanization, and the nutrition transition. Nutrition Bytes. 2002;**8**:1-7

[5] Roberts EA. Non-alcoholic fatty liver disease (NAFLD) in children. Frontiers in Bioscience. 2005;**10**:2306-2318

[6] Vos MB, McClain CJ. Nutrition and non-alcoholic fatty liver disease in children. Current Diabetes Reports. 2008;**8**:399-406

[7] Bellentani S, Scaglioni F, Marino M, Bedogni G. Epidemiology of non-alcoholic fatty liver disease. Digestive Diseases. 2010;**28**:155-161

[8] Younossi ZM, Koenig AB, Abdelatif D, Fazel Y, Henry L, Wymer M. Global epidemiology of non-alcoholic fatty liver disease-meta-analytic assessment of prevalence, incidence, and outcomes. Hepatology. 2016;**64**:73-84

[9] Martins IJ. Increased risk for obesity and diabetes with neurodegeneration in developing countries. Journal of Molecular and Genetic Medicine. 2013;**S1**:001

[10] Martins IJ. Unhealthy nutrigenomic diets accelerate NAFLD and adiposity in global communities. Journal of Molecular and Genetic Medicine. 2015;**9**:1-11

[11] Martins IJ. Appetite control with relevance to mitochondrial biogenesis and activation of post-prandial lipid metabolism in obesity linked diabetes. Annals of Obesity and Disorders. 2016;**1**:1-3

[12] Martins IJ. Diet and nutrition reverse type 3 diabetes and accelerated aging linked to global chronic diseases. Journal of Diabetes Research and Therapy. 2016;**2**:1-6

[13] Martins IJ. Food intake and caffeine determine amyloid beta metabolism with relevance to mitophagy in brain aging and chronic disease. European. Journal of Food Science and Technology. 2016;**4**:11-17

[14] Martins IJ. Caffeine consumption and induction of obesity in the developed world. Annals of Obesity Disorders. 2017;**2**:1-3

[15] Jensen KJ, Alpini G, Glaser S. Hepatic nervous system and neurobiology of the liver. Comprehensive Physiology. 2013;**3**:655-665

[16] Gimble JM, Sutton GM, Ptitsyn AA, Floyd ZE, Bunnell BA. Circadian rhythms in adipose tissue: An update. Current Opinion and Clinical Nutrition and Metabolic Care. 2011;**14**:554-561

[17] Buijs RM, Escobar C, Swaab DF. The circadian system and the balance of the autonomic nervous system. Handbook of Clinical Neurology. 2013;**117**:173-191

[18] Kennedy OJ, Roderick P, Poole R, Parkes J. Coffee, caffeine and non-alcoholic fatty liver disease? Therapeutic Advances in Gastroenterology. 2016;**9**:417-418

[19] Chen S, Teoh NC, Chitturi S, Farrell GC. Coffee and non-alcoholic fatty liver disease: Brewing evidence for hepatoprotection? Journal of Gastroenterology and Hepatology. 2014;**29**:435-441

[20] Patell R, Dosi R, Joshi H, Sheth S, Shah P, Sarfaraz S. Non-alcoholic fatty liver disease (NAFLD) in obesity. Journal of Clinical and Diagnostic Research. 2014;**8**:62-66

[21] Wong RJ, Ahmed A. Obesity and non-alcoholic fatty liver disease: Disparate associations among Asian populations. World Journal of Hepatology. 2014;**6**:263-273

[22] Targher G, Byrne CD. Obesity: Metabolically healthy obesity and NAFLD. Nature Reviews Gastroenterology and Hepatology. 2016;**13**:442-444

[23] Ezzat WM, Ragab S, Ismail NA, Elhosary AY, AM NEAEB, et al. Frequency of non-alcoholic fatty liver disease in overweight/obese children and adults: Clinical, sonographic picture and biochemical assessment. Journal of Genetic Engineering and Biotechnology. 2012;**10**:221-227

[24] Suano de Souza FI, Silverio Amancio OM, Saccardo Sarni RO, Sacchi Pitta T, Fernandes AP, Affonso Fonseca FL, et al. Non-alcoholic fatty liver disease in overweight children and its relationship with retinol serum levels. International Journal of Vitamin Nutrition Research. 2008;**78**:27-32

[25] Kim NH, Kim JH, Kim YJ, Yoo HJ, Kim HY, Seo JA, et al. Clinical and metabolic factors associated with development and regression of non-alcoholic fatty liver disease in non-obese subjects. Liver International. 2014;**34**:604-611

[26] Acheson KJ, Gremaud G, Meirim I, Montigon F, Krebs Y, Fay LB, et al. Metabolic effects of caffeine in humans: Lipid oxidation or futile cycling? American Journal of Clinical Nutrition. 2004;**79**:40-46

[27] Martins IJ. Caffeine consumption with relevance to type 3 diabetes and accelerated brain aging. Research and Reviews: Neuroscience. 2016;**1**:1-5

[28] Ricchi M, Odoardi MR, Carulli L, Anzivino C, Ballestri S, Pinetti A, et al. Differential effect of oleic and palmitic acid on lipid accumulation and apoptosis in cultured hepatocytes. Journal of Gastroenterology and Hepatology. 2009;**24**:830-840

[29] Gambino R, Bugianesi E, Rosso C, Mezzabotta L, Pinach S, Alemanno N, et al. Different serum free fatty acid profiles in NAFLD subjects and healthy controls after oral fat load. International Journal of Molecular Science. 2016;17:479

[30] Puri P, Wiest MM, Cheung O, Mirshahi F, Sargeant C, Min HK, et al. The plasma lipidomic signature of non-alcoholic steatohepatitis. Hepatology. 2009;50:1827-1838

[31] French MA, Sundram K, Clandinin MT. Cholesterolaemic effect of palmitic acid in relation to other dietary fatty acids. Asia Pacific Journal of Clinical Nutrition. 2002;11(Suppl. 7):S401-S407

[32] Clandinin MT, Cook SL, Konard SD, French MA. The effect of palmitic acid on lipoprotein cholesterol levels. International Journal of Food Science Nutrition. 2000;51(Suppl):S61-S71

[33] Miyoshi T, Lönnfors M, Peter Slotte J, Kato S. A detailed analysis of partial molecular volumes in DPPC/cholesterol binary bilayers. Biochimica et Biophysica Acta. 2014;1838:3069-3077

[34] Kheyfets BB, Mukhin SI. Simple model of local ordering of DPPC lipids in contact with cholesterol. Biochemistry (Moscow) Supplement Series A. 2015;9:77-83

[35] Davis CH, Berkowitz ML. Interaction between amyloid-beta (1-42) peptide and phospholipid bilayers: A molecular dynamics study. Biophysical Journal. 2009;96:785-797

[36] Ege C, Lee KY. Insertion of Alzheimer's A beta 40 peptide into lipid monolayers. Biophysical Journal. 2004;87:1732-1740

[37] Martins IJ, Fernando WMADB. High fibre diets and Alzheimer's disease. Food and Nutrition Sciences. 2014;5:410-424

[38] Cao C, Cirrito JR, Lin X, Wang L, Verges DK, Dickson A, et al. Caffeine suppresses amyloid-beta levels in plasma and brain of Alzheimer's disease transgenic mice. Journal of Alzheimer's Disease. 2009;17:681-697

[39] Arendash GW, Mori T, Cao C, Mamcarz M, Runfeldt M, Dickson A, et al. Caffeine reverses cognitive impairment and decreases brain amyloid-beta levels in aged Alzheimer's disease mice. Journal of Alzheimer's Disease. 2009;17:661-680

[40] Martins IJ, Lenzo NP, Redgrave TG. Phosphatidylcholine metabolism after transfer from lipid emulsions injected intravenously into rats. Implications for high density lipoprotein metabolism. Biochimica et Biophysica Acta. 1989;1005:217-224

[41] Dubrez L, Coll JL, Hurbin A, Solary E, Favrot MC. Caffeine sensitizes human H358 cell line to p53-mediated apoptosis by inducing mitochondrial translocation and conformational change of BAX protein. Journal of Biological Chemistry. 2001;276:38980-39807

[42] He Z, Ma WY, Hashimoto T, Bode AM, Yang CS, Dong Z. Induction of apoptosis by caffeine is mediated by the p53, Bax, and caspase 3 pathways. Cancer Research. 2003;63:4396-4401

[43] Hansen MK, Connolly TM. Nuclear receptors as drug targets in obesity, dyslipidaemia and atherosclerosis. Current Opinion in Investigational Drugs. 2008;**9**:247-255

[44] Harrison C. Neurodegenerative disorders: A neuroprotective role for sirtuin 1. Nature Reviews Drug Discovery. 2012;**11**:108

[45] Kawada T, Goto T, Hirai S, Kang MS, Uemura T, Yu R. Dietary regulation of nuclear receptors in obesity-related metabolic syndrome. Asia Pacific Journal of Clinical Nutrition. 2008;**17**:126-130

[46] Swanson HI, Wada T, Xie W, Renga B, Zampella A, Distrutti E. Role of nuclear receptors in lipid dysfunction and obesity-related diseases. Drug Metabolism & Disposition. 2013;**41**:1-11

[47] Cakir I, Perello M, Lansari O, Messier NJ, Vaslet CA, Nillni EA. Hypothalamic sirt1 regulates food intake in a rodent model system. PloS One. 2009;**4**:e8322

[48] Kitamura T, Sasaki T. Hypothalamic sirt1 and regulation of food intake. Diabetology International. 2012;**3**:109-112

[49] Wei D, Tao R, Zhang Y, White MF, Dong XC. Feedback regulation of hepatic gluconeogenesis through modulation of SHP/Nr0b2 gene expression by Sirt1 and FoxO1. American Journal of Physiology Endocrinology and Metabolism. 2011;**300**:E312-E320

[50] Li X. SIRT1 and energy metabolism. Acta Biochimica et Biophysica Sinica (Shanghai). 2013;**45**:51-60

[51] Chang HC, Guarente L. SIRT1 and other sirtuins in metabolism. Trends in Endocrinology and Metabolism. 2014;**25**:138-145

[52] Mayoral R, Osborn O, McNelis J, Johnson AM, DY O, Izquierdo CL, Chung H, et al. Adipocyte SIRT1 knockout promotes PPARγ activity, adipogenesis and insulin sensitivity in chronic-HFD and obesity. Molecular Metabolism. 2015;**4**:378-391

[53] Picard F, Kurtev M, Chung N, Topark-Ngarm A, Senawong T, Machado De Oliveira R, et al. Sirt1 promotes fat mobilization in white adipocytes by repressing PPAR-gamma. Nature. 2004;**429**:771-776

[54] Bordone L, Motta MC, Picard F, Robinson A, Jhala US, Apfeld J, et al. Sirt1 regulates insulin secretion by repressing UCP2 in pancreatic beta cells. PLoS Biology. 2006;**4**:e31

[55] Xu C, Bai B, Fan P, Cai Y, Huang B, Law IK, et al. Selective overexpression of human SIRT1 in adipose tissue enhances energy homeostasis and prevents the deterioration of insulin sensitivity with ageing in mice. American Journal of Translational Research. 2013;**5**:412-426

[56] Choi Y, Um SJ, Park T. Indole-3-carbinol directly targets SIRT1 to inhibit adipocyte differentiation. International Journal of Obesity (London). 2013;**37**:881-884

[57] Siersbaek R, Nielsen R, Mandrup SPPAR. Gamma in adipocyte differentiation and metabolism—Novel insights from genome-wide studies. FEBS Letters. 2010;**584**:3242-3249

[58] Körner A, Wabitsch M, Seidel B, Fischer-Posovszky P, Berthold A, Stumvoll M, et al. Adiponectin expression in humans is dependent on differentiation of adipocytes and down-regulated by humoral serum components of high molecular weight. Biochemical and Biophysical Research Communications. 2005;**337**:540-550

[59] Lee MJ, Wu Y, Fried SK. Adipose tissue re-modeling in pathophysiology of obesity. Current Opinion and Clinical Nutrition and Metabolic Care. 2010;**13**:371-376

[60] Qiao L, Shao J. SIRT1 regulates adiponectin gene expression through Foxo1-C/enhancer-binding protein alpha transcriptional complex. Journal of Biological Chemistry. 2006;**281**:39915-39924

[61] Qiang L, Wang H, Farmer SR. Adiponectin secretion is regulated by SIRT1 and the endoplasmic reticulum oxidoreductase Ero1-L alpha. Molecular and Cellular Biology. 2007;**27**:4698-4707

[62] Shen Z, Liang X, Rogers CQ, Rideout D, You M. Involvement of adiponectin-SIRT1-AMPK signaling in the protective action of rosiglitazone against alcoholic fatty liver in mice. American Journal of Physiology. Gastrointestinal and Liver Physiology. 2010;**298**:G364-G374

[63] Lancaster GI, Febbraio MA. Adiponectin sphings into action. Nature Medicine. 2011;**17**:37-38

[64] Samad F, Badeanlou L, Shah C, Yang G. Adipose tissue and ceramide biosynthesis in the pathogenesis of obesity. Advances in Experimental Medicine and Biology. 2011;**721**:67-86

[65] Błachnio-Zabielska AU, Pułka M, Baranowski M, Nikołajuk A, Zabielski P, Górska M, et al. Ceramide metabolism is affected by obesity and diabetes in human adipose tissue. Journal of Cellular Physiology. 2012;**227**:550-557

[66] Matsuura F, Oku H, Koseki M, Sandoval JC, Yuasa-Kawase M, Tsubakio-Yamamoto K, et al. Adiponectin accelerates reverse cholesterol transport by increasing high density lipoprotein assembly in the liver. Biochemical and Biophysical Research Communications. 2007;**358**:1091-1095

[67] Toth PP. Adiponectin and high-density lipoprotein: A metabolic association through thick and thin. European Heart Journal. 2005;**26**:1579-1581

[68] Bullen JW, Bluher S, Kelesidis T, Mantzoros CS. Regulation of adiponectin and its receptors in response to development of diet-induced obesity in mice. American Journal of Physiology: Endocrinology and Metabolism. 2007;**292**:E1079-E1086

[69] Polyzos SA, Kountouras J, Zavos C, Tsiaousi E. The role of adiponectin in the pathogenesis and treatment of non-alcoholic fatty liver disease. Diabetes Obesity and Metabolism. 2010;**12**:365-383

[70] Finelli C, Tarantino G. What is the role of adiponectin in obesity related non-alcoholic fatty liver disease? World Journal of Gastroenterology. 2013;**19**:802-812

[71] Pagano C, Soardo G, Esposito W, Fallo F, Basan L, Donnini D, et al. Plasma adiponectin is decreased in non-alcoholic fatty liver disease. European Journal of Endocrinology. 2005;**152**:113-118

[72] Oku H, Matsuura F, Koseki M, Sandoval JC, Yuasa-Kawase M, Tsubakio-Yamamoto K, et al. Adiponectin deficiency suppresses ABCA1 expression and ApoA-I synthesis in the liver. FEBS Letters. 2007;**581**:5029-5033

[73] Badman MK, Pissios P, Kennedy AR, Koukos G, Flier JS, Maratos-Flier E. Hepatic fibroblast growth factor 21 is regulated by PPARalpha and is a key mediator of hepatic lipid metabolism in ketotic states. Cell Metabolism. 2007;**5**:426-437

[74] Zhu S, Wu Y, Ye X, Ma L, Qi J, Yu D, et al. FGF21 ameliorates non-alcoholic fatty liver disease by inducing autophagy. Molecular and Cellular Biochemistry. 2016;**420**:107-119

[75] Dushay J, Chui PC, Gopalakrishnan GS, Varela-Rey M, Crawley M, Fisher FM, et al. Increased fibroblast growth factor 21 in obesity and non-alcoholic fatty liver disease. Gastroenterology. 2010;**139**:456-463

[76] Liu J, Xu Y, Hu Y, Wang G. The role of fibroblast growth factor 21 in the pathogenesis of non-alcoholic fatty liver disease and implications for therapy. Metabolism. 2015;**64**:380-390

[77] Tao C, Sifuentes A, Holland WL. Regulation of glucose and lipid homeostasis by adiponectin: Effects on hepatocytes, pancreatic β cells and adipocytes. Best Practice & Research: Clinical Endocrinology and Metabolism. 2014;**28**:43-58

[78] Pagadala M, Kasumov T, McCullough AJ, Zein NN, Kirwan JP. Role of ceramides in non-alcoholic fatty liver disease. Trends in Endocrinology and Metabolism. 2012;**23**:365-371

[79] Kasumov T, Li L, Li M, Gulshan K, Kirwan JP, Liu X, et al. Ceramide as a mediator of non-alcoholic fatty liver disease and associated atherosclerosis. PloS One 2015;**10**:e0126910

[80] Luukkonen PK, Zhou Y, Sädevirta S, Leivonen M, Arola J, Orešič M, et al. Hepatic ceramides dissociate steatosis and insulin resistance in patients with non-alcoholic fatty liver disease. Journal of Hepatology. 2016;**64**:1167-1175

[81] Yu C, Alterman M, Dobrowsky RT. Ceramide displaces cholesterol from lipid rafts and decreases the association of the cholesterol binding protein caveolin-1. Journal of Lipid Research. 2005;**46**:1678-1691

[82] Ali MR, Cheng KH, Huang J. Ceramide drives cholesterol out of the ordered lipid bilayer phase into the crystal phase in 1-palmitoyl-2-oleoyl-sn-glycero-3-phosphocholine/cholesterol/ceramide ternary mixtures. Biochemistry. 2006;**45**:12629-12638

[83] Castro BM, Silva LC, Fedorov A, de Almeida RF, Prieto M. Cholesterol-rich fluid membranes solubilize ceramide domains: Implications for the structure and dynamics of mammalian intracellular and plasma membranes. Journal of Biological Chemistry. 2009;**284**:22978-22987

[84] Martins IJ, Creegan R. Links between insulin resistance, lipoprotein metabolism and amyloidosis in Alzheimer's disease. Health. 2014;**6**:1549-1579

[85] Martins IJ. The role of clinical proteomics, lipidomics, and genomics in the diagnosis of Alzheimer's disease. Proteomes. 2016;**4**:1-19

[86] Puig KL, Floden AM, Adhikari R, Golovko MY, Combs CK. Amyloid precursor protein and proinflammatory changes are regulated in brain and adipose tissue in a murine model of high fat diet-induced obesity. PloS One. 2012;**7**:e30378

[87] Lee YH, Martin JM, Maple RL, Tharp WG, Pratley RE. Plasma amyloid-beta peptide levels correlate with adipocyte amyloid precursor protein gene expression in obese individuals. Neuroendocrinology. 2009;**90**:383-390

[88] Vanitha S, Martin JM, Dixon AE, Ades PA, Savage PD, Spaulding L, et al. Overexpression of amyloid precursor protein in adipose tissue of obese diabetic vs. obese non-diabetic individuals. Diabetes. 2007;**56**:363

[89] Lee YH, Tharp WG, Maple RL, Nair S, Permana PA, Pratley RE. Amyloid precursor protein expression is up-regulated in adipocytes in obesity. Obesity (Silver Spring). 2008;**16**:1493-1500

[90] Freeman LR, Zhang L, Dasuri K, Fernandez-Kim SO, Bruce-Keller AJ, Keller JN. Mutant amyloid precursor protein differentially alters adipose biology under obesogenic and non-obesogenic conditions. PloS One. 2012;**7**:e43193

[91] Puig KL, Floden AM, Adhikari R. Golovko. The role of adiponectin in the pathogenesis and treatment of non-alcoholic fatty liver disease. Diabetes Obesity and Metabolism. 2010;**12**:365-383

[92] Bahceci M, Gokalp D, Bahceci S, Tuzcu A, Atmaca S, Arikan S. The correlation between adiposity and adiponectin, tumor necrosis factor alpha, interleukin-6 and high sensitivity C-reactive protein levels. Is adipocyte size associated with inflammation in adults? Journal of Endocrinological Investigation. 2007;**30**:210-214

[93] Bhaktha G, Nayak BS, Mayya S, Shantaram M. Relationship of caffeine with adiponectin and blood sugar levels in subjects with and without diabetes. Journal of Clinical and Diagnostic Research. 2015;**9**:BC01-BC03

[94] Yamashita K, Yatsuya H, Muramatsu T, Toyoshina H, Murohara T, Tamakoshi K. Association of coffee consumption with serum adiponectin, leptin, inflammation and metabolic markers in Japanese workers: A cross-sectional study. Nutrition and Diabetes. 2012;**2**:e33

[95]   Seidel C, Schnekenburger M, Dicato M, Diederich M. Histone deacetylase modulators provided by mother nature. Genes and Nutrition. 2012;**7**:357-367

[96]   SH S, Shyu HW, Yeh YT, Chen KM, Yeh H, Su SJ. Caffeine inhibits adipogenic differentiation of primary adipose-derived stem cells and bone marrow stromal cells. Toxicology In Vitro. 2013;**27**:1830-1837

[97]   Kim AR, Yoon BK, Park H, Seok JW, Choi H, JH Y, et al. Caffeine inhibits adipogenesis through modulation of mitotic clonal expansion and the AKT/GSK3 pathway in 3T3-L1 adipocytes. BMB Reports. 2016;**49**:111-115

[98]   Sinha RA, Farah BL, Singh BK, Siddique MM, Li Y, Wu Y, et al. Caffeine stimulates hepatic lipid metabolism by the autophagy-lysosomal pathway in mice. Hepatology. 2014;**59**:1366-1380

[99]   Horrigan LA, Kelly JP, Connor TJ. Immunomodulatory effects of caffeine: Friend or foe? Pharmacology and Therapeutics. 2006;**111**:877-892

[100] Meli R, Mattace Raso G, Calignano A. Role of innate immune response in non-alcoholic fatty liver disease: Metabolic complications and therapeutic tools. Frontiers in Immunology. 2014;**5**:177

[101] Kong S, McBurney MW, Fang D. Sirtuin 1 in immune regulation and autoimmunity. Immunology and Cell Biology. 2012;**90**:6-13

[102] Chen X, Lu Y, Zhang Z, Wang J, Yang H, et al. Intercellular interplay between Sirt1 signalling and cell metabolism in immune cell biology. Immunology. 2015;**145**:455-467

[103] Martins IJ, Tran JML, Redgrave TG. Food restriction normalizes chylomicron remnant metabolism in murine models of obesity as assessed by a novel stable isotope breath test. Journal of Nutrition. 2002;**132**:176-181

[104] Martins IJ, Redgrave TG. A 13CO2 breath test for the assessment of remnant metabolism in mice. Journal of Lipid Research. 1998;**39**:693-699

[105] Martins IJ, Sainsbury AJ, Mamo JCL, Redgrave TG. Lipid and apolipoprotein B48 transport in mesenteric lymph and the effect of hyperphagia on chylomicron clearance in insulin-deficient rats. Diabetologia. 1994;**37**:238-246

[106] Dane-Stewart CA, Watts GF, Barrett PH, Stuckey BG, Mamo JC, Martins IJ, et al. Chylomicron remnant metabolism studied with a new breath test in postmenopausal women with and without type 2 diabetes mellitus. Clinical Endocrinology. 2003;**58**:15-20

[107] Martins IJ, Redgrave TG. Obesity and post-prandial lipid metabolism. Feast or famine? The Journal of Nutritional Biochemistry. 2004;**15**:130-141

[108] Xu F, Gao ZG, Zhang J, Rivera CA, Yin J, Weng JP, et al. Lack of SIRT1 (mammalian Sirtuin 1) activity leads to liver steatosis in the SIRT1+/− mice: A role of lipid mobilization and inflammation. Endocrinology. 2010;**151**:2504-2514

[109] Purushotham A, Xu Q, Li XL. Systemic SIRT1 insufficiency results in disruption of energy homeostasis and steroid hormone metabolism upon high-fat-diet feeding. FASEB Journal. 2012;**26**:656-667

[110] Bordone L, Cohen D, Robinson A, Motta MC, Van Veen E, Czopik A, et al. SIRT1 transgenic mice show phenotypes resembling calorie restriction. Aging Cell. 2007;**6**:759-767

[111] Ideally how many grams of fat should you consume daily. Available from: http://healthyeating.sfgate.com/ideally-many-grams-fat-should-consume-daily-5501.html

[112] Martins IJ. Nutrition therapy regulates caffeine metabolism with relevance to NAFLD and induction of type 3 diabetes. Journal of Diabetes and Metabolic Disorders. 2017;**4**:19

[113] Blanchard J. Protein binding of caffeine in young and elderly males. Journal of Pharmaceutical Sciences. 1982;**71**:1415-1418

[114] Martins IJ. Unhealthy diets determine benign or toxic amyloid beta states and promote brain amyloid beta aggregation. Austin Journal of Clinical Neurology. 2015;**2**:1060-1066

[115] Sharma B, Paul S. Action of caffeine as an amyloid inhibitor in the aggregation of Aβ16-22 peptides. Journal of Physical Chemistry B. 2016;**120**:9019-9033

[116] Martins IJ. Magnesium therapy prevents senescence with the reversal of diabetes and Alzheimer's disease. Health. 2016;**8**:694-710

[117] Kynast-Gales SA, Massey LK. Effect of caffeine on circadian excretion of urinary calcium and magnesium. Journal of the American College of Nutrition. 1994;**13**:467-472

[118] Shen H, Rodriguez AC, Shiani A, Lipka S, Shahzad G, Kumar A, et al. Association between caffeine consumption and non-alcoholic fatty liver disease: A systemic review and meta-analysis. Therapeutic Advances in Gastroenterology. 2016;**9**:113-120

[119] Shen C, Dou X, Ma Y, Ma W, Li S, Song Z. Nicotinamide protects hepatocytes against palmitate-induced lipotoxicity via SIRT1-dependent autophagy induction. Nutrition Research. 2017;**40**:40-47

[120] Tong X, Zhang D, Arthurs B, Li P, Durudogan L, Gupta N, et al. Palmitate inhibits SIRT1-dependent BMAL1/CLOCK interaction and disrupts circadian gene oscillations in hepatocytes. PloS One. 2015;**10**:e0130047

[121] Chen JX, Yan SS. Role of mitochondrial amyloid-beta in Alzheimer's disease. Journal of Alzheimer's Disease. 2010;**20**(Suppl. 2):S569-S578

[122] Koczor CA, White RC, Zhao P, Zhu L, Fields E, Lewis W. p53 and mitochondrial DNA, their role in mitochondrial homeostasis and toxicity of anti-retrovirals. American Journal of Pathology. 2012;**180**:2276-2283

[123] Park J-H, Zhuang J, Li J, Hwang PM. p53 as guardian of the mitochondrial genome. FEBS Letters. 2016;**590**:924-934

[124] Safdar A, Little JP, Stokl AJ, Hettinga BP, Akhtar M, Tarnopolsky MA. Exercise increases mitochondrial PGC-1alpha content and promotes nuclear-mitochondrial

cross-talk to coordinate mitochondrial biogenesis. Journal of Biology Chemistry. 2011;**286**:10605-10617

[125] Sen N, Satija YK, Das S. PGC-1α, a key modulator of p53, promotes cell survival upon metabolic stress. Molecular Cell. 2011;**44**:621-634

[126] Aquilano K, Baldelli S, Pagliei B, Cannata SM, Rotilio G, Ciriolo MR. p53 orchestrates the PGC-1α-mediated antioxidant response upon mild redox and metabolic imbalance. Antioxidants and Redox Signalling. 2013;**18**:386-399

[127] Martins IJ. Type 3 diabetes with links to NAFLD and other chronic diseases in the Western World. International Journal of Diabetes. 2016;**1**:1-5

[128] Martins IJ. Heat shock gene Sirtuin 1 regulates post-prandial lipid metabolism with relevance to nutrition and appetite regulation in diabetes. International Journal of Diabetes and Clinical Diagnosis. 2016;**3**:20

[129] Martins IJ. Calorie sensitive anti-aging gene regulates hepatic amyloid beta clearance in diabetes and neurodegenerative diseases. EC Nutrition. 2017;**ECO. 01**:30-32

[130] Martins IJ. Heat shock gene dysregulation and inactivation of drug therapy. EC Pharmacology and Toxicology. 2017;**ECO.01**:13-15

[131] Martins IJ. Regulation of core body temperature and the immune system determines species longevity. Current Updates in Gerontology. 2017;**1**:1-6

[132] Martins IJ. Induction of NAFLD with increased risk of obesity and chronic diseases in developed countries. Open Journal of Endocrine and Metabolic Diseases. 2014;**4**:90-110

[133] Martins IJ. Nutritional diets accelerate amyloid beta metabolism and prevent the induction of chronic diseases and Alzheimer's disease. In: The Journal for Endocrinology and Metabolism, Imprint: Photon, Peer Reviewed Indexed International Journal. Photon ebooks; 2017. p. 1-48

[134] Martins IJ. Apelinergic system defects with relevance to mental disorders in diabetes. World Journal of Psychiatry and Mental Health Research. 2017;**1**:1001

[135] Martins IJ. Defective interplay between adipose tissue and immune system induces non-alcoholic fatty liver disease. Updates in Nutritional Disorders and Therapy. 2017;**1**:3.1

[136] Pénicaud L. Relationships between adipose tissues and brain: What do we learn from animal studies? Diabetes and Metabolism. 2010;**36**(Suppl. 3):S39-S44

[137] Ramachandran A, Snehalatha C, Shetty AS, Nanditha A. Trends in prevalence of diabetes in Asian countries. World Journal of Diabetes. 2012;**3**:110-117

[138] Farrell GC, Wong VW, Chitturi S. NAFLD in Asia—As common and important as in the west. Nature Reviews Gastroenterology and Hepatology. 2013;**10**:307-318

[139] Amarapurkar D, Kamani P, Patel N, Gupte P, Kumar P, Agal S, et al. Prevalence of non-alcoholic fatty liver disease: Population based study. Annals of Hepatology. 2007;**6**:161-163

[140] LaBrecque DR, Abbas Z, Anania F, Ferenci P, Khan AG, Goh KL, et al. World gastroenterology organisation global guidelines: Non-alcoholic fatty liver disease and non-alcoholic steatohepatitis. Journal of Clinical Gastroenterology. 2014;**48**:467-473

[141] Hu FB. Globalization of diabetes: The role of diet, lifestyle, and genes. Diabetes Care. 2011;**34**:1249-1257

[142] Shi X, Xue W, Liang S, Zhao J, Zhang X. Acute caffeine ingestion reduces insulin sensitivity in healthy subjects: A systematic review and meta-analysis. Nutrition Journal. 2016;**15**:103

[143] Dewar L, Heuberger R. The effect of acute caffeine intake on insulin sensitivity and glycemic control in people with diabetes. Diabetes and Metabolic Syndrome: Clinical. Research and Reviews. 2017; Available online 23 April 2017. In Press, Accepted Manuscript. https://doi.org/10.1016/j.dsx.2017.04.017

[144] Martins IJ. Bacterial lipopolysaccharides change membrane fluidity with relevance to phospholipid and amyloid beta dynamics in Alzheimer's disease. Journal of Microbiology and Biochemical Technology. 2016;**8**:322-324

[145] Martins IJ. The future of genomic medicine involves the maintenance of sirtuin 1 in global populations. International Journal of Molecular Biology. 2017;**2**:00013

[146] How Much Fat Per Day—How Many Grams of Fat Should You Eat? http://www.acaloriecounter.com/diet/how-much-fat-per-day, Accessed 06072017, Copyright © 2007 - 2017 A Calorie Counter. All Rights Reserved. Terms Of Use

[147] Martins IJ. In: Atta-ur-Rahman, editor Nutritional and Genotoxic Stress Contributes to Diabetes and Neurodegenerative Diseases such as Parkinson's and Alzheimer's Diseases. Frontiers in Clinical Drug Research-CNS and Neurological Disorders 2015 3. pp. 158-192

[148] Tahara Y, Shibata S. Circadian rhythms of liver physiology and disease: Experimental and clinical evidence. Nature Reviews. Gastroenterology & Hepatology. 2016;**13**:217-226

[149] Burke TM, Markwald RR, McHill AW, Chinoy ED, Snider JA, Bessman SC, et al. Effects of caffeine on the human circadian clock in vivo and in vitro. Science Translational Medicine. 2015;**7**:305ra146

[150] Martins IJ. Geriatric medicine and heat shock gene therapy in global populations. Current Updates in Gerontology. 2016;**1**:1-5

[151] Scorletti E, Bhatia L, McCormick KG, Clough GF, Nash K, Hodson L, et al. WELCOME Study. Effects of purified eicosapentaenoic and docosahexaenoic acids in nonalcoholic fatty liver disease: Results from the Welcome* study. Hepatology. 2014;**60**:1211-1221

[152] Alkhouri N, Dixon LJ, Feldstein AE. Lipotoxicity in non-alcoholic fatty liver disease: Not all lipids are created equal. Expert Review in Gastroenterology and Hepatology. 2009;**3**:445-451

[153] Martins IJ, Gupta V, Wilson AC, Fuller SJ, Martins RN. Interactions between Apo E and amyloid beta and their relationship to nutriproteomics and neurodegeneration. Current Proteomics. 2014;**11**:173-183

[154] Martins IJ. Over-nutrition determines LPS regulation of mycotoxin induced neuro-toxicity in neurodegenerative diseases. International Journal of Molecular Science. 2015;**16**:29554-29573

[155] Tong X, Yin L. Circadian rhythms in liver physiology and liver diseases. Comparative Physiology. 2013;**3**:917-940

[156] Gnanou JV, Caszo BA, Khalil KM, Abdullah SL, Knight VF, Bidin MZ. Effects of Ramadan fasting on glucose homeostasis and adiponectin levels in healthy adult males. Journal of Diabetes and Metabolic Disorders. 2015;**14**:55

[157] Martins IJ. The global obesity epidemic is related to stroke, dementia and Alzheimer's disease. JSM Alzheimer's Disease and Related Dementia. 2014;**1**:1010

[158] Cassidy A, Skidmore P, Rimm EB, Welch A, Fairweather-Tait S, Skinner J, et al. Plasma adiponectin concentrations are associated with body composition and plant-based dietary factors in female twins. Journal of Nutrition. 2009;**139**:353-358

[159] Markaki A, Kyriazis J, Stylianou K, Fragkiadakis GA, Perakis K, Margioris AN, et al. The role of serum magnesium and calcium on the association between adiponectin levels and all-cause mortality in end-stage renal disease patients. PloS One. 2012;**7**:e52350

[160] Sierksma A, Patel H, Ouchi N, Kihara S, Funahashi T, Heine RJ, et al. Effect of moderate alcohol consumption on adiponectin, tumor necrosis factor-alpha, and insulin sensitivity. Diabetes Care. 2004;**27**:184-189

[161] Burg VK, Grimm HS, Rothhaar TL, Grösgen S, Hundsdörfer B, Haupenthal VJ, et al. Plant sterols the better cholesterol in Alzheimer's disease? A mechanistical study. Journal of Neuroscience. 2013;**33**:16072-16087

[162] Sodhi K, Puri N, Favero G, Stevens S, Meadows C, Abraham NG, et al. Fructose mediated non-alcoholic fatty liver is attenuated by HO-1-SIRT1 module in murine hepatocytes and mice fed a high fructose diet. PloS One. 2015;**10**:e0128648

[163] Rebollo A, Roglans N, Baena M, Sánchez RM, Merlos M, Alegret M, et al. Liquid fructose down-regulates Sirt1 expression and activity and impairs the oxidation of fatty acids in rat and human liver cells. Biochimica et Biophysica Acta. 2014;**1841**:514-524

[164] Martins IJ. Magnesium deficiency and induction of NAFLD and Type 3 diabetes in Australasia. Australasian Medical Journal. 2017;**10**:235-237

[165] Martins IJ. Drug therapy for obesity with anti-aging genes modification. Annals of Obesity and Disorders. 2016;**1**:1001

[166] Martins IJ. Inactivation of anti-aging genes is related to defective drug metabolism in diabetes. International Journal of Drug Discovery. 2017;**1**:3

[167] Martins IJ. Early diagnosis of neuron mitochondrial dysfunction may reverse global metabolic and neurodegenerative disease. Global Journal of Medical Research. 2016;**2**:1-8

4

Molecular Mechanisms of Hepatocellular Carcinoma Related to Aflatoxins

Xi-Dai Long, Yan Deng, Xiao-Ying Huang,
Jin-Guang Yao, Qun-Ying Su, Xue-Min Wu,
Juan Wang, Qun-Qing Xu, Xiao-Ying Zhu,
Chao Wang, Bing-Chen Huang and Qiang Xia

Abstract

Hepatocellular carcinoma (hepatocarcinoma) is a major type of primary liver cancer and one of the most frequent human malignant neoplasms. Aflatoxins are I-type chemical carcinogen for hepatocarcinoma. Increasing evidence has shown that hepatocarcinoma induced by aflatoxins is the result of interaction between aflatoxins and hereditary factor. Aflatoxins can induce DNA damage including DNA strand break, adducts formation, oxidative DNA damage, and gene mutation and determine which susceptible individuals feature cancer. Inheritance such as alterations may result in the activation of proto-oncogenes and the inactivation of tumor suppressor genes and determine individual susceptibility to cancer. Interaction between aflatoxins and genetic susceptible factors commonly involve in almost all pathologic sequence of hepatocarcinoma: chronic liver injury, cirrhosis, atypical hyperplastic nodules, and hepatocarcinoma of early stages. In this review, we discuss the biogenesis, toxification, and epidemiology of aflatoxins and signal pathways of aflatoxin-induced hepatocarcinoma. We also discuss the roles of some important genes related to cell apoptosis, DNA repair, drug metabolism, and tumor metastasis in hepatocarcinogenesis related to aflatoxins.

Keywords: hepatocellular carcinoma, molecular mechanism, aflatoxin

1. Introduction

Hepatocellular carcinoma (also called hepatocarcinoma or liver carcinoma) is a major type of primary liver cancer and one of the most frequent human malignant neoplasms. This malignancy has been proved to correlate with aflatoxins, especially aflatoxin B1 (AFB1) [1–3].

Increasing evidence has exhibited that several mechanisms, including the toxic production from metabolism, the accumulation of DNA damage and genic mutation–induced aflatoxins, the decreasing DNA repair capacity, and dysregulation of signal pathways may play a central role in the tumorigenesis of aflatoxin-induced hepatocarcinoma [4–6]. In this review, we discuss the biogenesis, metabolism, and genic toxification of aflatoxins. We also discuss the molecular mechanisms of aflatoxin-induced hepatocarcinoma, involving in aflatoxin toxification, abnormal change of tumor relative genes, the interaction of aflatoxins and genetic factors, and signal pathway for tumorigenesis. The roles of some important genes related to cell apoptosis, DNA repair, drug metabolism, and tumor metastasis in hepatocarcinogenesis related to aflatoxins are further emphasized.

2. Aflatoxin biosynthesis, metabolism, and toxification

2.1. Aflatoxin biosynthesis

The biosynthesis of aflatoxins has been fully summarized in several previous reviews [7, 8]. In brief, aflatoxins are an important type of mycotoxins, which were the most early identified in the *Aspergillus flavus* (*A. flavus*) and regarded as causative agents of "turkey X" disease in the late 1950s and early 1960s. Thus, these toxins were named as "aflatoxins (namely *A. flavus* toxins)" according to their origin fungus [9]. Until now, 17 related aflatoxin isoforms and aflatoxin metabolites have been identified, and 4 of them often contaminated a number of agricultural commodities [10]. According to the amounts and fluorescent reactions, four aflatoxins primarily identified in foodstuffs are named as AFB1, aflatoxin B2 (AFB2), aflatoxin G1 (AFG1), and aflatoxin G2 (AFG2). Among these four known aflatoxins, AFB1 and AFB2 are named as B-type aflatoxins because they are attached to a pentanone and can produce blue-color fluorescent under UV light, whereas AFG1 and AFG2 are termed as G-type aflatoxins because of their attachment to a 6-membered lactone and producing green fluorescent color feature. These aflatoxins are mainly produced by *A. flavus*, *Aspergillus parasiticus* (*A. parasiticus*), *Aspergillus nidulans* (*A. nidulans*), *Aspergillus pseudotamarii* (*A. pseudotamarii*), and *Aspergillus bombycis* (*A. bombycis*) [7, 8].

Toxigenic strains of *A. flavus* produce only B-type aflatoxins, but do not synthesize G-type aflatoxins due to the deletion of an unstable microsome enzyme and a-220 kDa cytosolic protein. The other aflatoxigenic species including *A. parasiticus*, *A. nidulans*, *A. pseudotamarii*, and *A. bombycis* can produce all four aflatoxins [8].

Numeral synthetical genes, such as aflatoxin regulatory protein gene (aflR), are required for aflatoxin biosynthesis and act as a huge neighbor gene cluster consisting of about 60–70 kb in original fungi (**Figure** 1) [8–10]. All corresponding gene-encoding enzymes and transcription factors produce aflatoxin production and regulate biosynthesis. Increasing evidence has proved that aflatoxin biosynthesis involves in at least 3 stages and 18 enzyme steps (**Figures 2–4**). The first stage, including the first (R01) to eighth reaction (R08) of biosynthesis, refers from acetyl CoA to hydroxyversicolorone. The primary product hydroxyversicolorone will be formed and regulated by transcription factors aflR and aflJ (**Figure 2**) [8, 10]. The second (biosynthesis

Aflatoxin Gene Cluster (AFGC)

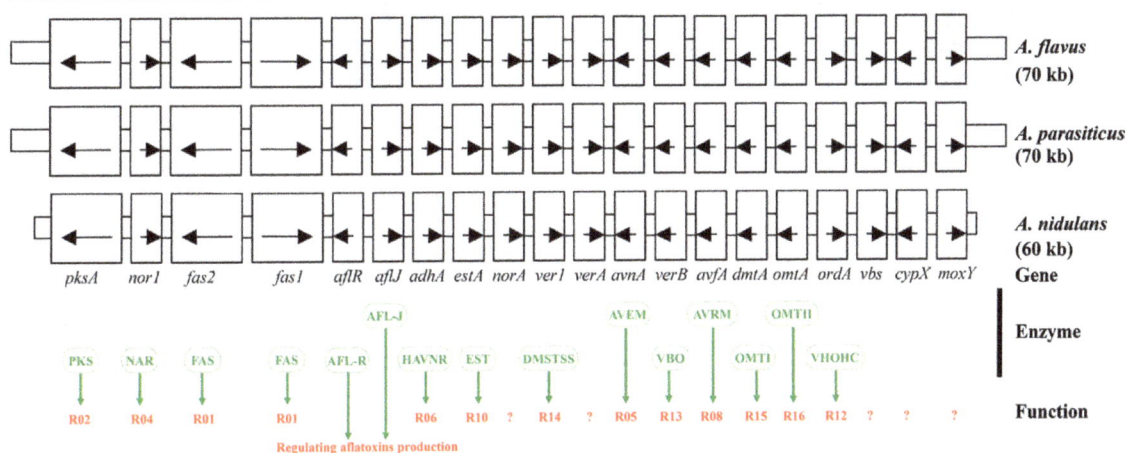

Figure 1. The aflatoxin gene cluster and their expression productions and functions. In the fungus-producing aflatoxins including *A. nidulans*, *A. parasiticus*, and *A. flavus*, genes encoding the enzymes and the transcription factors involving in aflatoxin biosynthesis commonly locate within a huge gene cluster of about 60–70 kb in the genomes. These genes, except for aflR and aflJ, involve in the 18 enzyme reaction steps (R01–R18) of aflatoxin biosynthesis, whereas aflR and aflJ expressing proteins are two important transcription factors and can regulate enzyme-related gene expression. "?" shows that the function of the corresponding gene is unknown (Note: adapted from Yabe and Nakajima [7]). *Abbreviations*. MCA, malonyl CoA; HAS, hexanoate synthase (also termed fatty acid synthase); PKS, polyketide synthase; NAS, Norsolorinic acid (NA) synthase; NAR, norsolorinic acid (NA) reductase; AVN, averantin; AVNM, averantin (AVN) monooxygenase; HAVN, 5′-hydroxyaverantin; HAVNR, 5′-hydroxyaverantin reductase; OVENC, 5′-oxoaverantin (OAVN) cyclase; AVRM, averufin (AVR) monooxygenase; VHAS, versiconal hemiacetal acetate (VHA) synthase; VHOHC, versiconal (VHOH) cyclase (also called versicolorin B synthase); VHAR, versiconal hemiacetal acetate (VHA) reductase; VBD, versicolorin B (VB) desaturase; DMSTSS, demethylsterigmatocystin (DMST) synthase system; OMTI, *O*-methyltransferase I; OMTII, *O*-methyltransferase II; OAE, OrdA enzyme.

reaction: R09–R12) (**Figure 3**) and third stages (biosynthesis reaction: R13–R18) (**Figure 4**) refer from hydroxyversicolorone to versicolorin B and from versicolorin B (VB) to the formation of ultimate products, respectively. These two stages involve in the formation of hydroxy- and non–hydroxy-versicolorone, and toxins. During the aflatoxin synthesis, more than 10 nicotin-amide-adenine dinucleotide phosphate reduced form (NAPDH), one nicotinamide-adenine dinucleotide (NAD), and 2S-adenosylmethionine (SAM) are required. These cofactors may play a critical role in the control of aflatoxin biosynthesis [7–10].

2.2. The metabolism of aflatoxins in liver

Aflatoxins synthesized in the mycelia are finally excreted into such mediums as cereals (maize, wheat, sorghum, rice, and millet), nuts (peanuts, pistachios, walnuts, Brazil nut, and coco-nut), spices (chili, turmeric, paprika, black pepper, and ginger), and seeds. Epidemiological studies have exhibited that AFB1 is the most common in contaminated human foods [8, 10]. Once this aflatoxin in the mediums is taken into body, it is metabolized via two-stage reac-tions in the liver. The first-stage metabolisms include reduction reaction (ketoreduction to aflatoxicol), oxidative reaction (O-dealkylation to aflatoxin P1), and hydrolytic reactions (hydroxylation to aflatoxin M1, aflatoxin Q1, and aflatoxin B2). This stage reaction involves numerous enzymes such as cytochromes P450 (CYP450), monooxygenases, amino-oxidases, alcohol dehydrogenases, epoxide-hydrolases, aldehyde-reductases, and ketone-reductases. The second-stage reaction mainly comprises covalent binding reaction (toxic produces) and conjugation reaction (excretion and detoxification). Through these metabolites, aflatoxins ultimately transform into nontoxic secretions and toxic products [10, 11].

2.3. The toxification of aflatoxins in liver

Toxification of aflatoxins in liver is mainly divided into acute and chronic toxic effects. Data from epidemiological, experimental, and clinical studies have shown that above 6000 mg exposure of aflatoxin through digestion will cause acute severe liver damage and subsequent

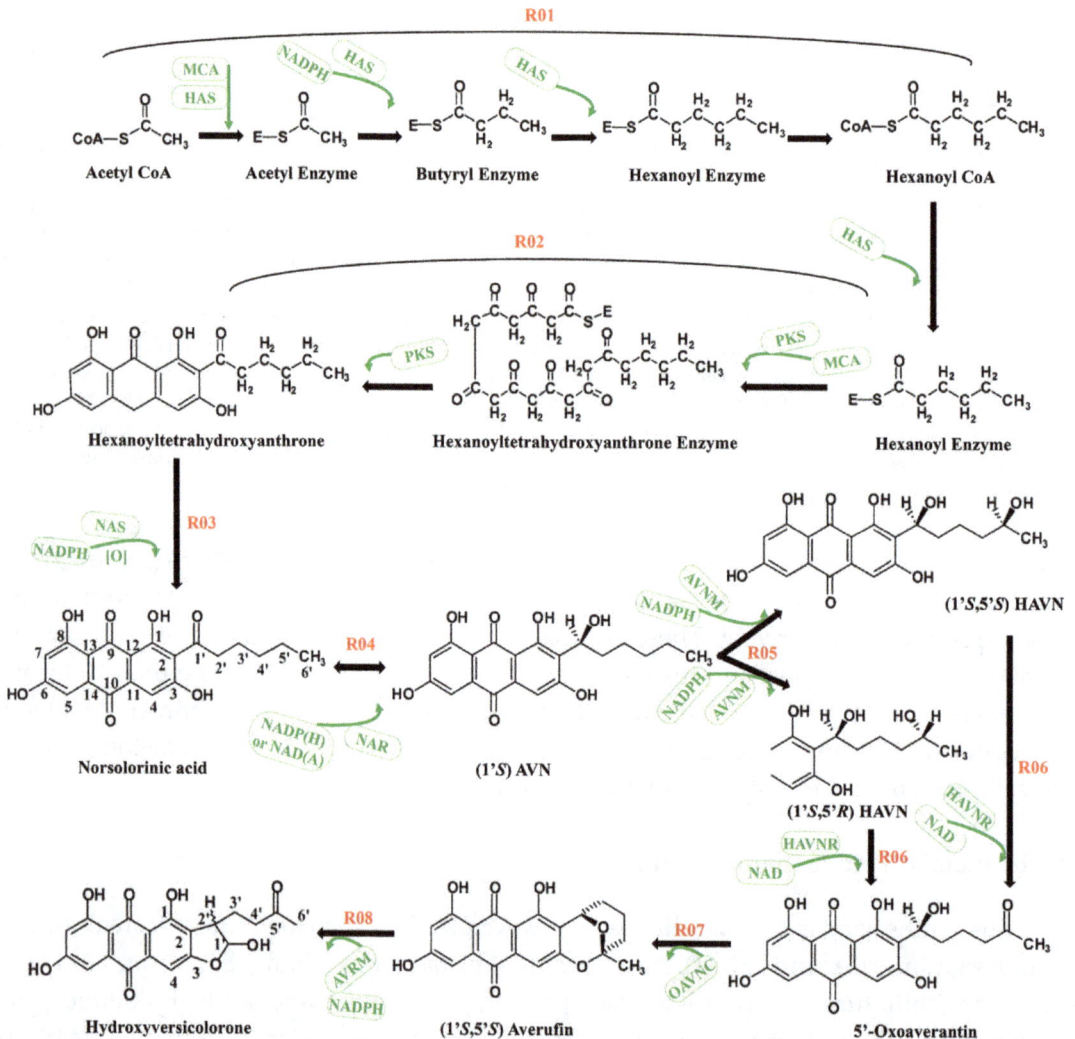

Figure 2. The first stage of aflatoxin biosynthesis. The first stage of aflatoxin biosynthesis, including the first (R01) to eighth reaction (R08) of biosynthesis, refers from acetyl CoA to hydroxyversicolorone. *Abbreviations.* MCA, malonyl CoA; HAS, hexanoate synthase (also termed fatty acid synthase); PKS, polyketide synthase; NAS, norsolorinic acid (NA) synthase; NAR, norsolorinic acid (NA) reductase; AVN, averantin; AVNM, averantin (AVN) monooxygenase; HAVN, 5'-hydroxyaverantin; HAVNR, 5'-hydroxyaverantin reductase; OVENC, 5'-oxoaverantin (OAVN) cyclase; AVRM, averufin (AVR) monooxygenase; NADP, nicotinamide adenine dinucleotide phosphate; NADPH, nicotinamide-adenine dinucleotide phosphate (reduced form); CoA, coenzyme A. *Noted:* adapted from Yabe and Nakajima [7].

illness or death. This kind of acute effect is mainly associated with malfunction of the liver induced by toxic metabolic products. For chronic toxic effects, chronic exposure of aflatoxins can induce DNA damage and produce genotoxicity and carcinogenicity. In the past decades, increasing evidence has proved that AFB1 as aflatoxins often induce genic mutations such as TP53 and are among the most carcinogenic substances known and the major cancerous hepatocarcinoma risk factor.

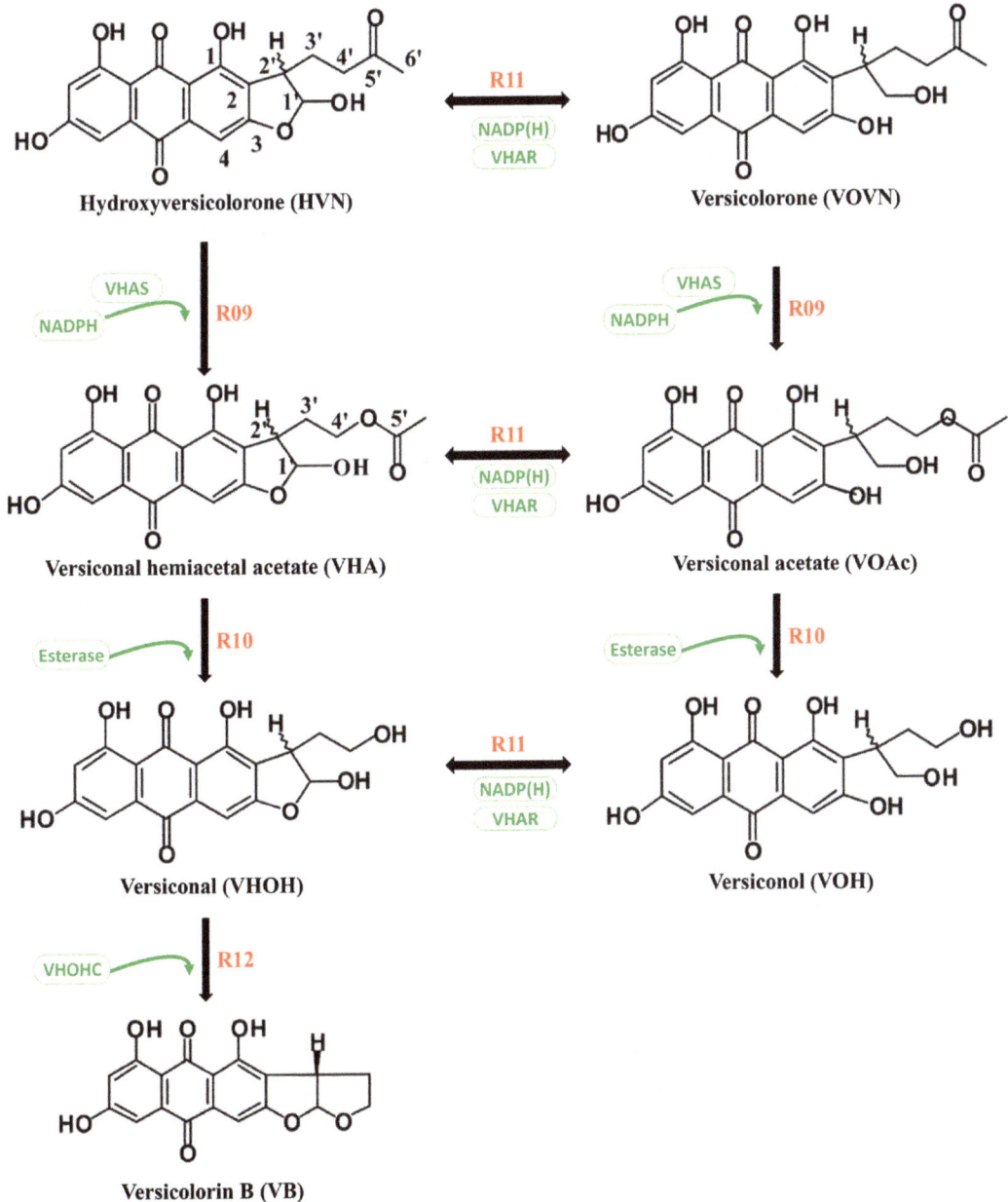

Figure 3. The second stage of aflatoxin biosynthesis. The second stage of aflatoxin biosynthesis, including the ninth (R09) to twelfth reaction (R12) of biosynthesis, refers from hydroxyversicolorone to versicolorin B (VB). *Abbreviations.* VHAS, versiconal hemiacetal acetate (VHA) synthase; VHOHC, versiconal (VHOH) cyclase (also called versicolorin B synthase); VHAR, versiconal hemiacetal acetate (VHA) reductase; NADP, nicotinamide adenine dinucleotide phosphate; NADPH, nicotinamide-adenine dinucleotide phosphate (reduced form). *Noted:* adapted from Yabe and Nakajima [7].

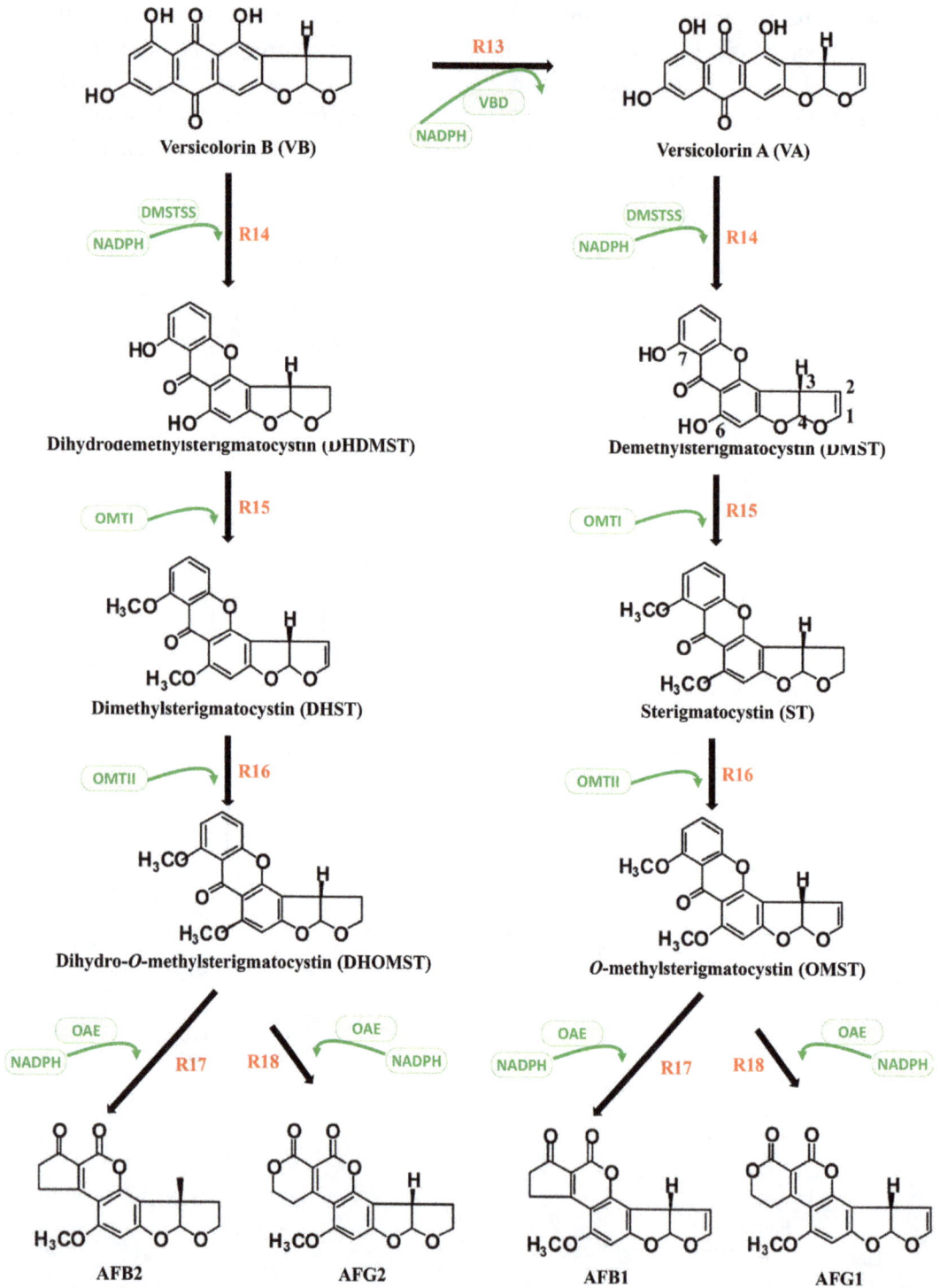

Figure 4. The third stage of aflatoxin biosynthesis. The third stage of aflatoxin biosynthesis, including the 13th (R13) to 18th reaction (R18) of biosynthesis, refers from versicolorin B (VB) to the formation of aflatoxin B1 (AFB1), aflatoxin B2 (AFB2), aflatoxin G1 (AFG1), and aflatoxin G2 (AFG2). *Abbreviations.* VBD, versicolorin B (VB) desaturase; DMSTSS, demethylsterigmatocystin (DMST) synthase system; OMTI, *O*-methyltransferase I; OMTII, *O*-methyltransferase II; OAE, OrdA enzyme; NADP, nicotinamide adenine dinucleotide phosphate; NADPH, nicotinamide-adenine dinucleotide phosphate (reduced form). *Noted:* adapted from Yabe and Nakajima [7].

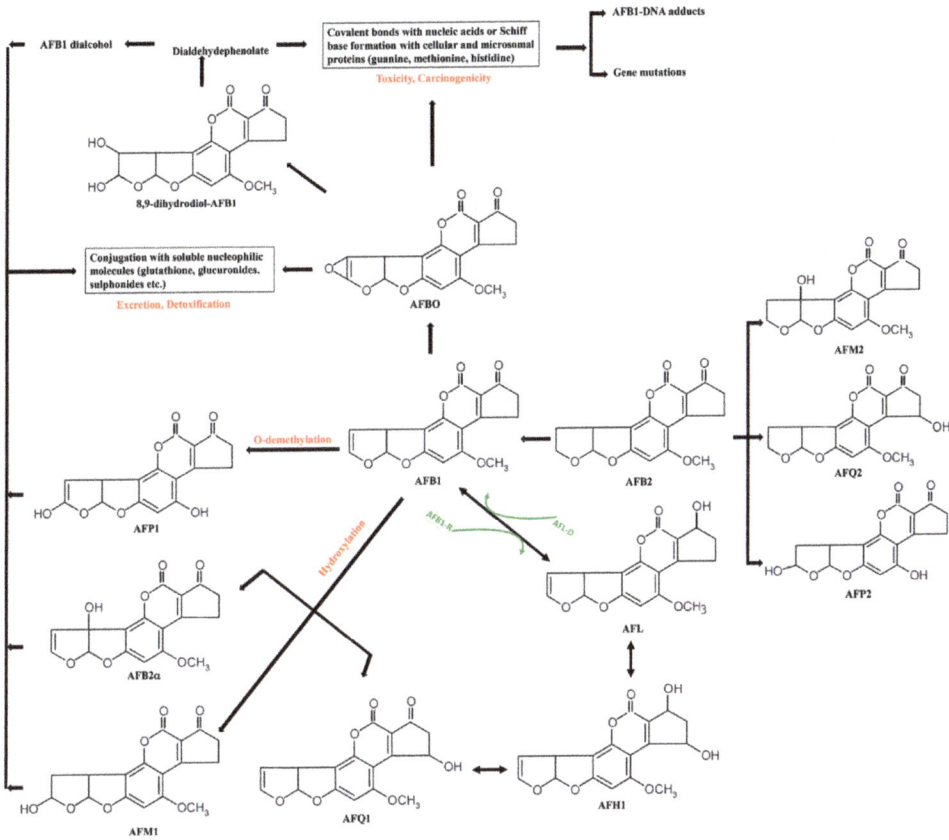

Figure 5. The metabolite of aflatoxins in the liver. Aflatoxins are metabolized via four metabolic pathways: O-dealkylation to aflatoxin P1 (AFP1), ketoreduction to aflatoxicol (AFL), epoxidation to AFB1-8,9-epoxide (AFBO, highly toxic, mutagenic, and carcinogenic), and hydroxylation to aflatoxin M1 (AFM1, highly toxic), AFP1, aflatoxin Q1 (AFQ1), or aflatoxin B2a (AFB2a). *Abbreviations.* AFM2, aflatoxin M2; AFP2, aflatoxin P2; AFQ2, aflatoxin Q2; AFL-D, aflatoxicol dehydrogenase; AFB1-R, aflatoxin B1 reductase. *Noted:* adapted from Wu and Jezkova [10].

3. The molecular mechanisms of aflatoxin-induced hepatocarcinoma

As described earlier, the main chronic toxification of aflatoxins is chronic liver damage and induced tumorigenesis of hepatocarcinoma. AFB1 has been proved as an I-type chemical carcinogen. Mechanisms of AFB1-induced hepatocarcinoma mainly involve in DNA damage and repair, the inactivation of tumor suppressor genes and the activation of oncogenes from genic mutations, abnormal immunoreaction, and inheritance alterations.

3.1. Aflatoxin-induced DNA damage

Increasing evidence has shown that the carcinogenicity of aflatoxins results from aflatoxin-induced DNA damage, including the formation of DNA adducts, DNA single strand breaks (SSBs) or double strand breaks (DSBs), chromosomal aberration damage (CAD), unscheduled DNA synthesis (USDS), abnormal chromatid exchange (ACE), the formation of micronuclei and macronuclei, and oxidation DNA damage. Of these DNA damages, AFB1-DNA adducts are the most common damage types and consist of 8,9-dihydro-8-(N^7-guanyl)-9-hydroxy–AFB1 adduct (AFB1-GA) and ring-opened formamidopyrimidine AFB1 adduct (AFB1-FAPYA). The formation of AFB1-GA begins from AFB1 covalent binding to DNA and its product 8,9-epoxide-AFB1 (AFBE) by CYP450 [12, 13]. This adduct can automatically not only give rise to AFB1-FAYPA, which is accumulated using a time-dependence and nonenzyme pathway, but also be transferred into AFP1, AFM1, AFQ1, and other products by metabolic enzymes.

Additionally, AFB1 also induces oxidation DNA damage such as 8-oxodeoxyguanosine (8-$_{oxyG}$). These damages induced by aflatoxins, if not timely repaired, can cause subsequent repair-resistant adducts and depurination or lead to error-prone DNA repair resulting in DSBs, SSBs, USDs, CAD, ACE, and frame shift mutations. Interestingly, the accumulation of DNA damages is positively associated with the time and the levels of aflatoxin exposure and modifies the risk of hepatocarcinoma through regulating the expression of some genes such as a disintegrin and metalloproteinase with thrombospondin motifs 5 (ADAMTS5) [14], X-ray repair complementing 4 (XRCC4) [15], microRNA-4651 [16], and so on (**Table 1**). For example, Huang et al. [14] investigated the association between AFB1-DNA adducts via a hospital-based case control study and found increasing AFB1-DNA adducts negatively correlated with ADAMTS5 expression. It is known that ADAMTS5 may act as a tumor suppressor gene via decreasing vascular endothelial growth factor (VEGF) expression and inhibiting tumor angiogenesis and metastasis [17]. The downregulation of XRCC4 by increasing AFB1-DNA adducts decreases repair capacity for SSBs and DSBs and increases risk of tumor suppressor gene TP53 mutation and tumors [15, 18–22]. These genes progress the tumorigenesis and progression of hepatocarcinoma via regulating DNA repair capacity and angiogenesis. Although AFB1-DNA adducts are mainly produced in liver cells, they are also found in the immune cells and may regulate the immune function. Thus, DNA damage may be an important molecular event and may play a crucial role in the carcinogenesis of hepatocarcinoma caused by aflatoxins.

3.2. The mutagenesis of aflatoxins

Aflatoxin-induced DNA adducts can produce depurination, DSBs, the substitution of DNA bases, and frame shift mutations. In the past decades, the *in vivo* and *in vitro* studies have shown that the mutagenesis of aflatoxins can induce the mutation from GC to TA. As previously shown, mispairing of the aflatoxin-DNA adducts can cause both transition and transversion mutations [25–27]. In an *in vitro* non-sense analysis, Foster et al. found that the action form of AFB1 (namely AFBE) can induce more than 90% of GC to TA mutation [28]. This

Gene	Expression change	Role of change in the hepatocarcinoma carcinogenesis	Ref
ADAMTS5	Down	Angiogenesis, metastasis, prognosis	[14]
XRCC4	Down	Low DNA repair capacity, gene mutation	[15]
MicroRNA-4651	Up	Angiogenesis, metastasis, prognosis	[16]
MicroRNA-24	Up	Angiogenesis, metastasis, prognosis	[23]
MicroRNA-429	Up	Angiogenesis, metastasis, prognosis	[24]

Table 1. The change of gene expression related to DNA damage induced by aflatoxins.

mutation was further proved to locate in the GC-rich regions via the plasmid system identifying mutational target enzyme and named as hot-spot regions for aflatoxin-induced mutations [29–31]. Results from quantitative analyses based on the *in vitro* cell model, which was transfected by pS189 (a shuttle vector having mutative targets), also showed that more than 90% of mutative spectra caused by aflatoxins was GC to TA (about 50% of mutations) and GG to TC transversion (about 30% of mutations) [32]. It has been proved that the accumulation of these transversions will result in the mutations of some important genes such as TP53 and Ras and promote hepatocarcinogenesis [31, 33].

3.3. The abnormality of tumor suppressor genes induced by aflatoxins

Studies *in vivo* and *in vitro* have examined the abnormality of tumor suppressor genes by aflatoxin exposure (**Table 2**). Among these known genes, the abnormality of TP53 induced by aflatoxins has been proved to be an important molecule change [34, 35]. In high aflatoxin-exposure areas, the mutations of TP53 gene, especially hot-spot mutation at codon 249, are present among more than 40% of patients with AFB1-related hepatocarcinoma, whereas this kind of mutation is very rare among cases with null or low AFB1 exposure [14, 36, 37]. Therefore, the mutation at codon 249 of TP53 gene has been defined as a molecular symbol for hepatocarcinoma caused by AFB1 exposure. Results from clinical sample and experimental studies further display that consistent exposure of aflatoxins may result in the accumulation of TP53 mutant protein and abnormal DNA damage repair, apoptosis, and immunoreaction [38]. Other genes such as bcl2, p27, p16, and p21 are found to produce different expression or abnormal structural change under the conditions of aflatoxin expression (**Table 2**). Taken together, inactivation of tumor suppressor genes from mutation and increasing mutant expression may be a crucial step of malignant transformation for liver cells.

3.4. The abnormality of oncogenes induced by aflatoxins

In the past decades, the abnormality of oncogenes induced by aflatoxins has mainly been focused on c-myc and ras genes, involving in the activation, expression, and mutation of proto-oncogenes (**Table 3**). For example, Tashiro et al. investigated the effects of AFB1 exposure on oncogenes based on rat model with AFB1-induced hepatomas and found that the expression of both c-myc and c-Ha-ras was upregulated in all the tumors [65]. They also observed c-Ha-ras amplification and rearrangement [65]. In Fischer rat models with AFB1- and AFG1-induced liver tumors, Sinha et al. observed that aflatoxins can induce activation of N-ras and spot mutation of G to A at codon 12 of Ki-ras [66]. This type of activation and mutation will increase in the tissues with liver cancer than those with noncancers [66–69]. Results from *in vitro* studies have further proved that aflatoxins can induce gene mutations of oncogenes [70]. Together, these data suggest that aflatoxins may activate proto-oncogenes by inducing gene mutations and promote the carcinogenesis of hepatocarcinoma.

3.5. The interaction of aflatoxins and hepatitis B virus promoting hepatocarcinogenesis

The interaction of aflatoxins and hepatitis B virus (HBV) has been proved in the carcinogenesis of hepatocarcinoma by molecular epidemiological and clinicopathological studies and sys-

Gene	Study design	Change	Significance	Ref
TP53	Mice model with HNP	Expression ↑	DNA damage ↑	[39]
bcl2	Mice model with HNP	Expression ↓	DNA damage ↑	[39]
p27	Hepatocytes *in vitro*	Expression ↓	DNA damage ↑	[40]
p21	Hepatocytes *in vitro*	Expression ↓	DNA damage ↑	[40]
TP53	HCCs (n = 223)	Expression ↑, multiplot mutation	Carcinogenesis	[41]
TP53	HCCs (n = 124)	Mutation at codon 249: 60%	Carcinogenesis	[42]
H2AX	HCC cells *in vitro*	Phosphorylation	Carcinogenesis	[43]
BP1	HCC cells *in vitro*	Phosphorylation	Carcinogenesis	[43]
TP53	HCCs (n = 52)	Mutation at codon 249: 50%	Carcinogenesis	[44]
p16	HCCs (n = 40)	Methylation	Carcinogenesis	[45]
p53	HCCs (n = 40)	Multiplot mutation	Carcinogenesis	[45]
p53	AFB1-induced mutation *in vitro*	Multiplot mutation at CpG	Carcinogenesis	[46]
TP53	HCCs (n = 64) plus a meta-analysis	Mutation at codon 249: 36%, protein accumulation: 50%	Carcinogenesis	[47]
TP53	Mice model with HNP	Multiplot mutation	Carcinogenesis	[48]
TP53	HCC cells *in vitro*	AFB1-induced mutation at codon 249 promoting IGF-II expression	Carcinogenesis	[49]
TP53	Atcc-Ccl13 *in vitro*	Mutation at codon 249	Carcinogenesis	[50]
TP53	HCCs (n = 36)	Mutation at codon 249	Carcinogenesis	[51]
TP53	Mice model	Mutation at codon 249 and 346, mutant protein increasing	Carcinogenesis	[52–57]
TP53	HCCs (n = 60)	Mutation at codon 249: 69%	Carcinogenesis	[58, 59]
TP53	Hepatocytes *in vitro*	Multiplot mutation	Carcinogenesis	[60]
TP53	HCCs (n = 110)	Mutation at codon 249: 69%	DNA damage, carcinogenesis	[61]
TP53	HCCs (n = 15)	Mutation at codon 249 and 254	Carcinogenesis	[62]
TP53	HCC cells *in vitro*	AFB1-induced Mutation at codon 249	Carcinogenesis	[63]
TP53	HCCs (n = 18)	Mutation at codon 249: 53%	Carcinogenesis	[64]

Abbreviations. HNP, hepatic neoplasms; HCC, hepatocarcinoma.

Table 2. The change information of tumor suppressor genes induced by aflatoxins in hepatic cells and hepatocarcinoma cells.

Gene	Study design	Change	Significance	Ref
N-ras	HCCs (n = 36)	Mutation at codon 61	Carcinogenesis	[51]
c-myc	Mice model with HNP	Expression ↑, amplification, rearrangement	Carcinogenesis	[65]
c-Ha-ras	Mice model with HNP	Expression ↑, amplification, rearrangement	Carcinogenesis	[65]
Ki-ras	Mice model with HNP	Activation	Carcinogenesis	[69]
N-ras	Mice model with HNP	Activation	Carcinogenesis	[66]
Ki-ras	Mice model with HNP	Mutation at codon 12	Carcinogenesis	[66]
N-ras	Mice model with HCC	Activation	Carcinogenesis	[67]
Ki-ras	Mice model with HCC	Activation	Carcinogenesis	[67]
c-Ha-ras	Mice model with HNP	Mutation at codon 61: 40–60%	Carcinogenesis	[71, 72]

Abbreviations. HNP, hepatic neoplasms; HCC, hepatocarcinoma.

Table 3. The change information of oncogenes induced by aflatoxins.

tematically reviewed by several studies [73–75]. In brief, the first clinicopathological evidence of aflatoxins interacting with HBV was provided by Yeh et al. [76]. Through a case-control study design conducted in Guangxi Area, they found that these HBV-positive individuals with high AFB1 exposure consumption featured 10-times the mortality rate compared with those with low exposure consumption. Results from multivariable interactive analyses have further convinced that AFB1 multiplicatively interacted with HBV status for promoting hepatocarcinoma risk [77–80]. For example, Williams et al. reported that the risk of developing hepatocarcinoma was 6.37 for aflatoxin exposure, 11.3 for HBV infection, and 73.0 for the combination of aflatoxin and HBV [77]. The following several molecular epidemiological studies with large-size samples from areas with high aflatoxin exposure and high HBV infection in China showed remarkably multiplicative effect for hepatocarcinoma risk (multiplicative interaction: $63.2_{(both\ positive)} > 1.9_{(AFB1\ positive)} \times 9.5_{(HBV\ positive)}$ [78–80].

This interaction of two hepatocarcinogenic causes has been proved in the transgenic mice models with overexpressing HBV large envelope polypeptide [81]. Results from this study exhibited that animals will produce more rapid and extensive hepatic dysplasia and hepatocarcinoma under the conditions with aflatoxin consumption [81]. Similar findings have also shown in the studies based on woodchuck and duck models [82–84].

The aflatoxins interacting with HBV infection promoting hepatocarcinoma development mechanically involve in the following aspects. First, HBV infection directly or indirectly increases the sensitivity of hepatocytes on the toxification of aflatoxins. Evidence from observation studies have displayed that HBV-positive carriers have more amount of aflatoxin adducts than those with negative HBV status, although they are from the same high aflatoxin exposure area [85, 86]. The active product of aflatoxin AFBE is found to significantly increase the risk of viral DNA integrating into damaged DNA strand [87]. This promotes malignant transformation of damaged hepatocytes by aflatoxins. Second, HBV infection increases the mutation frequency at codon 249 of TP53 gene and coordinates with aflatoxins for abrogating the normal functions of TP53 (such as the control of cell cycle, DNA damage repair, and cell apoptosis), which contributes to multisteps of hepatic carcinogenesis [64, 88]. Third, the HBV X gene–expressing protein inhibits base excision repair potential and results in an increasing accumulation of aflatoxin-DNA adducts [89]. Finally, HBV infections can cause hepatocytic necrosis, inflammatory proliferation, and oxygen/nitrogen active products, which may increase the likelihood of aflatoxin-induced mutations and the cellular clonal expansion containing mutations [90–92].

3.6. The interaction of aflatoxins and inheritance alterations promoting hepatocarcinogenesis

Increasing evidence has exhibited that the genetic alterations in DNA repair genes increase the amount of AFB1-DNA adducts and the frequency of hot-spot mutation at codon 249 of TP53 gene and may promote hepatic toxification of aflatoxins [1, 19, 20, 22, 37, 93–98]. Joint analyses based on meta-analyses further showed this kind of toxic effects (**Table 4**) [1, 22]. The genetic variants in other genes, such as CYP450, glutathione S-transferase T1 (GSTT1), glutathione S-transferase M1 (GSTM1), and microsomal epoxide hydrolase (HEHY), also display similar modificative effects on aflatoxin-induced hepatocarcinoma [98–101]. Interestingly, the multiplicatively interactive effects between aflatoxins and genetic alterations in these genes have been identified in the risk elucidation of hepatocarcinoma related to aflatoxins [22]. Taken together, genetic deficiency in the DNA repair and detoxification capacity may play a vital role in the carcinogenetic process of aflatoxin-induced hepatocarcinoma.

3.7. The aflatoxin-caused immunosuppression promoting hepatocarcinogenesis

Increasing evidence from in vitro and in vivo studies has proved that the immunosuppression induced by aflatoxins plays an important role in the carcinogenesis of hepatocarcinoma. Several known mechanisms may involve in this progression step. First, aflatoxins can significantly suppress the functions of macrophages via affecting the expression and secretions of cytokines such as tumor necrosis factor (TNF)-α, interleukin (IL)-1, IL-2, IL-3, IL-6, and reactive intermediates (including nitric oxide, hydrogen peroxide, and superoxide anion) [102, 103]. The suppression of macrophages by aflatoxins may be also correlated with the arrest in the G1/G0 phase [104] and altered expression of CD14 (a cell surface protein functionally regulating immunoreaction) [105]. This suppression may result in the dysregulation of the immune response and homeostasis, which contributes to the accumulation of abnormal cells with DNA damage and altered genome induced by aflatoxins, and ultimately progresses tumorigenesis. Second, aflatoxin exposure can decrease the secretion of antibody such as IgA [106]. For example, Turner et al. investigated effects of aflatoxin exposure on antibody production based on a large molecular epidemiological study [106]. In their study, they tested the levels of saliva secretory IgA (sIgA) in Gambian children (n = 472) with different degree exposure of aflatoxins and found that these individuals with high aflatoxin exposure featured lower level of sIgA in their saliva compared to those without high exposure (50.4 vs. 70.2 µg/mg protein). Finally, aflatoxins may alter T-cell functions (including decreased T-cell populations and suppressed CD4+ T-cell function) and increase individuals' susceptibility to other carcinogens [77, 107].

Gene	RS#	Genotype	TP53M			DNA adducts	
			%	Risk	P	Mean	P
XRCC1	rs25487	CC	46.51	Reference		3.276	
		CT	45.25	2.419	3.371×10^{-11}	3.264	0.899
		TT	8.24	5.028	6.651×10^{-6}	3.640	0.026
XRCC3	rs861539	GG	32.17	Reference		2.990	
		GA	43.55	1.380	0.018	3.216	0.025
		AA	24.28	1.524	0.011	3.897	4.962×10^{-14}
XRCC7	rs7003908	AA	21.24	Reference		2.879	
		AC	46.06	1.883	1.372×10^{-5}	3.347	1.663×10^{-5}
		CC	32.71	2.089	4.368×10^{-6}	3.550	1.751×10^{-8}
XRCC4	rs28383151	GG	67.03	Reference		3.308	
		GA	21.68	1.688	0.001	3.405	0.069
		AA	11.29	3.829	7.387×10^{-6}	3.721	2.867×10^{-4}
XRCC4	rs3734091	GG	72.31	Reference		3.229	
		GT	17.56	2.799	9.191×10^{-7}	3.439	0.095
		TT	10.13	5.104	3.826×10^{-6}	3.654	0.005
XPD	rs13181	TT	34.41	Reference		2.926	
		TG	41.85	1.458	0.005	3.253	0.011
		GG	23.75	1.744	0.001	4.062	4.265×10^{-6}
XPC	rs2228001	TT	34.05	Reference		3.083	
		TG	48.30	1.500	0.002	3.332	0.001
		GG	17.65	1.818	0.001	3.666	3.404×10^{-22}

Noted: Adapted from Refs. [13] and [84]. *Abbreviations.* TP53M, hot-spot mutation at codon 249 of TP53 gene; RS#, the number of polymorphism.

Table 4. Polymorphisms in DNA repair genes and HCC risk.

Altogether, the data available to date make it clear that aflatoxins can exert an immunosuppressive effect via different pathways. However, more detailed mechanisms by which this effect is mediated remain unknown.

4. Limitation and further direction

In the past decades, the advance in pathological mechanisms of aflatoxin-related hepatocarcinoma held great promise. However, we are still far from a comprehensive view of this kind of potentials. First, the detailed metabolic step and corresponding enzymes, especially the first-stage reaction and toxicity mechanisms, have not been elucidated. Second, although the activation of aflatoxins is found to act as a crucial step, it is unclear how the tumorigenesis of hepatocarcinoma is triggered by aflatoxins. Third, the vast literature for aflatoxin-induced hepatocarcinoma mainly focuses on the studies on AFB1, and some important information may have been lost. Fourth, in spite of some evidence of AFB1 inducing abnormal immunoreaction and interacting with hepatitis virus and genetic factors, they are at the primary stage and still far from elucidation. Therefore, the detailed toxicity mechanisms of aflatoxins and corresponding carcinogenesis mechanism will greatly benefit our understanding of aflatoxin-related hepatocarcinoma.

5. Summary

It has been shown that increasing exposure of aflatoxins may promote the carcinogenesis of hepatocarcinoma. Molecular mechanisms of aflatoxin-induced hepatocarcinoma involve in DNA damage, gene mutations, the inactivation of such tumor suppressor gene as TP53, the activation of proto-oncogenes, abnormal immunoreaction, and the interaction between aflatoxins and other carcinogens such as HBV. However, an understanding of aflatoxin-induced hepatocarcinoma is far from complete, and further research in this field is looked forward to elucidating more detailed mechanisms responsible for hepatocarcinoma related to aflatoxins in the future.

Conflicts of interest and source of funding

The authors declare no competing financial interests. This study was supported in part by the National Natural Science Foundation of China (Nos. 81760502, 81572353, 81372639, 81472243, 81660495, and 81460423), the Innovation Program of Guangxi Municipal Education Department (Nos. 201204LX674 and 201204LX324), Innovation Program of Guangxi Health Department (No. Z2013781), the Natural Science Foundation of Guangxi (Nos. 2017GXNSFGA198002, 2017JJF10001, 2017GXNSFAA198002, 2016GXNSFDA380003, 2015GXNSFAA139223, 2013GXNSFAA019251, 2014GXNSFDA118021, and 2014GXNSFAA118144), Research Program of Guangxi "Zhouyue Scholar" (No. 2017-38), Research Program of Guangxi Specially-invited Expert (No. 2017-6th), Research Program of Guangxi Clinic Research Center of Hepatobiliary Diseases (No. AD17129025), and Open Research Program from Molecular Immunity Study Room Involving in Acute & Severe Diseases in Guangxi Colleges and Universities (Nos. kfkt20160062 and kfkt20160063).

Abbreviations

AFB1	aflatoxin B1
AFB2	aflatoxin B2
AFG1	aflatoxin G1

AFG2	aflatoxin G2
AFP	α-fetoprotein
A. flavus	*Aspergillus flavus*
A. parasiticus	*Aspergillus parasiticus*
A. nidulans	*Aspergillus nidulans*
A. pseudotamarii	*Aspergillus pseudotamarii*
A. bombycis	*Aspergillus bombycis*
HBV	hepatitis virus B
HCV	hepatitis virus C
Hepatocarcinoma	hepatocellular carcinoma
NAPDH	nicotinamide-adenine dinucleotide phosphate reduced form
NAD	one nicotinamide-adenine dinucleotide
SAM	*S*-adenosylmethionine
CYP450	cytochromes P450

Author details

Xi-Dai Long[1,2,3*†], Yan Deng[4†], Xiao-Ying Huang[1†], Jin-Guang Yao[1†], Qun-Ying Su[1†], Xue-Min Wu[1†], Juan Wang[1†], Qun-Qing Xu[3], Xiao-Ying Zhu[3], Chao Wang[5], Bing-Chen Huang[1] and Qiang Xia[2]

*Address all correspondence to: sjtulongxd@263.net

1 Department of Pathology, the Affiliated Hospital of Youjiang Medical University for Nationalities, Baise, China

2 Department of Liver Surgery, Ren Ji Hospital, School of Medicine, Shanghai Jiao Tong University, Shanghai, China

3 Guangxi Clinic Research Center of Hepatobiliary Diseases, Baise, China

4 Department of Epidemiology, Youjiang Medical University for Nationalities, Baise, China

5 Department of Medicine, the Affiliated Hospital of Youjiang Medical University for Nationalities, Baise, China

† These authors contributed equally to this work.

References

[1] Long XD, Yao JD, Yang Q, Huang CH, Liao P, Nong LG, Tang YJ, Huang XY, Wang C, Wu XM, Huang BC, Ban FZ, Zeng LX, Ma Y, Zhai B, Zhang JQ, Xue F, Lu CX, Xia Q. Polymorphisms of DNA repair genes and toxicological effects of aflatoxin B1 exposure. In: Faulkner AG, editor. Aflatoxins: Food Sources, Occurrence and Toxicological Effects. 1st ed. New York: Nova Science Publishers; 2014. pp. 107-124. DOI: 978-1-63117-298-4

[2] Siegel RL, Miller KD, Jemal A. Cancer statistics, 2017. CA: A Cancer Journal for Clinicians. 2017;**67**:7-30. DOI: 10.3322/caac.21387

[3] Chen W, Zheng R, Baade PD, Zhang S, Zeng H, Bray F, Jemal A, Yu XQ, He J. Cancer statistics in China, 2015. CA: A Cancer Journal for Clinicians. 2016;**66**:115-132. DOI: 10.3322/caac.21338

[4] Umesha S, Manukumar HM, Chandrasekhar B, Shivakumara P, Shiva Kumar J, Raghava S, Avinash P, Shirin M, Bharathi TR, Rajini SB, Nandhini M, Vinaya Rani GG, Shobha M, Prakash HS. Aflatoxins and food pathogens: Impact of biologically active aflatoxins and their control strategies. Journal of the Science of Food and Agriculture. 2017;**97**:1698-1707. DOI: 10.1002/jsfa.8144

[5] Sarma UP, Bhetaria PJ, Devi P, Varma A. Aflatoxins: Implications on health. Indian Journal of Clinical Biochemistry. 2017;**32**:124-133. DOI: 10.1007/s12291-017-0649-2

[6] Kowalska A, Walkiewicz K, Koziel P, Muc-Wierzgon M. Aflatoxins: characteristics and impact on human health. Postepy Higieny i Medycyny Doświadczalnej (Online). 2017;**71**:315-327. DOI: 10.5604/01.3001.0010.3816

[7] Yabe K, Nakajima H. Enzyme reactions and genes in aflatoxin biosynthesis. Applied Microbiology and Biotechnology. 2004;**64**:745-755. DOI: 10.1007/s00253-004-1566-x

[8] Abrar M, Anjum FM, Butt MS, Pasha I, Randhawa MA, Saeed F, Waqas K. Aflatoxins: Biosynthesis, occurrence, toxicity, and remedies. Critical Reviews in Food Science and Nutrition. 2013;**53**:862-874. DOI: 10.1080/10408398.2011.563154

[9] Kensler TW, Roebuck BD, Wogan GN, Groopman JD. Aflatoxin: A 50-year odyssey of mechanistic and translational toxicology. Toxicological Sciences. 2011;**120**(Suppl 1):S28-S48. DOI: 10.1093/toxsci/kfq283

[10] Wu Q, Jezkova A, Yuan Z, Pavlikova L, Dohnal V, Kuca K. Biological degradation of aflatoxins. Drug Metabolism Reviews. 2009;**41**:1-7. DOI: 10.1080/03602530802563850

[11] Woloshuk CP, Shim WB. Aflatoxins, fumonisins, and trichothecenes: A convergence of knowledge. FEMS Microbiology Reviews. 2013;**37**:94-109. DOI: 10.1111/1574-6976.12009

[12] Essigmann JM, Croy RG, Nadzan AM, Busby WF Jr, Reinhold VN, Buchi G, Wogan GN. Structural identification of the major DNA adduct formed by aflatoxin B1 in vitro. Proceedings of the National Academy of Sciences of the United States of America. 1977; **74**:1870-1874. DOI: 10.1073/pnas.PMC431033

[13] Croy RG, Essigmann JM, Reinhold VN, Wogan GN. Identification of the principal aflatoxin B1-DNA adduct formed in vivo in rat liver. Proceedings of the National Academy of Sciences of the United States of America. 1978;75:1745-1749. DOI: 10.1073/pnas.PMC392416

[14] Huang XY, Yao JG, Huang BC, Ma Y, Xia Q, Long XD. Polymorphisms of a disintegrin and metalloproteinase with thrombospondin motifs 5 and aflatoxin B1-related hepatocellular carcinoma. Cancer Epidemiology, Biomarkers & Prevention. 2016;25:334-343. DOI: 10.1158/1055-9965.EPI-15-0774

[15] Lu J, Wang XZ, Zhang TQ, Huang XY, Yao JG, Wang C, Wei ZH, Ma Y, Wu XM, Luo CY, Xia Q, Long XD. Prognostic significance of XRCC4 expression in hepatocellular carcinoma. Oncotarget. 2017;8:87955-87970. DOI: 10.18632/oncotarget.21360

[16] Wu XM, Xi ZF, Liao P, Huang HD, Huang XY, Wang C, Ma Y, Xia Q, Yao JG, Long XD. Diagnostic and prognostic potential of serum microRNA-4651 for patients with hepatocellular carcinoma related to aflatoxin B1. Oncotarget. 2017;8:81235-81249. DOI: 10.18632/oncotarget.16027

[17] Li C, Xiong Y, Yang X, Wang L, Zhang S, Dai N, Li M, Ren T, Yang Y, Zhou SF, Gan L, Wang D. Lost expression of ADAMTS5 protein associates with progression and poor prognosis of hepatocellular carcinoma. Drug Design, Development and Therapy. 2015;9:1773-1783. DOI: 10.2147/DDDT.S77069

[18] Long XD, Ma Y, Huang YZ, Yi Y, Liang QX, Ma AM, Zeng LP, Fu GH. Genetic polymorphisms in DNA repair genes XPC, XPD, and XRCC4, and susceptibility to helicobacter pylori infection-related gastric antrum adenocarcinoma in Guangxi population. China Molecular Carcinogenesis. 2010;49:611-618. DOI: 10.1002/mc.20630

[19] Long XD, Yao JG, Zeng Z, Ma Y, Huang XY, Wei ZH, Liu M, Zhang JJ, Xue F, Zhai B, Xia Q. Polymorphisms in the coding region of X-ray repair complementing group 4 and aflatoxin B1-related hepatocellular carcinoma. Hepatology. 2013;58:171-181. DOI: 10.1002/hep.26311

[20] Long XD, Zhao D, Wang C, Huang XY, Yao JG, Ma Y, Wei ZH, Liu M, Zeng LX, Mo XQ, Zhang JJ, Xue F, Zhai B, Xia Q. Genetic polymorphisms in DNA repair genes XRCC4 and XRCC5 and aflatoxin B1-related hepatocellular carcinoma. Epidemiology. 2013;24:671-681. DOI: 10.1097/EDE.0b013e31829d2744

[21] Lin ZH, Chen JC, Wang YS, Huang TJ, Wang J, Long XD. DNA repair gene XRCC4 codon 247 polymorphism modified diffusely infiltrating astrocytoma risk and prognosis. International Journal of Molecular Sciences. 2014;15:250-260. DOI: 10.3390/ijms15010250

[22] Yao JG, Huang XY, Long XD. Interaction of DNA repair gene polymorphisms and aflatoxin B1 in the risk of hepatocellular carcinoma. International Journal of Clinical and Experimental Pathology. 2014;7:6231-6244. DOI: 10.2016/1936-2625.25337275

[23] Liu YX, Long XD, Xi ZF, Ma Y, Huang XY, Yao JG, Wang C, Xing TY, Xia Q. MicroRNA-24 modulates aflatoxin B1-related hepatocellular carcinoma prognosis and tumorigenesis. BioMed Research International. 2014;2014:482926. DOI: 10.1155/2014/482926

[24] Huang XY, Yao JG, Huang HD, Wang C, Ma Y, Xia Q, Long XD. MicroRNA-429 modulates hepatocellular carcinoma prognosis and tumorigenesis. Gastroenterology Research and Practice. 2013;**2013**:804128. DOI: 10.1155/2013/804128

[25] Hagiwara N, Mechanic LE, Trivers GE, Cawley HL, Taga M, Bowman ED, Kumamoto K, He P, Bernard M, Doja S, Miyashita M, Tajiri T, Sasajima K, Nomura T, Makino H, Takahashi K, Hussain SP, Harris CC. Quantitative detection of p53 mutations in plasma DNA from tobacco smokers. Cancer Research. 2006;**66**:8309-8317. DOI: 10.1158/0008-5472. CAN-06-0991

[26] Harris LC, Remack JS, Houghton PJ, Brent TP. Wild-type p53 suppresses transcription of the human O6-methylguanine-DNA methyltransferase gene. Cancer Research. 1996; **56**:2029-2032

[27] Harris CC. Tumour suppressor genes, multistage carcinogenesis and molecular epidemiology. IARC Scientific Publications. 1992:67-85 DOI: PMID1428103

[28] Foster PL, Eisenstadt E, Miller JH. Base substitution mutations induced by metabolically activated aflatoxin B1. Proceedings of the National Academy of Sciences of the U S A. 1983;**80**:2695-2698. DOI: PMC393894

[29] Qi LN, Bai T, Chen ZS, Wu FX, Chen YY, De Xiang B, Peng T, Han ZG, Li LQ. The p53 mutation spectrum in hepatocellular carcinoma from Guangxi, China: Role of chronic hepatitis B virus infection and aflatoxin B1 exposure. Liver International. 2014. DOI: 10.1111/liv.12460

[30] Golli-Bennour EE, Kouidhi B, Bouslimi A, Abid-Essefi S, Hassen W, Bacha H. Cytotoxicity and genotoxicity induced by aflatoxin B1, ochratoxin A, and their combination in cultured Vero cells. Journal of Biochemical and Molecular Toxicology. 2010;**24**:42-50. DOI: 10.1002/jbt.20310

[31] Paget V, Sichel F, Garon D, Lechevrel M. Aflatoxin B1-induced TP53 mutational pattern in normal human cells using the FASAY (functional analysis of separated alleles in yeast). Mutation Research. 2008;**656**:55-61. DOI: 10.1016/j.mrgentox.2008.07.009

[32] Levy DD, Groopman JD, Lim SE, Seidman MM, Kraemer KH. Sequence specificity of aflatoxin B1-induced mutations in a plasmid replicated in xeroderma pigmentosum and DNA repair proficient human cells. Cancer Research 1992;**52**:5668-5673. DOI: 10.1158/0008-5472. CAN-Published-October-1992

[33] Wang JS, Groopman JD. DNA damage by mycotoxins. Mutation Research. 1999;**424**:167-181. DOI: 10.1016/S0027-5107(99)00017-2

[34] Long XD, Yao JG, Zeng Z, Huang CH, Huang ZS, Huang YZ, Ban FZ, Huang XY, Yao LM, Fan LD, Fu GH. DNA repair capacity-related to genetic polymorphisms of DNA repair genes and aflatoxin B1-related hepatocellular carcinoma among Chinese population. In: Kruman I, editor. DNA Repair. Rijeka: InTech; 2011. pp. 505-524. DOI: 10.5772/20792

[35] Xia Q, Huang XY, Xue F, Zhang JJ, Zhai B, Kong DC, Wang C, Huang ZQ, Long XD. Genetic polymorphisms of DNA repair genes and DNA repair capacity related to aflatoxin

b1 (AFB1)-induced DNA damages. In: Chen C, editor. New Research Directions in DNA Repair. 1st ed. Rijeka: InTech; 2013. pp. 377-412. DOI: 10.5772/53967

[36] Chen BP, Long XD, Fu GH. Meta-analysis of XRCC1 codon 399 polymorphism and susceptibility of hepatocellular carcinoma. Journal of Shanghai Jiao Tong University (Medical Science). 2011;31:1588-1602. DOI: 10.3969/j.issn.1674-8115.2011.11.018

[37] Long XD, Huang HD, Huang XY, Yao JG, Xia Q. XPC codon 939 polymorphism is associated with susceptibility to DNA damage induced by aflatoxin B1 exposure. International Journal of Clinical and Experimental Medicine. 2015;8:1197-1204. DOI: PMC4358568

[38] Shen HM, Ong CN. Mutations of the p53 tumor suppressor gene and ras oncogenes in aflatoxin hepatocarcinogenesis. Mutation Research. 1996;366:23-44. DOI: 10.1016/S0165-1110(96)90005-6

[39] Alm-Eldeen AA, Basyony MA, Elfiky NK, Ghalwash MM. Effect of the Egyptian propolis on the hepatic antioxidant defense and pro-apoptotic p53 and anti-apoptotic bcl2 expressions in aflatoxin B1 treated male mice. Biomedicine & Pharmacotherapy. 2017;87:247-255. DOI: 10.1016/j.biopha.2016.12.084

[40] Ranchal I, Gonzalez R, Bello RI, Ferrin G, Hidalgo AB, Linares CI, Aguilar-Melero P, Gonzalez-Rubio S, Barrera P, Marchal T, Nakayama KI, de la Mata M, Muntane J. The reduction of cell death and proliferation by p27(Kip1) minimizes DNA damage in an experimental model of genotoxicity. International Journal of Cancer. 2009;125:2270-2280. DOI: 10.1002/ijc.24621

[41] Qi LN, Bai T, Chen ZS, Wu FX, Chen YY, De Xiang B, Peng T, Han ZG, Li LQ. The p53 mutation spectrum in hepatocellular carcinoma from Guangxi, China: Role of chronic hepatitis B virus infection and aflatoxin B1 exposure. Liver International. 2015;35:999-1009. DOI: 10.1111/liv.12460

[42] Chittmittrapap S, Chieochansin T, Chaiteerakij R, Treeprasertsuk S, Klaikaew N, Tangkijvanich P, Komolmit P, Poovorawan Y. Prevalence of aflatoxin induced p53 mutation at codon 249 (R249s) in hepatocellular carcinoma patients with and without hepatitis B surface antigen (HBsAg). Asian Pacific Journal of Cancer Prevention. 2013;14:7675-7679. DOI: PMID24460352

[43] Gursoy-Yuzugullu O, Yuzugullu H, Yilmaz M, Ozturk M. Aflatoxin genotoxicity is associated with a defective DNA damage response bypassing p53 activation. Liver International. 2011;31:561-571. DOI: 10.1111/j.1478-3231.2011.02474.x

[44] Pineau P, Marchio A, Battiston C, Cordina E, Russo A, Terris B, Qin LX, Turlin B, Tang ZY, Mazzaferro V, Dejean A. Chromosome instability in human hepatocellular carcinoma depends on p53 status and aflatoxin exposure. Mutation Research. 2008;653:6-13. DOI: 10.1016/j.mrgentox.2008.01.012

[45] Zhang YJ, Rossner P Jr, Chen Y, Agrawal M, Wang Q, Wang L, Ahsan H, Yu MW, Lee PH, Santella RM. Aflatoxin B1 and polycyclic aromatic hydrocarbon adducts, p53 mutations and p16 methylation in liver tissue and plasma of hepatocellular carcinoma patients. International Journal of Cancer. 2006;119:985-991. DOI: 10.1002/ijc.21699

[46] Chan KT, Hsieh DP, Lung ML. In vitro aflatoxin B1-induced p53 mutations. Cancer Letters. 2003;**199**:1-7. DOI: 10.1016/S0304-3835(03)00337-9

[47] Stern MC, Umbach DM, Yu MC, London SJ, Zhang ZQ, Taylor JA. Hepatitis B, aflatoxin B(1), and p53 codon 249 mutation in hepatocellular carcinomas from Guangxi, People's Republic of China, and a meta-analysis of existing studies. Cancer Epidemiology Biomarkers & Prevention. 2001;**10**:617-625. DOI: PMID11401911

[48] Park US, Su JJ, Ban KC, Qin L, Lee EH, Lee YI. Mutations in the p53 tumor suppressor gene in tree shrew hepatocellular carcinoma associated with hepatitis B virus infection and intake of aflatoxin B1. Gene. 2000;**251**:73-80. DOI: 10.1016/S0378-1119(00)00183-9

[49] Lee YI, Lee S, Das GC, Park US, Park SM, Lee YI. Activation of the insulin-like growth factor II transcription by aflatoxin B1 induced p53 mutant 249 is caused by activation of transcription complexes; implications for a gain-of-function during the formation of hepatocellular carcinoma. Oncogene. 2000;**19**:3717-3726. DOI: 10.1038/sj.onc.1203694

[50] Uwaifo O. P53 gene of chang-liver cells (Atcc-Ccl13) exposed to aflatoxin B1 (Afb): The effect of lysine on mutation at codon 249 of exon 7. African Journal of Medicine and Medical Sciences. 1999;**28**:71-75. DOI: PMID12953991

[51] Chao HK, Tsai TF, Lin CS, Su TS. Evidence that mutational activation of the ras genes may not be involved in aflatoxin B(1)-induced human hepatocarcinogenesis, based on sequence analysis of the ras and p53 genes. Molecular Carcinogenesis. 1999;**26**:69-73. DOI: 10.1002/(SICI)1098-2744(199910)26:2<69::AID-MC1>3.0.CO;2-A

[52] Ghebranious N, Sell S. The mouse equivalent of the human p53ser249 mutation p53ser246 enhances aflatoxin hepatocarcinogenesis in hepatitis B surface antigen transgenic and p53 heterozygous null mice. Hepatology. 1998;**27**:967-973. DOI: 10.1002/hep.510270411

[53] Ghebranious N, Sell S. Hepatitis B injury, male gender, aflatoxin, and p53 expression each contribute to hepatocarcinogenesis in transgenic mice. Hepatology. 1998;**27**:383-391. DOI: 10.1002/hep.510270211

[54] Liu YP, Lin Y, Ng ML. Immunochemical and genetic analysis of the p53 gene in liver preneoplastic nodules from aflatoxin-induced rats in one year. Annals of the Academy of Medicine of Singapore. 1996;**25**:31-36

[55] Hulla JE, Chen ZY, Eaton DL. Aflatoxin B1-induced rat hepatic hyperplastic nodules do not exhibit a site-specific mutation within the p53 gene. Cancer Research. 1993;**53**:9-11. DOI: PMID8380129

[56] Lilleberg SL, Cabonce MA, Raju NR, Wagner LM, Kier LD. Alterations in the structural gene and the expression of p53 in rat liver tumors induced by aflatoxin B1. Molecular Carcinogenesis. 1992;**6**:159-172. DOI: 10.1002/mc.2940060211

[57] Lilleberg SL, Cabonce MA, Raju NR, Wagner LM, Kier LD. Alterations in the p53 tumor suppressor gene in rat liver tumors induced by aflatoxin B1. Progress in Clinical and Biological Research. 1992;**376**:203-222

[58] Deng ZL, Ma Y. Aflatoxin sufferer and p53 gene mutation in hepatocellular carcinoma. World Journal of Gastroenterology. 1998;**4**:28-29. DOI: 10.3748/wjg.v4.i1.28

[59] Deng Z, Pan L, Ma Y. Sequence alterations in p53 gene of hepatocellular carcinoma from high aflatoxin risk area in Guangxi. Zhonghua Zhong Liu Za Zhi. 1997;**19**:18-21. DOI: PMID10743047

[60] Mace K, Aguilar F, Wang JS, Vautravers P, Gomez-Lechon M, Gonzalez FJ, Groopman J, Harris CC, Pfeifer AM. Aflatoxin B1-induced DNA adduct formation and p53 mutations in CYP450-expressing human liver cell lines. Carcinogenesis. 1997;**18**:1291-1297. DOI: PMID9230270

[61] Lunn RM, Zhang YJ, Wang LY, Chen CJ, Lee PH, Lee CS, Tsai WY, Santella RM. p53 mutations, chronic hepatitis B virus infection, and aflatoxin exposure in hepatocellular carcinoma in Taiwan. Cancer Reserch. 1997;**57**:3471-3477. DOI: PMID9270015

[62] Hollstein MC, Wild CP, Bleicher F, Chutimataewin S, Harris CC, Srivatanakul P, Montesano R. p53 mutations and aflatoxin B1 exposure in hepatocellular carcinoma patients from Thailand. International Journal of Cancer. 1993;**53**:51-55. DOI: 10.1002/ijc.2910530111

[63] Aguilar F, Hussain SP, Cerutti P. Aflatoxin B1 induces the transversion of G-->T in codon 249 of the p53 tumor suppressor gene in human hepatocytes. Proceedings of the National Academy of Sciences U S A. 1993;**90**:8586-8590. DOI: PMC47402

[64] Ozturk M. p53 mutation in hepatocellular carcinoma after aflatoxin exposure. Lancet. 1991;**338**:1356-1359. DOI: 10.1016/0140-6736(91)92236-U

[65] Tashiro F, Morimura S, Hayashi K, Makino R, Kawamura H, Horikoshi N, Nemoto K, Ohtsubo K, Sugimura T, Ueno Y. Expression of the c-Ha-ras and c-myc genes in aflatoxin B1-induced hepatocellular carcinomas. Biochemical and Biophysical Research Communications. 1986;**138**:858-864. DOI: 10.1016/S0006-291X(86)80575-7

[66] Sinha S, Webber C, Marshall CJ, Knowles MA, Proctor A, Barrass NC, Neal GE. Activation of ras oncogene in aflatoxin-induced rat liver carcinogenesis. Proceedings of the National Academy of Sciences U S A. 1988;**85**:3673-3677. DOI: PMC280280

[67] Soman NR, Wogan GN. Activation of the c-Ki-ras oncogene in aflatoxin B1-induced hepatocellular carcinoma and adenoma in the rat: Detection by denaturing gradient gel electrophoresis. Proceedings of the National Academy of Sciences U S A. 1993;**90**:2045-2049. DOI: PMC46017

[68] McMahon G, Hanson L, Lee JJ, Wogan GN. Identification of an activated c-Ki-ras oncogene in rat liver tumors induced by aflatoxin B1. Proceedings of the National Academy of Sciences U S A. 1986;**83**:9418-9422. DOI: PMC387149

[69] McMahon G, Davis EF, Huber LJ, Kim Y, Wogan GN. Characterization of c-Ki-ras and N-ras oncogenes in aflatoxin B1-induced rat liver tumors. Proceedings of the National Academy of Sciences U S A. 1990;**87**:1104-1108. DOI: PMC53419

[70] Riley J, Mandel HG, Sinha S, Judah DJ, Neal GE. In vitro activation of the human Harvey-ras proto-oncogene by aflatoxin B1. Carcinogenesis. 1997;**18**:905-910. DOI: PMID9163674

[71] Bauer-Hofmann R, Buchmann A, Wright AS, Schwarz M. Mutations in the Ha-ras proto-oncogene in spontaneous and chemically induced liver tumours of the CF1 mouse. Carcinogenesis. 1990;**11**:1875-1877. DOI: PMID2119910

[72] Wiseman RW, Stowers SJ, Miller EC, Anderson MW, Miller JA. Activating mutations of the c-Ha-ras protooncogene in chemically induced hepatomas of the male B6C3 F1 mouse. Proceedings of the National Academy of Sciences U S A. 1986;**83**:5825-5829. DOI: PMC386388

[73] Kew MC. Synergistic interaction between aflatoxin B1 and hepatitis B virus in hepatocar-cinogenesis. Liver International. 2003;**23**:405-409. DOI: 10.1111/j.1478-3231.2003.00869.x

[74] Kew MC. Aflatoxins as a cause of hepatocellular carcinoma. Journal of Gastrointestinal and Liver Diseases. 2013;**22**:305-310. DOI: PMID24078988

[75] Moudgil V, Redhu D, Dhanda S, Singh JA. Review of molecular mechanisms in the development of hepatocellular carcinoma by aflatoxin and hepatitis B and C viruses. Journal of Environmental Pathology, Toxicology and Oncology. 2013;**32**:165-175. DOI: 10.1615/JEnvironPatholToxicolOncol.2013007166

[76] Yeh FS, Mo CC, Yen RC. Risk factors for hepatocellular carcinoma in Guangxi, People's Republic of China. National Cancer Institute Monograph. 1985;**69**:47-48. DOI: PMID3010122

[77] Williams JH, Phillips TD, Jolly PE, Stiles JK, Jolly CM, Aggarwal D. Human aflatoxicosis in developing countries: A review of toxicology, exposure, potential health consequences, and interventions. The American Journal of Clinical Nutrition. 2004;**80**:1106-1122. DOI: PMID15531656

[78] Qian GS, Ross RK, Yu MC, Yuan JM, Gao YT, Henderson BE, Wogan GN, Groopman JD. A follow-up study of urinary markers of aflatoxin exposure and liver cancer risk in Shanghai, People's Republic of China. Cancer Epidemiology, Biomarkers & Prevention. 1994;**3**:3-10. DOI: PMID8118382

[79] Wang JS, Qian GS, Zarba A, He X, Zhu YR, Zhang BC, Jacobson L, Gange SJ, Munoz A, Kensler TW, et al. Temporal patterns of aflatoxin-albumin adducts in hepatitis B sur-face antigen-positive and antigen-negative residents of Daxin, Qidong County, People's Republic of China. Cancer Epidemiology, Biomarkers & Prevention: A publication of the American Association for Cancer Research, Cosponsored by the American Society of Preventive Oncology. 1996;**5**:253-261. DOI: PMID8722216

[80] Ross RK, Yuan JM, MC Y, Wogan GN, Qian GS, JT T, Groopman JD, Gao YT, Henderson BE. Urinary aflatoxin biomarkers and risk of hepatocellular carcinoma. Lancet. 1992;**339**:943-946. DOI: 10.1016/0140-6736(92)91528-G

[81] Sell S, Hunt JM, Dunsford HA, Chisari FV. Synergy between hepatitis B virus expression and chemical hepatocarcinogens in transgenic mice. Cancer Reserch. 1991;**51**:1278-1285. DOI: PMID1847661

[82] Bannasch P, Khoshkhou NI, Hacker HJ, Radaeva S, Mrozek M, Zillmann U, Kopp-Schneider A, Haberkorn U, Elgas M, Tolle T, et al. Synergistic hepatocarcinogenic effect of hepadnaviral infection and dietary aflatoxin B1 in woodchucks. Cancer Reserch. 1995;**55**:3318-3330. DOI: PMID7614467

[83] Li Y, Su JJ, Qin LL, Yang C, Ban KC, Yan RQ. Synergistic effect of hepatitis B virus and aflatoxin B1 in hepatocarcinogenesis in tree shrews. Annals of the Academy of Medicine Singapore. 1999;**28**:67-71. DOI: PMID10374028

[84] Cova L, Wild CP, Mehrotra R, Turusov V, Shirai T, Lambert V, Jacquet C, Tomatis L, Trepo C, Montesano R. Contribution of aflatoxin B1 and hepatitis B virus infection in the induction of liver tumors in ducks. Cancer Reserch. 1990;**50**:2156-2163. DOI: PMID2107970

[85] Allen SJ, Wild CP, Wheeler JG, Riley EM, Montesano R, Bennett S, Whittle HC, Hall AJ, Greenwood BM. Aflatoxin exposure, malaria and hepatitis B infection in rural Gambian children. Transactions of the Royal Society of Tropical Medicine and Hygiene. 1992;**86**: 426-430. DOI: PMID1440826

[86] Turner PC, Mendy M, Whittle H, Fortuin M, Hall AJ, Wild CP, Hepatitis B. Infection and aflatoxin biomarker levels in Gambian children. Tropical Medicine & International Health. 2000;**5**:837-841. DOI: 10.1046/j.1365-3156.2000.00664.x

[87] Groopman JD, Wang JS, Scholl P. Molecular biomarkers for aflatoxins: From adducts to gene mutations to human liver cancer. Canadian Journal of Physiology and Pharmacology. 1996;**74**:203-209. DOI: PMID8723033

[88] Coursaget P, Depril N, Chabaud M, Nandi R, Mayelo V, LeCann P, Yvonnet B. High prevalence of mutations at codon 249 of the p53 gene in hepatocellular carcinomas from Senegal. British Journal of Cancer. 1993;**67**:1395-1397. DOI: PMC1968506

[89] Kew MC, Hepatitis B. Virus x protein in the pathogenesis of hepatitis B virus-induced hepatocellular carcinoma. Journal of Gastroenterology and Hepatology. 2011;**26**(Suppl 1): 144-152. DOI: 10.1111/j.1440-1746.2010.06546.x

[90] Gomez-Moreno A, Garaigorta U, Hepatitis B. Virus and DNA damage response: Interactions and consequences for the infection. Virus. 2017;**9**. DOI: 10.3390/v9100304

[91] Castelli G, Pelosi E, Testa U. Liver cancer: Molecular characterization, clonal evolution and cancer stem cells. Cancers (Basel). 2017;**9**. DOI: 10.3390/cancers9090127

[92] Ghouri YA, Mian I, Rowe JH. Review of hepatocellular carcinoma: Epidemiology, etiology, and carcinogenesis. Journal of Carcinogenesis. 2017;**16**:1. DOI: 10.4103/jcar.JCar_9_16

[93] Long XD, Huang HD, Xia Q. The polymorphism of XRCC3 codon 241 and the hotspot mutation in the TP53 gene in hepatocellular carcinoma induced by aflatoxin B1. Journal of Tumor. 2014;**2**:272-277. DOI: 10.6051/j.issn.1819-6187.2014.02.57

[94] Long XD, Yao JG, Huang YZ, Huang XY, Ban FZ, Yao LM, Fan LDDNA. Repair gene XRCC7 polymorphisms (rs#7003908 and rs#10109984) and hepatocellular carcinoma related to AFB1 exposure among Guangxi population, China. Hepatology Research. 2011;**41**:1085-1093. DOI: 10.1111/j.1872-034X.2011.00866.x

[95] Long XD, Ma Y, Zhou YF, Ma AM, Fu GH. Polymorphism in xeroderma pigmentosum complementation group C codon 939 and aflatoxin B1-related hepatocellular carcinoma in the Guangxi population. Hepatology. 2010;**52**:1301-1309. DOI: 10.1002/hep.23807

[96] Long XD, Ma Y, Zhou YF, Yao JG, Ban FZ, Huang YZ, Huang BC. XPD Codon 312 and 751 polymorphisms, and AFB1 exposure, and hepatocellular carcinoma risk. BMC Cancer. 2009;**9**:400. DOI: 10.1186/1471-2407-9-400

[97] Long XD, Ma Y, Huang HD, Yao JG, Qu de Y, Lu YL. Polymorphism of XRCC1 and the frequency of mutation in codon 249 of the p53 gene in hepatocellular carcinoma among Guangxi population, China. Molecular Carcinogenesis 2008;**47**:295-300. doi: 10.1002/mc.20384

[98] Long XD, Ma Y, Wei YP, Deng ZL. The polymorphisms of GSTM1, GSTT1, HYL1*2, and XRCC1, and aflatoxin B1-related hepatocellular carcinoma in Guangxi population, China. Hepatology Research. 2006;**36**:48-55. DOI: 10.1016/j.hepres.2006.06.004

[99] Long XD, Ma Y, Deng ZL. GSTM1 and XRCC3 polymorphisms: Effects on levels of aflatoxin B1-DNA adducts. Chinese Journal of Cancer Research. 2009;**21**:177-184. DOI: 10.1007/s11670-009-0177-6

[100] Long XD, Ma Y, Wei YP, Deng ZL. A study about the association of detoxication gene GSTM1 polymorphism and the susceptibility to aflatoxin B1-related hepatocellular carcinoma. Zhonghua Gan Zang Bing Za Zhi. 2005;**13**:668-670. DOI: PMID16174455

[101] Long XD, Ma Y, Wei YP, Deng ZL. Study on the detoxication gene gstM1-gstT1-null and susceptibility to aflatoxin B1 related hepatocellular carcinoma in Guangxi. Zhonghua Liu Xing Bing Xue Za Zhi. 2005;**26**:777-781. DOI: PMID16536303

[102] Moon EY, Rhee DK, Pyo S. In vitro suppressive effect of aflatoxin B1 on murine perito-neal macrophage functions. Toxicology. 1999;**133**:171-179. DOI: PMID10378483

[103] Moon EY, Rhee DK, Pyo S. Inhibition of various functions in murine peritoneal macro-phages by aflatoxin B1 exposure in vivo. International Journal of Immunopharmacology. 1999;**21**:47-58. DOI: 10.1016/S0192-0561(98)00069-1

[104] Bianco G, Russo R, Marzocco S, Velotto S, Autore G, Severino L. Modulation of mac-rophage activity by aflatoxins B1 and B2 and their metabolites aflatoxins M1 and M2. Toxicon. 2012;**59**:644-650. DOI: 10.1016/j.toxicon.2012.02.010

[105] Bruneau JC, Stack E, O'Kennedy R, Loscher CE. Aflatoxins B(1), B(2) and G(1) modulate cytokine secretion and cell surface marker expression in J774A.1 murine macrophages. Toxicology In Vitro. 2012;**26**:686-693. DOI: 10.1016/j.tiv.2012.03.003

[106] Turner PC, Moore SE, Hall AJ, Prentice AM, Wild CP. Modification of immune func-tion through exposure to dietary aflatoxin in Gambian children. Environmental Health Perspectives. 2003;**111**:217-220. DOI: PMC1241353

[107] Oswald IP, Marin DE, Bouhet S, Pinton P, Taranu I, Accensi F. Immunotoxicological risk of mycotoxins for domestic animals. Food Additives and Contaminants. 2005;**22**:354-360. DOI: 10.1080/02652030500058320

5

Management of Ascites Associated with Severe Hyponatremia

Andra Iulia Suceveanu, Roxana Popoiag,
Laura Mazilu, Irinel Raluca Parepa,
Andreea Gheorghe, Anca Stoian, Felix Voinea,
Claudia Voinea and Adrian Paul Suceveanu

Abstract

Advanced liver cirrhosis requiring hospitalization is frequently associated with electro-lytic disturbances, the most common finding being serum hyponatremia. The goal of treatment in patients with decompensated liver cirrhosis complicated with severe hypo-natremia is to normalize the increased amount of water in the body and to improve the sodium concentration. Fluid restriction is recommended at 1.5 L/day to prevent sodium depletion in the serum, but the lack of efficacy is probably due to a poor patient com-pliance. Discontinuation or adjustments of diuretic dosages are sometimes required. Albumin associated with vasoconstrictors as midodrine can increase the effective arte-rial blood volume and seems to improve the serum sodium concentration. A promis-ing therapeutic option targeting the pathophysiological mechanism of hyponatremia consists of improving solute-free water excretion, which is markedly impaired in these patients. The use of agents such as k opioid agonists has been attempted, but has been dropped due to the severe side effects. Recently, a new therapeutic class called vaptans has taken an important place in the treatment of hypervolemic hyponatremia. The main side effects during the administration of these drugs in patients with liver cirrhosis are reversible after discontinuing therapy. Therefore, it is recommended to use vaptans for short periods of time.

Keywords: hypervolemia, hyponatremia, liver cirrhosis, fluid restriction, vasopressin receptor antagonists, vaptans

1. Introduction

Ascites is the most common complication of cirrhosis, approximately 60% of patients develop ascites within 10 years of disease progression. The mechanism of production is the development of portal hypertension and renal retention of sodium. This inability to excrete an adequate amount of sodium in the urine occurs due to arterial splanchnic vasodilatation. Therefore, arterial and pulmonary cardio vascular receptor activation occurs with homeostatic activation of vasoconstrictor and sodium retention systems, resulting in a decrease in the required arterial blood volume. Renal sodium retention increases the volume of extracellular fluid leading to ascites and edema [1–5].

At approximately 75% of patients from Western Europe and USA, the main cause of ascites is represented by cirrhosis. Other causes of ascites may be malignancy, heart failure, tuberculosis, pancreatic disease, or other causes.

Hyponatremia is one of the complications that occurs in end stage cirrhosis due to the impossibility of renal clearance of free water, which leads to a higher water retention than sodium with the occurrence of hyposomolarity, with an increase in mortality and morbidity. In the pathogenesis of hyponatremia, the main factor involved is hypersecretion of antidiuretic hormone (ADH). Hyponatremia is a risk factor for both hepatic encephalopathy and liver transplantation because it is associated with an increased frequency of complications and a short-term survival [6].

2. Definition

Patients with liver cirrhosis show two types of hyponatremia: hypovolemic and hypervolemic.

Hypervolemic hyponatremia is the most common form and is characterized by low levels of serum sodium and increased volume of extracellular fluid, ascites, and edema. It may appear secondary to bacterial infections, excessive hypotonic fluids or may occur spontaneously. Hypovolemic hyponatremia is less common, with low levels of sodium, without ascites and edema as a consequence of excessive diuretic administration.

Hyponatremia is defined when serum sodium levels fall below 130 mmol/L but according to the recent guidelines, reductions below 135 mmol/L should also be considered as hyponatremia [7].

3. Prevalence

A study made over an Asian population following 997 patients with cirrhosis and ascites over 28 days in 28 centers showed that hyponatremia is present in more than half of the patients [8].

4. Pathophysiology

The mechanism by which ascites fluid is formed is the excess water and sodium retention in the body. Several theories have been developed to understand pathophysiology, and in turn, it has been shown that much of it would arise as a result of portal hypertension. The three proposed theories are three distinct mechanisms named: filling, oversaturation, and peripheral arterial vasodilatation. The first theory of filling is determined by portal hypertension and decreased circulating volume that produces vascular fluid retention. Since cirrhotic patients have a higher percentage of hypervolemia than hypovolemia, the second overload theory is determined by the retention of water and sodium in the absence of volume exhaustion. And the third theory uses the first two theories. This indicates that vasodilation occurs as a result of portal hypertension and favors the increase in arterial blood volume. Also, several factors are involved in ascites fluid formation: hypoalbuminemia and oncotic low plasma pressure, elevated levels of epinephrine and norepinephrine.

The main mechanism of hyponatremia is represented by arterial vasodilation. By reducing effective blood volume, several neurohumoral systems such as the renin-angiotensin-aldosterone system and the sympathetic nervous system are stimulated and lead to the release of ADH.

Activation of those trigger systems causes sodium retention and may lead to renal vasoconstriction. Vasopressin 2 receptors affected by the ADH play an important role in rate of excretion of solute-free water. In the end, water excretion occurs with the appearance of serum dilution and hypo-osmolality [6].

Under normal circumstances, there is a synchronous increase in serum osmolarity and ADH secretion, and reabsorption of water occurs when activating the aquaporin channels in the renal collection tubes. In opposite, the inactivation of aquaporin channels occurs when a decrease in osmolarity appears, resulting in urine dilution as a mechanism in maintaining serum osmolarity. Thus, the good functioning of osmoreceptors in the anterior hypothalamus, the release of ADH and the mutual action between ADH and AQP-2 compete to adapt the release of free water.

ADH is secreted into the supraoptic and paraventricular nuclei of the hypothalamus and maintained in the posterior pituitary gland. Vasopressin secretion is stimulated by increased plasma osmolarity and hypovolemia. The release of ADH is conditioned by osmotic and nonosmotic stimulation. The osmoreceptors in the anterior hypothalamus, near the supraoptic nuclei mediate the osmotic pathway. These receptors detect intracellular water content in neurons and respond to changes in plasma osmolarity. The main nonosmotic pathway delivers an ADH release through the autonomic nervous system mediated by baroreceptors located in the atrium, ventricle, aortic arch, and carotid sinus. Through the parasympathetic pathway, these baroreceptors stimulate the hypothalamus to release ADH in response to hypovolemia [9].

Most patients with cirrhosis present low serum osmolarity and sodium levels, and it is expected to produce inhibition of ADH release if stimulation was achieved by osmoreceptors [10]. Because of the activation of the neurohumoral mechanisms that retain sodium, the levels of ADH, aldosterone, norepinephrine, and renin activity were significantly higher in patients with cirrhosis and ascites after the water loading test. Effective arterial uptake would result from a decrease in systemic vascular resistance and would result in nonosmotic stimulation due to baroreceptors of ADH and other vasoconstriction systems. These cause the activation of the neurohumoral mechanisms that produce sodium retention in order to restore the perfusion pressure [11].

It is suggested that hypoosmotic stimuli are suppressed by nonosmotic stimuli to suppress ADH release. That is why the body sacrifices osmolar homeostasis and releases ADH following nonosmotic stimulation of endogenous vasoconstrictors, and thus impairs vascular collapse by exhausting effective circulatory volume. It results in an inability to release sodium and water to replenish the circulation volume. All of these things happen despite the increase in cardiac output, plasma volume, and total body volume. To eliminate the extra amount of water, it is necessary to suppress adherence and the ability of the kidneys to remove water. The presence of nonosmotic adherence leads to the occurrence of a hyponatremia of dilution or hypervolemic hyponatremia. Therefore, in this category of patients, hyponatremia is only dilute and does not represent a sodium deficiency [12].

In a prospective cohort study of patients with ascites, it was demonstrated that the occurrence of hyponatremia is preceded by refractory ascites and subsequently by hepatorenal syndrome. Each of these steps was associated with a progressive Child Pugh score and Model for End Stage Liver Disease (MELD) indicating a worsening of liver function. Therefore, hyponatremia is an intermediate stage between ascites progression and hepatorenal syndrome [13].

5. Prognostic value

Hyponatremia in patients with cirrhosis is chronic, therefore, allows the brain to adapt to the hypo extracellular fluid osmolality. In conclusion, patients are less likely to have severe neurological symptoms. However, hyponatremia can aggravate cerebral edema and swollen astrocytes by adding to their dysfunction created by increased intracellular glutamine concentration, speeding up the appearance of hepatic encephalopathy [6].

Due to the severe restriction of fluid consumption, the quality of life of patients with cirrhosis and hyponatremia is poor [14]. Several studies have shown that the severity of hyponatremia and ascites is a prognostic factor of the disease [15, 16]. In one study, it was demonstrated that the serum sodium level prior to the occurrence of spontaneous bacterial peritonitis (SBP) was an independent predictor of renal insufficiency produced by SBP [17]. It is also a predictive marker with a higher sensitivity than serum creatinine to predict the occurrence of circulatory dysfunction resulting in renal insufficiency or death. Although patients with hyponatremia are susceptible to the hepatorenal syndrome, there is not only an increased level of ADH involved, but there is a decrease in glomerular filtration rate (GFR) and proximal sodium reabsorption [18].

Sodium concentration was included in the MELD model to indicate the need for liver transplantation and patient priority on waiting lists in order to improve prognosis [19]. It was found that the MELD-Na score indicated an anticipation of short-term mortality of transplant patient candidates much better than the initial MELD score [20].

6. Clinical presentation

Symptoms of hyponatremia are caused by the damage to the nervous system, with cerebral edema due to the migration of water from the intravascular space in the brain [21]. As a rapid adaptive mechanism, there is an increase in electrolytes in brain cells. As a slow adaptation mechanism, organic osmoliths are extruded. Finally, these mechanisms help return the water to the intravascular space and prevent brain edema [22].

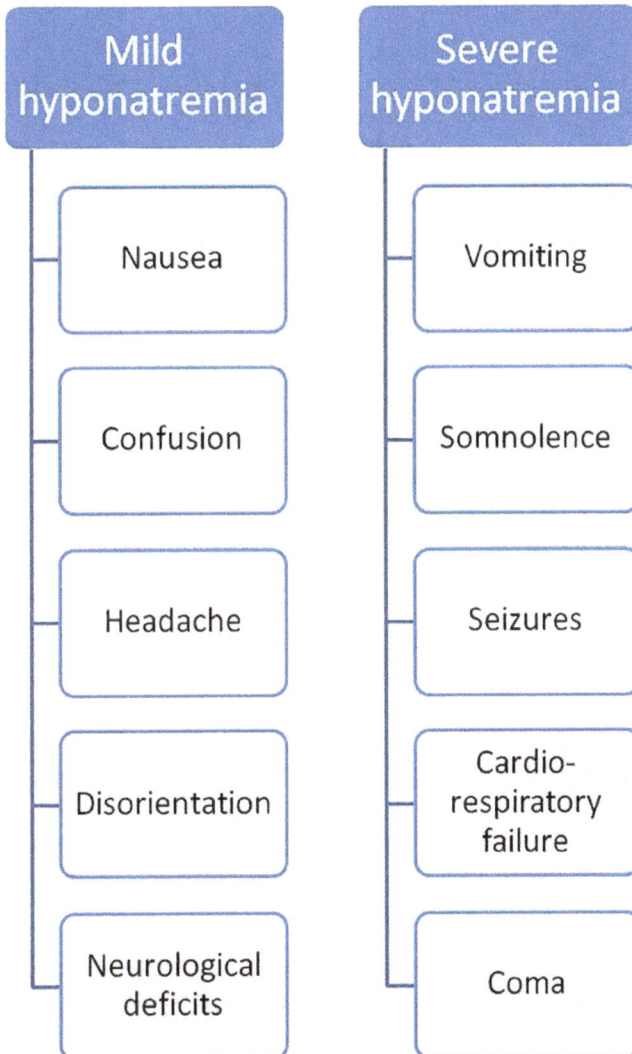

Figure 1. Clinical manifestations of hyponatremia.

In patients without hepatic impairment, hyponatremia manifests with: headache, disorientation, confusion, and neurological deficits. In contrast, in cirrhotic patients, hyponatremia develops slowly and at a value of 125 mEq/L is asymptomatic due to adaptive mechanisms. However, a rapid drop in sodium concentration may overcome adaptive mechanisms and serious symptoms may occur such as coma, seizures, brain-stern herniation, respiratory failure, and death [23] (**Figure 1**).

Hyponatremia usually occurs in the final stage of liver disease and is difficult to differentiate if the symptoms are within it or are part of liver encephalopathy occurrence. Both hyponatremia and hyperammonemia cause an alteration in brain metabolism of myoinositol [24].

Some theories show that hyponatremia can cause the appearance of a minimal cerebral edema that occurs by swelling of astrocytes and may cause the appearance of hepatic encephalopathy. This minimal brain edema occurs by increasing the concentration of glutamine resulting from the metabolism of ammonia and leads to a series of neurological changes to the appearance of hepatic encephalopathy [25].

7. Complications

Central pontine myelinolysis (CPM) is a complication of severe hyponatremia and occurs when its correction has been achieved very quickly. It is a neurological disorder that consists of a demyelination that occurs in a region called pons [26].

The mechanism by which this affection occurs is not fully known. One theory claims that this demyelination occurs by compressing fibrous structures as a result of cerebral edema arising from an osmotic fluctuation. Currently accepted theory supports the fact that brain cells adjust their osmolarity with certain osmolites, like inositol, betaine, and glutamine. In case of chronic hyponatremia, there is a decrease in these osmoliths in the brain, preventing fluid absorption [27, 28]. Clinical manifestations depend on the affected brain region, initially manifested by symptoms of hyponatremic encephalopathy such as nausea, vomiting, headache, confusion, and seizures. These symptoms can be reversed when adjusting the sodium concentration. Later signs of myelinolysis such as walking disturbances and respiratory dysfunction can occur [29]. Among the risk factors for this condition are: sodium concentration < 120 mEq/L for 48 hours, aggressive correction with saline solution and the occurrence of hypernatremia during treatment. If post liver transplant patients develop symptoms as confusion or weakness, CPM should be suspected because it may complicate a liver transplant [30].

Although the prognosis is poor with the occurrence of numerous neurological complications such as spastic quadriparesis and blocked syndrome, recovery is possible although it has a long duration [31].

Diagnosis can be done clinically and imagistically. The preferred imaging method is MRI, although lesions appear late and often initially may be normal [32]. The most common images are T2 weighted with hyperintense areas where demyelination was performed [33].

8. Management of hyponatremia

There are no data to recommend optimal serum sodium to initiate the treatment, but is generally recommended at a value of 130 mmol/L.

The identification and adjustment of excessive diuretic dosages and the addition of sodium are the main treatment requirements in the setting of hypovolemic hyponatremia. In case of hypervolemic hyponatremia, the most important issue is to decrease the amount of water to improve the sodium concentration.

When patients experience neurological symptoms due to hyponatremia or have a sodium concentration of less than 120 mEq/L, fluid restriction is indicated. In the case of mild and asymptomatic hyponatremia, fluid restriction is not indicated. Increasing sodium concentration in the first 24–48 hours is an important parameter that suggests an adequate fluid restriction. If this increase does not occur, either the restriction has to be more severe or the patient is not compliant. Fluid restriction is useful, but ineffective. Because the fluid restriction is severe, most patients cannot be compliant.

If patients have severe hyponatremia, there have been no responses to fluid restriction; it is indicated to administer the hypertonic saline. However, caution should be exercised in order not to cause a rapid increase in sodium concentration, which predisposes to the occurrence of numerous complications such as: central myelinolysis, quadriplegia, coma, or death [6].

The efficacy of using hypertonic sodium chloride in severe hypervolemic hyponatremia is partial, short-lived and aggravates ascites and edema. Instead, administration of albumin appears to have benefits, helps to increase the sodium concentration, but is not fully studied [34].

An important issue in patients with cirrhosis and hyponatremia is the correction of hypokalemia. Hypokalemia favors the appearance of hepatic encephalopathy because it increases the kidney synthesis of ammonium. By correcting it, there is also an increase in sodium concentration because both sodium and potassium are osmotically active [35].

In the past, the use of k-opiod agonist therapy has been attempted due to side effects [36]. According to recent studies, a new class of therapy, called vaptans, has been discovered in the treatment of hypervolemic hyponatremia. Vaptans selectively block the V2-receptors of AVP. They can be used in diseases like syndrome of inappropriate antidiuretic hormone secretion (SIADH), heart failure and cirrhosis, having the role of improving sodium concentration. The benefits of their administration over a short period of time are the increasing of urine volume and solute-free water excretion, and also, the improvement of the low serum sodium levels in 45–82% of patients [37] (**Figure 2**).

Hypernatremia, dehydration, renal impairment, and osmotic demyelination syndrome owing to a very rapid increase in serum sodium concentration could be the side effects of the administration of vaptans in patients with liver cirrhosis. Therefore, treatment should be initiated in the hospital and patients should be closely monitored to avoid hypernatremia.

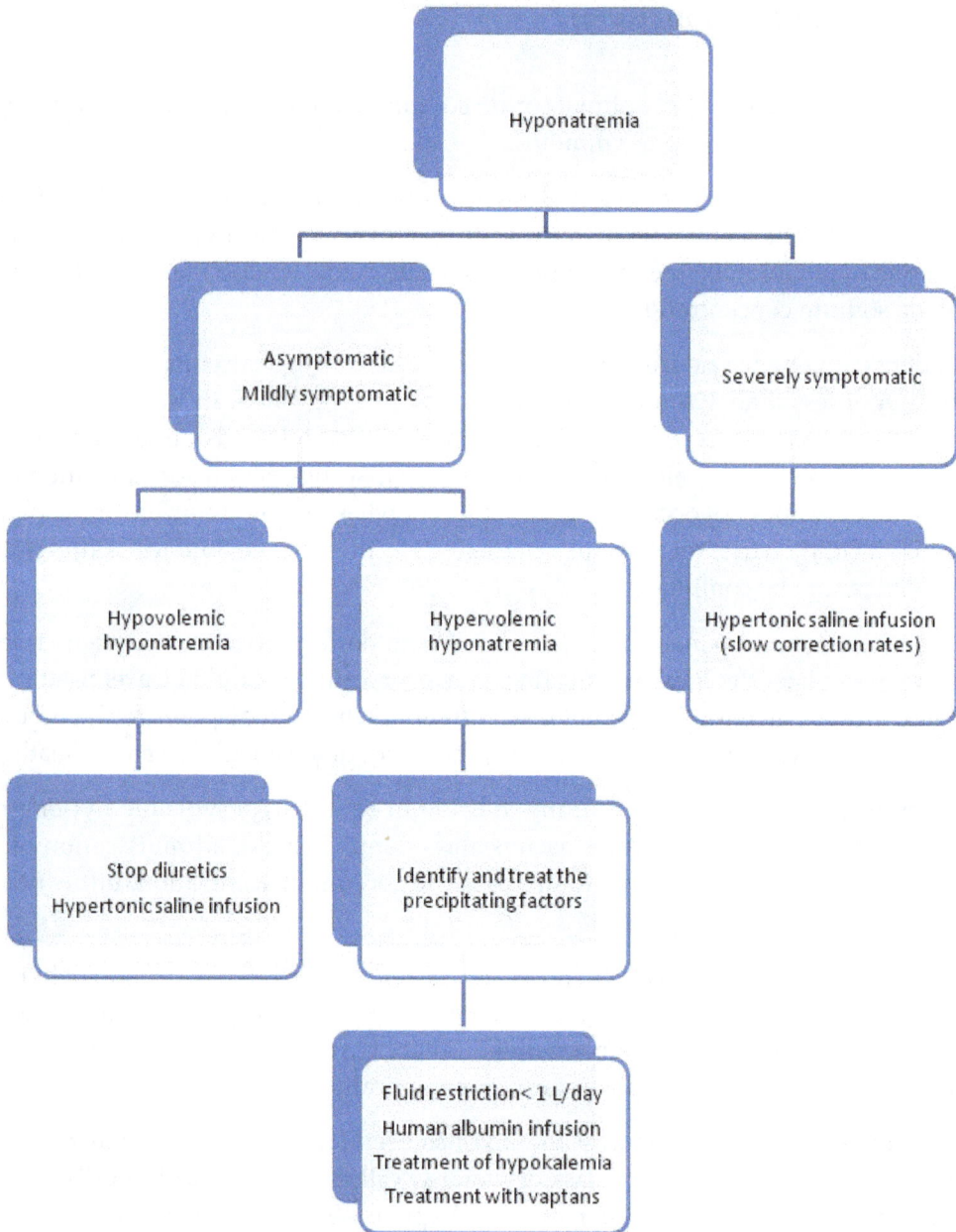

Figure 2. Management of hyponatremia.

Due to the risk of dehydration and hypernatremia, vaptans are also contraindicated in patients with an inappropriate consciousness state, unable to measure the volumes of fluid consumed.

The metabolism of vaptans is achieved in the liver by CYP3A enzymes. Therefore, CYP3A inhibitory drugs should be avoided because they increase the concentration of vaptans and may lead to the increase of serum sodium concentration. Also, drugs that are inducers of the CYP3A should be avoided because those drugs can reduce the concentration of vaptans.

Tolvaptan and conivaptan are recently approved in the USA for the treatment of severe hypervolemic hyponatremia from diseases such as cirrhosis, heart failure and SIADH. Treatment is started at a dose of 15 mg/day and can be increased progressively depending on the sodium concentration. In Europe, tolvaptan is authorized only for the treatment of SIADH. As an alternative option, conivaptan can be used to treat hypervolemic hyponatremia for short periods of time, especially when cirrhosis is associated with various conditions [38, 39].

Tolvaptan should be initiated without taking into account the period of meals, but initially it is advisable not to suppress the consumption of fluids to avoid rapid correction of sodium concentration. If, on completion of tolvaptan therapy, hyponatremia recurs, it should be corrected in a hospital unit. There may be no need for hospitalization, if treatment can be monitored to prevent excessive sodium concentration [40].

In randomized trials, the only side effects of tolvaptan treatment were gastrointestinal bleeding, but slightly increased incidence compared to placebo. It should be taken into account that the treatment was administered over a short period of time and new studies of the safety of long-term treatment are needed [41].

Treatment with conivaptan is contraindicated in patients who are allergic to constituents, in hyponatremia or hypovolaemia because it can induce from renal failure to shock. CYP3a4 inhibitors should not be administered concomitantly [42]. In general, the treatment was tolerated and adverse reactions were reported: local reactions (pain and erythema at the administration level), orthostatic hypotension, peripheral edema, headache, nausea, vomiting, urinary tract infections, and insomnia [43]. Effective treatment of hyponatremia should be initiated promptly to prevent irreversible neurological damage, but rapid correction may cause osmotic demyelination syndrome that can lead to death [44].

Domecycline favors the increase in free water excretion as an ADH antagonist, but cannot be used in cirrhosis due to nephrotoxicity [45].

The use of vasoconstrictors in hyponatremia is not tested, but studies of the hepatorenal syndrome have shown an improvement in sodium concentration [46].

The use of vasoconstrictors in hepatorenal syndrome has the following benefits: it improves the effective blood volume, vascular or systemic vasodilation, and renal perfusion. They are usually used in concomitant albumin administration. The most commonly used are: terlipressin, norepinephrine, vasopressin, and octeotrid, in combination with midodrine.

This combination can be used without supervision in a medical unit and is safe. Octreotide produces decreased splanchnic vasodilatation and midodrine improves renal perfusion and in combination with albumin improves kidney function, but there are still insufficient studies in this regard.

The octreotide is administered subcutaneously at the dose of 100 micrograms, 3 times per day, and the dose can be increased to 200 µg, 3 times per day. Midodrine is given orally 7.5 mg, 3 times per day and the dose can also be increased up to 12.5 mg, 3 times per day [47].

Treatment with terlipressin should be avoided in patients with cirrhosis, as it may cause severe hyponatremia, reversible upon discontinuation of treatment. Terlipresin acts on the vasopressin V1 receptor, but is also a partial vasopressin V2 receptor agonist. This is beneficial in the treatment of bleeding caused by portal hypertension, but also in hepatorenal syndrome [48].

By correcting hyponatremia in patients with cirrhosis, there are number of advantages: avoiding fluid restriction, administering effective doses of diuretics, especially in the treatment of refractory ascites, reducing the risk by developing hepatic encephalopathy, and improving the quality of life. It can also help reduce neurological complications after transplantation [49, 50].

9. Conclusions

Hyponatremia is a complication of cirrhosis, associated with an increased risk of mortality and morbidity in patients on the waiting list for a liver transplant. It also increases the risk of complications, such as hepatic encephalopathy, renal failure, and spontaneous bacterial peritonitis.

Hyponatremia occurred during cirrhosis evolution has as a pathophysiological mechanism arterial vasodilation that produces inadequate AVP secretion and a reduction in glomerular filtration rate with impairment of free water clearance. Clinical presentation does not differ from that of patients without hepatic impairment, but the symptoms of hyponatremia in cirrhosis are sometimes associated and difficult to differentiate from those in hepatic encephalopathy. As a dilutional hyponatremia, its treatment is not indicated if it is asymptomatic. Conversely, at a concentration of Na <120 mEq/L and on the occurrence of neurological symptoms, treatment can be initiated. An exception is the situation where patients are about to receive a liver transplant in a short time and the Na concentration is <130 mEq/L. In this case, its treatment is indicated to prevent the occurrence of serious neurological complications such as osmotic demyelination syndrome as a result of a rapid correction in the operating room. An important role is the differentiation of hypovolemic hyponatremia from the hypervolemic hyponatremia to initiate a suitable therapeutic scheme. In hypovolemic hyponatremia, it is necessary to identify the trigger factor and its treatment, usually discontinuation of diuretic treatment and administration of salt solution represents optimal methods in the correction of this. In hypervolemic hyponatremia, therapeutic methods are limited. Fluid restriction to about 1 L/day is important in improving Na concentration, but a small number of patients may be compliant with this therapy. Administration of saline solution in this case is only recommended if hyponatremia is severe because it usually favors the growth of ascites fluid and edema. Administration of albumin appears to be beneficial, but there is not enough data to confirm this.

A novelty in hyponatremic therapy is the treatment with vaptans. Treatment with tolvaptan should be given in the hospital to avoid a sudden increase in Na concentration, in oral administration, and with the possibility to increase the dose progressively to achieve the desired effects. Concomitant administration with vaptans of saline solution or fluid restriction is contraindicated to prevent osmotic demyelination syndrome. Medications that are inhibitors or inducers of CYP3A are also contraindicated. Conivaptan is given intravenously. Both conivaptan and tolvaptan can be administered for a short period of time, and hyponatremia may reappear when the treatment is stopped. Although treatment with vaptans is effective in relieving hyponatremia, their use requires additional data.

Author details

Andra Iulia Suceveanu[1]*, Roxana Popoiag[1], Laura Mazilu[1], Irinel Raluca Parepa[1], Andreea Gheorghe[1], Anca Stoian[2], Felix Voinea[1], Claudia Voinea[1] and Adrian Paul Suceveanu[1]

*Address all correspondence to: andrasuceveanu@yahoo.com

1 Ovidius University, Faculty of Medicine, Constanta, Romania

2 Carol Davila University, Bucharest, Romania

References

[1] Gins P, Quintero E, Arroyo V, et al. Compensated cirrhosis: Natural history and prognostic factors. Hepatology. 1987;7:122128

[2] Ripoll C, Groszmann R, Garcia-Tsao G, et al. Hepatic venous gradient predicts clinical decompensation in patients with compensated cirrhosis. Gastroenterology. 2007;133: 481488

[3] Schrier RW, Arroyo V, Bernardi M, et al. Peripheral arterial vasodilation hypothesis: A proposal for the initiation of renal sodium and water retention in cirrhosis. Hepatology. 1988;8:11511157

[4] Mller S, Henriksen JH. The systemic circulation in cirrhosis. in: Gins P, Arroyo V, Rods J, Schrier RW, editors. Ascites and renal dysfunction in liver disease. Malden: Blackwell; 2005:139155

[5] Henriksen JH, Mller S. Alterations of hepatic and splanchnic microvascular exchange in cirrhosis: Local factors in the formation of ascites. In: Gins P, Arroyo V, Rods J, Schrier RW, editors. Ascites and Renal Dysfunction in Liver Disease. Malden: Blackwell; 2005:174185

[6] Ginès P, Guevara M. Hyponatremia in cirrhosis: Pathogenesis, clinical significance, and management. Hepatology. 2008;48:1002

[7] Gins P, Berl T, Bernardi M, et al. Hyponatremia in cirrhosis: From pathogenesis to treatment. Hepatology. 1998;28:851864

[8] Angeli P, Wong F, Watson H, Ginès P, CAPPS Investigators. Hyponatremia in cirrhosis: Results of a patient population survey. Hepatology. 2006 Dec;44(6):1535-1542

[9]   Oliet SH, Bourque CW. Mechanosensitive channels transduce osmosensitivity in supra-optic neurons. Nature. 1993 Jul 22;**364**(6435):341-343

[10] Ginés P, Berl T, Bernardi M, Bichet DG, Hamon G, Jiménez W, Liard JF, Martin PY, Schrier RW. Hyponatremia in cirrhosis: From pathogenesis to treatment. Hepatology. 1998 Sep;**28**(3):851-864

[11] Schrier RW, Arroyo V, Bernardi M, Epstein M, Henriksen JH, Rodés J. Peripheral arterial vasodilation hypothesis: A proposal for the initiation of renal sodium and water retention in cirrhosis. Hepatology. 1988 Sep-Oct; **8**(5):151-1157

[12] Schrier RW. Water and sodium retention in edematous disorders: Role of vasopressin and aldosterone. American Journal of Medicine. 2006 Jul;**119**(7 Suppl 1):S47-S53

[13] Jalan R, Mookerjee R, Cheshire L, Williams R, et al. Albumin infusion for severe hyponatremia in patients with refractory ascites: A randomized clinical trial. Journal of Hepatology. 2007;**46**:232A (Abstract)

[14] Solà E, Watson H, Graupera I, Turón F, Barreto R, Rodríguez E, Pavesi M, Arroyo V, Guevara M, Ginès P. Factors related to quality of life in patients with cirrhosis and ascites: Relevance of serum sodium concentration and leg edema. Journal of Hepatology. 2012 Dec;**57**(6):1199-1206

[15] Arroyo V, Rodés J, Gutiérrez-Lizárraga MA, Revert L. Prognostic value of spontaneous hyponatremia in cirrhosis with ascites. American Journal of Digestive Diseases. 1976 Mar; **21**(3):249-256

[16] Heuman DM, Abou-Assi SG, Habib A, Williams LM, Stravitz RT, Sanyal AJ, Fisher RA, Mihas AA. Persistent ascites and low serum sodium identify patients with cirrosis and low MELD scores who are at high risk for early death. Hepatology. 2004 Oct; **40**(4):802-810

[17] Follo A, Llovet JM, Navasa M, Planas R, Forns X, Francitorra A, Rimola A, Gassull MA, Arroyo V, Rodés J. Renal impairment after spontaneous bacterial peritonitis in cirrhosis: Incidence, clinical course, predictive factors and prognosis. Hepatology. 1994 Dec;**20**(6):1495-1501

[18] Ginès P, Guevara M. Hyponatremia in cirrhosis: Pathogenesis, clinical significance, and management. Hepatology. 2008 Sep;**48**(3):1002-1010

[19] Kamath PS, Wiesner RH, Malinchoc M, Kremers W, Therneau TM, Kosberg CL, D'Amico G, Dickson ER, Kim WR. A model to predict survival in patients with end-stage liver disease. Hepatology. 2001;**33**:464-470

[20] Kim WR, Biggins SW, Kremers WK, Wiesner RH, Kamath PS, Benson JT, Edwards E, Therneau TM. Hyponatremia and mortality among patients on the liver-transplant waiting list. The New England Journal of Medicine. 2008;**359**:1018-1026

[21] Adrogué HJ, Madias NE. Hyponatremia. The New England Journal of Medicine. 2000 May 25;**342**(21):1581-1589

[22] Hyponatremia Treatment Guidelines 2007. Expert Panel Recommendations. American Journal of Medicine. 2007;**120**:S1S21

[23] Adrogué HJ, Madias NE. Hyponatremia. The New England Journal of Medicine. 2000;**342**:1581-1589

[24] Córdoba J, García-Martinez R, Simón-Talero M. Hyponatremic and hepatic encephalopathies: Similarities, differences and coexistence. Metabolic Brain Disease. 2010;**25**:73-80

[25] Häussinger D. Low grade cerebral edema and the pathogenesis of hepatic encephalopathy in cirrhosis. Hepatology. 2006 Jun;**43**(6):1187-1190

[26] Singh TD, Fugate JE, Rabinstein AA. Central pontine and extrapontine myelinolysis: A systematic review. European Journal of Neurology. 2014 Dec;**21**(12):1443-1450

[27] Karp BI, Laureno R. Pontine and extrapontine myelinolysis: A neurologic disorder following rapid correction of hyponatremia. Medicine (Baltimore). 1993 Nov;**72**(6):359-373

[28] Laureno R, Karp BI. Myelinolysis after correction of hyponatremia. Annals of Internal Medicine. 1997 Jan 1;**126**(1):57-62

[29] Odier C, Nguyen DK, Panisset M. Central pontine and extrapontine myelinolysis: From epileptic and other manifestations to cognitive prognosis. Journal of Neurology. July 2010;**257**(7):1176-1180

[30] Crivellin C, Cagnin A, Manara R, Boccagni P, Cillo U, Feltracco P, et al. Risk factors for central pontine and extrapontine myelinolysis after liver transplantation: A single-center study. Transplantation. 2015 Jun;**99**(6):1257-1264

[31] Bose P, Kunnacherry A, Maliakal P. Central pontine myelinolysis without hyponatraemia. The Journal of the Royal College of Physicians of Edinburgh.. 19 September 2011;**41**(3):211-214

[32] Graff-Radford J, Fugate JE, Kaufmann TJ, Mandrekar JN, Rabinstein AA. Clinical and radiologic correlations of central pontine myelinolysis syndrome. Mayo Clinic Proceedings. 2011 Nov;**86**(11):1063-1067

[33] DeWitt LD, Buonanno FS, Kistler JP, et al. Central pontine myelinolysis: Demonstration by nuclear magnetic resonance. Neurology. 1984 May;**34**(5):570-576

[34] McCormick PA, Mistry P, Kaye G, Burroughs AK, McIntyre N. Intravenous albumin infusion is an effective therapy for hyponatraemia in cirrhotic patients with ascites. Gut. 1990;**31**:204207

[35] Rose BD. New approach to disturbances in the plasma sodium concentration. American Journal of Medicine. 1986 Dec;**81**(6):1033-1040

[36] Planas R, Montoliu S, Balleste B, Rivera M, Miquel M, Masnou H, et al. Natural history of patients hospitalized for management of cirrhotic ascites. Clinical Gastroenterology and Hepatology. 2006;**4**:1385-1394

[37] Quittnat F, Gross P. Vaptans and the treatment of water-retaining disorders. Seminars in Nephrology. 2006;**26**:234243

[38] Schrier RW, Gross P, Gheorghiade M, Berl T, Verbalis JG, Czerwiec FS, et al. Tolvaptan, a selective oral vasopressin V2-receptor antagonist, for hyponatremia. The New England Journal of Medicine. 2006;**355**:20992112

[39] OLeary JG, Favis G. Conivaptan increases serum sodium in hyponatremic patients with end stage liver disease. Liver Transplantation. 2009;**15**:13251329

[40] Berl T, Quittnat-Pelletier F, Verbalis JG, Schrier RW, Bichet DG, Ouyang J, Czerwiec FS, SALTWATER investigators. Oral tolvaptan is safe and effective in chronic hyponatremia. Journal of the American Society of Nephrology. 2010 Apr;**21**(4):705-712

[41] Afdhal N, Cardenas A, Gins P, et al. Randomized, placebo-controlled trial of tolvaptan, a novel V2-receptor antagonist, in hyponatremia: Results of the SALT 2 trial with emphasis on efficacy and safety in cirrhosis. Hepatology. 2005;**42**:LB19A ([Abstract])

[42] Vaprisol [package insert] Deerfield, IL: Astellas Pharma US, Inc; 2006

[43] Goldsmith SR, Elkayam U, Haught WH, Barve A, He W. Efficacy and safety of the vasopressin V1A/V2-receptor antagonist conivaptan in acute decompensated heart failure: A dose-ranging pilot study. Journal of Cardiac Failure. 2008 Oct;**14**(8):641-647

[44] Sterns RH, Cappuccio JD, silver SM, Cohen EP. Neurologic sequelae after treatment of severe hyponatremia: A multicenter perspective. Journal of the American Society of Nephrology. 1994 Feb;**4**(8):1522-1530

[45] Miller PD, Linas SL, Schrier RW. Plasma demeclocycline levels and nephrotoxicity. Correlation in hyponatremic cirrhotic patients. JAMA. 1980 Jun 27;**243**(24):2513-2515

[46] Garcia-Tsao G, Parikh CR, Viola A. Acute kidney injury in cirrhosis. Hepatology. 2008;**48**(6):2064-2077

[47] Kalambokis G, Economou M, Fotopoulos A, et al. The effects of chronic treatment with octreotide versus octreotide plus midodrine on systemic hemodynamics and renal hemodynamics and function in nonazotemic cirrhotic patients with ascites. The American Journal of Gastroenterology. 2005;**100**(4):879-885

[48] Solà E, Lens S, Guevara M, Martín-Llahí M, Fagundes C, Pereira G, Pavesi M, Fernández J, González-Abraldes J, Escorsell A, Mas A, Bosch J, Arroyo V, Ginès P. Hyponatremia in patients treated with terlipressin for severe gastrointestinal bleeding due to portal hypertension. Hepatology. 2010 Nov;**52**(5):1783-1790

[49] Jalan R, Elton RA, Redhead DN, Simpson KJ, Finlayson NDC, Hayes PC, et al. Analysis of prognostic variables in the prediction of shunt failure, variceal rebleeding, early mortality and encephalopathy following the transjugular intrahepatic portosystemic stent-shunt (TIPSS). Journal of Hepatology. 1995;**23**:123-128

[50] Baccaro ME, Guevara M, Torre A, Arcos E. Martı'n-Llahı'M, Terra C, et al. Hyponatremia predisposes to hepatic encephalopathy in patients with cirrhosis. Results of a prospective study with time-dependent analysis [abstract]. Hepatology. 2006;**233A**:44

6

Nutrition and Lifestyle Modifications in the Prevention and Treatment of Non-Alcoholic Fatty Liver Disease

Kingsley Asare Kwadwo Pereko, Jacob Setorglo,
Matilda Steiner-Asiedu and
Joyce Bayebanona Maaweh Tiweh

Abstract

Non-alcoholic fatty liver disease (NAFLD) is a burgeoning health problem worldwide. NAFLD is an umbrella term for a range of liver conditions affecting people who drink little to no alcohol Different methods are employed in the diagnosis of NAFLD. Certain drugs, genetics, lifestyle factors have been implicated in the development of NAFLD. NAFLD symptoms are asymptomatic but indicated when there is unexplained persistent elevation of liver enzyme levels. Nutrition and lifestyle modifications are widely prescribed as helpful in the prevention and treatment of Non-Alcoholic Fatty Liver disease (NAFLD). Dietary and lifestyle modifications are apparent measures considering the disease association with obesity, diabetes, and cardiovascular disease which many reviews have linked to the condition. Reduction in body weight, involvement in both aerobic and anaerobic exercises, conscious intake in the types of fat and carbohydrates are helpful in the management of NAFLD. This chapter highlights the various theories and principles underlying nutrition and lifestyle modifications in the prevention and treatment of NAFLDs.

Keywords: fatty liver, obesity, non-alcoholic, dietary, lifestyle

1. Introduction

Non-alcoholic fatty liver disease (NAFLD) is a burgeoning health problem worldwide and is a risk factor for both hepatic and cardiometabolic mortality [1, 2]. A meta-analysis of prevalence, incidence and outcome of NAFLD following publications on pubmed from 1989 to 2015 estimated global prevalence at 25.24% (95% CI: 22.10–28.65) with highest prevalence in the Middle East 31.79% (13.48–58.23) and South America 30.45% (22.74–39.44) and lowest in Africa 13.48% (5.69–28.69) [2]. NAFLD describes a range of conditions caused by a build-up of fat within liver cells and can be divided into four stages namely:

1. Simple fatty liver (hepatic steatosis). Under normal conditions, very little fat is stored in liver cells of humans. Hepatic steatosis therefore refers to a situation where excess fat accumulates in the hepatic cells. Sometimes simple fatty liver does not cause any harm to the liver or pose health risks. However, in some instances it leads to NAFLD and its severe forms and that is where the problem arises.

2. Non-alcoholic steatohepatitis (NASH). This expression is much less common than NAFLD. Here, the excess fat stored in the liver cells is associated with inflammation of the liver.

3. Fibrosis: This is associated with persistent hepatitis, including steatohepatitis and may lead to scarring of the liver tissue (fibrosis). This is not life threatening since when fibrosis some of the liver cells that continue to perform its functions.

4. Cirrhosis: This stage of a liver disease can be life threatening because normal liver tissues are replaced by a lot of fibrosis. The structure and function of the liver are therefore modified. There are different scientific means of detecting liver diseases.

2. Diagnosis

There are different methods of diagnosing NAFLD. The test ranges from metabolic syndrome assessment, detecting metabolites in the blood as well as enzymes such as Alanine transaminase (ALT) and Aspartate Aminotransferase (AST) [3]. Medical imaging and sonographic techniques are also performed to create an image of the liver. Further tests such as fibroscan and biopsy may be conducted apart from those listed earlier to determine the stage of the liver disease [4].

3. Risk factors

A wide range of diseases and conditions can predispose one to non-alcoholic fatty liver disease (NAFLD). Non-alcoholic steatohepatitis expresses itself among some sub-populations such as older people, diabetics and the obese. Certain drugs and hepatitis have been implicated in the development of NAFLD as well. Some risks are usually from lifestyle origin. These include:

- High cholesterol and triglycerides levels,
- Metabolic syndrome,

- Central adiposity,

- Polycystic ovary syndrome,

- Sleep apnea,

- Genetics,

- Hypothyroidism,

- Hypopituitarism [5].

Nutritional factors have also been cited as risks in the development of the disease. These include rapid weight loss, total parenteral nutrition, starvation and protein-calorie malnutrition [6]. The most common risk factor associated with NAFLD is the presence of the metabolic syndrome. The metabolic syndrome is defined by the presence of 3 or more of the following criteria (**Table 1**): (1) increased waist circumference, (2) hypertriglyceridemia, (3) hypertension, (4) high fasting glucose, and (5) a low high-density lipoprotein (HDL) level.

Parameter*	Value
Impaired glucose tolerance	Fasting blood glucose level ≥ 110 mg/dL
High blood pressure	≥130/85 mm Hg
Elevated triglyceride levels	>250 mg/dL
Low high-density lipoprotein level	<40 mg/dL for men; <50 mg/dL for women
Abdominal obesity	Waist: >102 cm (40 inches) for men; >88 cm (35 inches) for women

*Metabolic syndrome is diagnosed by the presence of 2 or more of these parameters.
Source: [2].

Table 1. Diagnostic criteria for metabolic syndrome.

4. Signs and symptoms and management

Nonalcoholic fatty liver disease occurs in every age group but especially in people in their 40s and 50s. The condition is also closely linked to metabolic syndrome, which is a cluster of abnormalities including increased abdominal fat, poor ability to use the hormone insulin, high blood pressure and high blood levels of triglycerides. NAFLD symptoms are asymptomatic but indicated when there is unexplained persistent elevation of liver enzyme levels after hepatitis and other chronic liver diseases have been excluded. However, at certain stages of the disease, patients are malaise, fatigue, and right upper quadrant or diffuse abdominal discomfort. Hepatomegaly is found on clinical examination. When there is cirrhosis there may be; spider angiomata, ascites, splenomegaly, hard liver border, ascites, portal hypertension and jaundice or pruritus [7].

Clinical evaluation includes a careful history and physical examination. It is relevant to inquire about excess alcohol consumption which is defined as intakes greater than 30 g/day for men and greater than 20 g/day for women within the past 5 years. A drink is 350 mL (12 oz) of beer, 120 mL (4 oz) of wine, and 45 mL (1.5 oz) of hard liquor each contain 10 g of alcohol.

There are several approaches to managing NAFLD. Hepatoprotective therapy, antioxidants insulin-sensitizing agents and treatment of obesity are part of these. However, this text limits itself to the nutritional management of the NAFLD. Key to nutritional therapeutic procedures are lifestyle changes in diet and improving exercise habits in addition to the control of comorbidities which are secondary to the development of NAFLD [8]. For instance, bile acid derivatives and associated compounds that influence bile acid related are becoming prominent therapeutic agents for NAFLD [9, 10, 11]. The immediate associated lifestyle causes of NAFLD are targeted in the management of the disease condition.

5. Obesity and genetics

Obesity when combined with physical inactivity and genetic predisposition, has been directly associated with metabolic syndrome and NAFLD among some adult populations [12, 2]. Obesity itself is the failure of normal homeostatic regulation of energy utilization [9]. NAFLD can be a precursor to developing metabolic syndrome or insulin resistance [10]. Data suggest that about 80% of adults who are class 1 and/or 2 obese and 90% morbid obese according to the World Health Organization classification are at risk of having NAFLD [13]. Body weight loss can alter the cellular activity of adipose tissue and reverse many of the negative consequences of NAFLD. The excess fat and energy content of a meal has been associated with NAFLD development in healthy populations [14, 15]. Insulin resistance, oxidative stress, and cytokine toxicity results due to obesity and these factors have been implicated in the pathogenesis of NAFLD [16]. Among these factors, central adiposity and insulin resistance have direct association with hepatic fat content and visceral adiposity [17–19]. Polymorphisms (genetic variations) in the single-nucleotide polymorphisms (SNPs) T455C and C482T in APOC3 are associated with fatty liver disease. The carriers of T-455C, C-482 T, or both (not additive) had a 30% increase in fasting plasma apolipoprotein C3, 60% increase in fasting plasma triglyceride and 46% reduction in plasma triglyceride clearance. Oxidative stress, hormonal imbalances, and mitochondrial abnormalities can be potential causes.

6. Total fat

Dietary composition of a meal in terms of the macro-molecule distribution has a positive relation with the development of NAFLD. The amount and type of dietary fat may directly affect liver fat content, with high-fat diets being potentially harmful [20]. It has also been shown that a high ratio of omega-6 to omega-3 polyunsaturated fatty acids (PUFAs) and an increased intake of saturated and trans fatty acids are associated with NAFLD [21–23]. It was noted that when severely obese patients were fed diets containing higher percentage of total fat beyond recommended ranges, the risk of developing NALFD increased [24]. The deduction therefore was that the type of fat ingested rather than the amount is associated with NAFLD in obese individuals.

7. Saturated fatty acids

Saturated fatty acid component in meals has been shown to induce insulin resistance especially among the obese [25–27]. In epidemiologic studies, both total fat and saturated fat in the diet had significant correlation with triglyceride content in hepatic cells [28, 29]. In a double-blind randomized controlled trial of two reduced-fat diets, compared with a control diet both reduced-fat diets decreased amount of low density lipoprotein cholesterol (LDLc) in healthy males [30]. There was a decrease in high density lipoprotein cholesterol (HDLc) and increase in triglyceride levels increased with the reduced-fat diets. The authors concluded that reduced saturated fat intake (below 10%) may benefit patients with NAFLD. It was also observed that, low total fat and low saturated fat diet (23% fat and 7% saturated fat) predicted changes in HDLc and LDLc but not the amount of fat in the hepatocytes [31].

8. *Trans* fatty acids

Trans fatty acids are positively associated with an increase in inflammatory processes, plasma triglycerides, and cholesterol as well as a reduction in HDLc level [32, 33]. Animal studies have shown positive relationships between the increased consumption of trans fatty acids from oxidized oils and liver inflammation [34, 35].

9. Polyunsaturated fatty acids (PUFAs)

Essential fatty acid, Omega-3 (which is a type of polyunsaturated fatty acids) PUFA levels are decreased in the hepatic tissue of people with NAFLD [22, 36] A higher omega-6 to omega-3 PUFA ratio may contribute to the development of a fatty liver within the hepatocytes of people NAFLD [36].

10. High carbohydrate intake

High carbohydrate intake especially the amount and type of carbohydrate consumed have an important impact on the development of NAFLD [37]. Simple carbohydrates intakes can lead to the development of NAFLD [38]. Meals high in carbohydrates lead to increased amounts of circulating insulin, which contribute to elevated triglyceride concentrations even under isocaloric conditions [39, 40]. A higher carbohydrate intake more than the recommended daily values has been positively associated with liver inflammation and NAFLD [24].

Coupled with a low-fat meal, high-carbohydrate meal promotes the development of a NAFLD through increased de novo fatty acid and triglyceride synthesis [41].

11. High-fructose corn syrup intake

Epidemiological data suggest that dietary pattern and an increased intake of simple sugars, especially fructose is associated with the development of NAFLD [42, 43]. The link is not too clear although it is assumed that the carbohydrates components increased risk of fatty infiltration of the liver or muscle. Therefore it was hypothesized that the link is through both indirect and direct mechanisms [44, 45]. Indirect association manifest itself through the adverse metabolic effects that can increase the risk of developing NAFLD. Fructose may cause hepatotoxic damage as a form of direct route link with NAFLD. Studies [46–49] have suggested that increased fructose consumption augments fat mass, de novo lipogenesis, and inflammation. There is also induction of insulin resistance and fasting and postprandial triglycerides, which in turn, can result in liver steatosis. In other studies [50, 51], sugar-sweetened beverage consumption was found to be associated with fatty liver independent of body mass index of the individuals. Direct positive association was found between the amount of fructose consumed and the development of NAFLD [52, 53]. Age and frequency of consuming fructose-based food was also found to be related to liver inflammation and NAFLD [54].

12. Physical inactivity

Physical activity has been documented to improve health and hence the World Health Organization recommendations for aerobic an anaerobic exercises across the life span. Physical inactivity however, has been associated with NAFLD. Using matched controls for age and gender, only about one-fifth of individuals with NAFLD met recommendations for physical activity [55, 56]. Among 349 individuals studied, the NAFLD group engaged in less physical activity, including total, aerobic, and resistance [55].

It has been noted that decreased physical activity correlates with intra-hepatic fat, decreased cellular insulin sensitivity, and increased central adiposity [57, 58]. Sedentary time alone is associated with metabolic status. Sedentary times predicted higher levels of fasting insulin, independent of the amount of time spent engaging in moderate- or vigorous-intensity activity [59]. Therefore to improve metabolic health it is generally important to reduce sedentary lifestyle even when one meets the requirements for physical activity.

13. Treatments

Aggressive pursuit of modified lifestyle modifications coupled with dietary changes are critical in treating NAFLD when body weight is the underlying cause. That is because dietary macronutrient composition, physical activity, and all play critical roles in successful weight reduction. Weight loss is effective for improving NAFLD as it positively influences insulin sensitivity and dyslipidemia.

14. Body weight loss

It was found that about 9% body weight loss significantly improves NAFLD [60]. The result was thought to be due to improvements in inflammation and steatosis. Reduction in body weight through lowering of daily caloric intake of about 200 kcal/day improved liver cellular structure histology and enzymes function. A 10% body weight reduction resulted in a 45% reduction in liver fat content [61]. Lifestyle modification through dietary intake, exercise, and behavior modification with the guidelines from health experts has been show to lead to resolution in NALFD [62]. A weight reduction of about 7% was therefore recommended [63]. A combination of diet and exercise reduces fibrosis and amount of liver fat by an average of 40% [64–66]. The degree of hepatic fat reduction is related to the intensity of the lifestyle mediation and normally required a weight loss range of 5–10% is suggested.

15. Bariatric surgery

Among persons with higher grades of obesity, physical remedy such as reduction in dietary intake and physical activities does not result in resolution of NAFLD. Other means such as bariatric surgery is the most effective strategy to achieve and maintain weight loss [67]. Results from several uncontrolled studies [68–70] and controlled studies [71, 72] indicated that body weight loss achieved through bariatric surgery reduces amount of liver enzymes and improves NAFLD.

A study found an association between bariatric surgery and lower serum alanine transferase and aspartate aminotransferase levels at two and 10 years follow-up [73] and histological improvements [74]. Steatosis, steatohepatitis, and fibrosis improved among majority of patients that have undergone surgery [75]. It is worth noting that hepatic decompensation can occur after gastric bypass so decision to opt for this should be taken with great care [3].

16. Nutrient content and healthful fats

Dietary composition can directly manipulate NAFLD progress. Changing either the composition of the macronutrient or micronutrient content can directly affect the level of inflammation, amount of serum lipids and insulin resistance [49]. Inverse association was found between Mediterranean diet consumption and cardiovascular disease risk [76]. Among obese women and overweight men, a low-fat diet decreased hepatic fat compared with a high-fat diet [64, 77]. The dietary recommendation is that the diet contain less than 7% saturated fats, less than 1% of trans fats and 25–35% of the calorific intake should be total fat among which is polyunsaturated fatty acid.

17. Monounsaturated fats

It was found that replacing carbohydrate intake with monounsaturated fatty acids (MUFAs) to about 32 g/day increases triglyceride-rich lipoprotein catabolism [30]. This can lead to resolution of NAFLD. This finding is supported by epidemiological studies [31, 78]. Olive oil which contains about 73% MUFAs appears to provide a direct benefit in improving plasma lipids and possible NAFLD [79]. In randomized trials, [80, 81] isocaloric low-fat/high-carbohydrate diet improved hepatic fat and improved insulin sensitivity. The diet was composed of 50% MUFAs and 18% omega-3 PUFAs, 40% from carbohydrate, and 20% protein. These findings were independent of body weight loss of patients.

18. Omega-3 Omega-6 PUFAs

Evidence from epidemiologic and randomized controlled trials indicate that supplementation with omega-3 PUFAs lowers triglyceride levels and reduces the risk of coronary heart disease and mortality.94,95 High consumption of omega-3 PUFAs derived from fish diminishes hepatic triglyceride lipoprotein secretion and inhibits de novo lipogenesis. [82]. Using the Therapeutic Lifestyle Change diet criteria with a diet high in fish-derived omega-3 fatty acid (1.23 g/day EPA + DHA) vs. a low fish diet (0.27 g/day EPA + DHA) for 24 weeks, the higher fish diet decreased plasma triglycerides by 24%. Three human clinical trials support these findings by showing that giving patients with NAFLD omega-3 PUFAs (1 to 2.7 g/day for six to 12 months) improved hepatic steatosis, inflammation, and fibrosis [82, 83]. Capanni and Spadaro both demonstrated that triglyceride levels decreased 25 to 37 mg/dL when patients' diets were supplemented with 1 to 2 g of omega-3 PUFAs per day for six and 12 months, respectively. This was thought to be through diminishes hepatic triglyceride lipoprotein secretion and inhibition de novo lipogenesis [82–84]. Diets based on therapeutic lifestyle change criteria supports improvements in NAFLD as the diet improves liver steatosis, inflammation, and fibrosis [85]. In a non-controlled trial, omega-6 PUFAs (15% of energy as linoleic acid) reduced liver fat compared with a diet high in saturated fatty acids in abdominally obese patients [86]. A diet consisting of mainly reduced simple carbohydrate may confer similar benefits among NALFD patients [87, 88].

19. Low sugar intake

Diet designed to produce a caloric deficit of 500 to1000 kcal/day is advised. Reduction of dietary carbohydrates, in particular dietary fructose, is the most beneficial and has been found to improve the lipid profile in overweight patients. Diets with less carbohydrate and more fat have relatively greater benefits in NAFLD management [89, 90]. Hypocaloric diet made up from 40% carbohydrate and 45% fat decreased serum alanine transaminase concentration than did a higher-carbohydrate (60%), low-fat diet (25% fat) [91]. Low-carbohydrate caloric restriction significantly improved hepatic insulin sensitivity. Diets with less carbohydrate and more fat have relatively greater benefits for insulin levels, triglycerides, and HDL cholesterol concentrations than do hypocaloric, low-fat diets. A hypocaloric diet moderately lower in carbohydrate (40% carbohydrate and 45% fat) decreased serum alanine transaminase concentrations to a greater degree than did a higher-carbohydrate, low-fat diet (60% carbohydrate and 25% fat).106 For individuals with NAFLD who were glucose intolerant, the low-carbohydrate caloric restriction significantly improved hepatic insulin sensitivity compared with the low-fat diet. In contrast, changes in visceral fat mass and insulin sensitivity were similar between a low-calorie, reduced-carbohydrate diet (fewer than 90 g of carbohydrate) and a reduced-fat diet (less than 20% fat). The World Health Organization recommends that the daily intake of added sugars makes up no more than 10% of total energy. The American Heart Association recommends limiting the amount of added sugars to no more than one-half of daily discretionary calories, which for women is approximately 100 kcal/day (6 tsp. of sugar) and for men is 150 kcal/day (9 tsp. of sugar).

20. Physical activity therapy

Physical activity enhances insulin sensitivity and favorably modifies lipids independent of weight loss [92, 93] Data suggest that there is improvement in cellular liver characteristics when NALFD individuals become active [94]. Exercise can lead to improvement in insulin sensitivity which intends contributes to the fatty acid delivery to the liver [95]. Improvement in insulin resistance and may decrease hepatic steatosis, inflammation, and disease progression in NAFLD [96, 97]. Four studies have investigated the effects of exercise without dietary modification on hepatic steatosis. Exercise can independently results in reduction in the fat in the hepatocytes without a significant weight change [98–101].

21. Exercise intensity and duration

Both intermittent and daily exercise helps achieve weight loss and improve insulin sensitivity [102]. Intensity and duration contribute to energy expenditure and therefore can lead to insulin sensitivity, triglycerides, and serum glucose amount [103]. Vigorous exercise and doubling the duration of vigorous exercise was associated with decreased odds of developing fat in the liver [104]. Increased exercise by 60 minutes or more per week significantly reduced body weight and all liver enzymes [105]. Regular aerobic exercise for half an hour at least per day at 60–70% max heart rate for least 5 days per week reduces liver alanine transaminase levels [106].

22. Aerobic and resistance exercises

Increased aerobic exercise has been associated with improvement in the metabolic parameters associated with NAFLD [61, 94, 106]. Combined aerobic and resistance exercises have been shown to be more effective than aerobic exercise alone for resolving inflammation and cardio-vascular risk factors [107]. An intervention of 30 minutes of aerobic exercise and 20 minutes of resistance exercise three times per week was found to be associated with improvements in hepatic fat among NAFLD patients [108]. This combination activity improves hepatic insulin sensitivity [100] reduction in liver fat [109]. Both findings were independent of body weight reduction. Antioxidant treatments such as vitamins and minerals supplementation have been mentioned to decrease oxidative stress and improve oxidative injury among NAFLD patients.

23. Vitamin E

In theory, vitamin E and other vitamins called antioxidants could help protect the liver by reducing or neutralizing the damage caused by inflammation. But more research is needed. Some evidence suggests vitamin E supplements may be helpful for people with liver damage caused by nonalcoholic fatty liver disease [110]. But vitamin E has been linked with increased risk of death and, in men, an increased risk of prostate cancer. Several small trials in humans with NAFLD have supported an effect of tocopherol (vitamin E) on the improvement of trans-aminase levels but there have been discordant results in histologic improvement [111]. There was a significant improvement in hepatic steatosis with vitamin E intakes at levels of 800 to 1000 IU/day [112, 113] Higher intakes of the vitamin can be fatal in most cases [114, 115].

24. Vitamin D

Vitamin D may play an important role in modifying the risk of cardio metabolic outcomes [116, 117]. Serum 25-hydroxy vitamin D concentrations were correlated with NAFLD in terms of liver steatosis, inflammation and fibrosis [118].

25. EPA + DHA

The evidence supporting the use of omega-3 PUFAs for treating NAFLD have consisted of small sample sizes and laden with errors [118, 119].

26. Probiotics

Gut microbiota has been associated with the development of obesity-related NAFLD [120]. Probiotics may improve liver enzymes and decrease markers of lipid peroxidation [121, 122]. The use of prebiotics and probiotics is to modify the microbiota as preventive or therapeutic strategies [123]. Their beneficial effects on NAFLD have been limited human studies [124]. Consuming a tablet containing 500 million *Lactobacillus bulgaricus* and *Streptococcus thermophilus* for 3 months improved levels of liver enzyme in patients with NAFLD [124].

27. Other nutrients

Ginger (*Zingiber officinale*) can improve insulin sensitivity and reduce hepatic fat content [125]. In studies of people with non-alcoholic fatty liver disease, those who reported drinking coffee had less liver damage than those who drank little or no coffee. It's not clear how coffee may influence liver damage or how much coffee you'd need to drink in order to benefit. **Table 2** summarizes the nutritional guidelines in the management and treatment of NAFLD.

Weight loss	10% of initial body weight over 6 months Maintenance of weight loss Bariatric surgery when individuals qualify
Calorie intake	1200 to 1500 daily *Energy deficit of 500 kcal/day based on Mifflin-St Jeor formula*
Total fat	≤ 35% of total calories
Monounsaturated fatty acids	15–25% of total calories
Polyunsaturated fatty acids	5–10% of total calories Omega-3 fatty acids
Saturated fatty acids	7–10% of total calories
Carbohydrate	50% of total calories > 50% carbohydrate sources from whole grains Avoid high-fructose corn syrup Added sugars <10% of total calories
Protein	15% of total calories Lean and vegetable protein
Antioxidants	None
Physical activity	≥ 150 minutes/week at moderate intensity or ≥75 minutes/week at vigorous intensity Cardiovascular exercise five times weekly Resistance training two or more times weekly Decrease time spent sedentary

Source: [65, 81, 83].

Table 2. Guidelines in the management and treatment of NAFLD.

Author details

Kingsley Asare Kwadwo Pereko[1]*, Jacob Setorglo[2], Matilda Steiner-Asiedu[3] and Joyce Bayebanona Maaweh Tiweh[4]

*Address all correspondence to: kpereko@gmail.com

1 School of Medical Sciences, University of Cape Coast, Cape Coast, Ghana

2 School of Allied Health Sciences, University of Cape Coast, Cape Coast, Ghana

3 Department of Nutrition and Food Science, University of Ghana, Legon, Ghana

4 Eye Unit, Manhyia Government Hospital, Kumasi, Ghana

References

[1] McCulough AJ. The clinical features, diagnosis and natural history of nonalcoholic fatty liver disease. Clinics in Liver Disease. Aug 2004;**8**(3):521-533. DOI: 10.1016/j.cld.2004.04.004. PMID 15331061

[2] Chalasani N, Younossi Z, Lavine JE, et al. The diagnosis and management of non-alcoholic fatty liver disease: Practice guideline by the American Association for the Study of Liver Diseases, American College of Gastroenterology, and the American Gastroenterological Association. Hepatology. 2012;**55**(6):2005-2023

[3] Chalasani N et al. The diagnosis and management of non-alcoholic fatty liver disease: Practice guideline by the American Association for the Study of Liver Diseases, American College of Gastroenterology, and the American Gastroenterological Association. American Journal of Gastroenterology. 2012;**107**(6):811-826

[4] Brunt EM. Pathology of non-alcoholic fatty liver disease. Nature Reviews. Gastroenterology & Hepatology. 2010;(4):195-203. Epub 2010 Mar 2

[5] Rinella ME. Nonalcoholic fatty liver disease: A systematic review. JAMA (Systematic Review). 2015;**313**(22):2263-2273. DOI: 10.1001/jama.2015.5370. PMID 26057287

[6] Allocca M, Selmi C. Emerging nutritional treatments for nonalcoholic fatty liver disease. In: Preedy VR, Lakshman R, Rajaskanthan RS, editors. Nutrition, Diet Therapy, and the Liver. Florida, USA: CRC Press; 2010. pp. 131-146. ISBN 1420085492

[7] Clark JM, Diehl AM. Nonalcoholic fatty liver disease: An underrecognized cause of cryptogenic cirrhosis. Journal of the American Medical Association. 2003;**289**(22):3000-3004. DOI: 10.1001/jama.289.22.3000. PMID 12799409

[8] Loria P, Adinolfi LE, Bellentani S, et al. Practice guidelines for the diagnosis and management of nonalcoholic fatty liver disease. A decalogue from the Italian Association for the study of the liver (AISF) expert committee. Digestive and Liver Disease. 2010;**42**(4):272-282

[9] Dandona P, Aljada A, Bandyopadhyay A. Inflammation: The link between insulin resistance, obesity and diabetes. Trends in Immunology. 2004;**25**(1):4-7

[10] Vanni E, Bugianesi E, Kotronen A, De Minicis S, Yki-Järvinen H, Svegliati-Baroni G. From the metabolic syndrome to NAFLD or vice versa? Digestive and Liver Disease. 2010;**42**(5):320-330

[11] Capristo E, Miele L, Forgione A, et al. Nutritional aspects in patients with non-alcoholic steatohepatitis (NASH). European Review for Medical and Pharmacological Sciences. 2005;**9**(5):265-268

[12] Marchesini G, Bugianesi E, Forlani G, et al. Nonalcoholic fatty liver, steatohepatitis, and the metabolic syndrome. Hepatology. 2003;**37**(4):917-923

[13] Gholam PM, Flancbaum L, Machan JT, Charney DA, Kotler DP. Nonalcoholic fatty liver disease in severely obese subjects. The American Journal of Gastroenterology. 2007;**102**(2):399-408

[14] Sobrecases H, Lê KA, Bortolotti M, et al. Effects of short-term overfeeding with fructose, fat and fructose plus fat on plasma and hepatic lipids in healthy men. Diabetes & Metabolism. 2010;**36**(3):244-246

[15] Ngo Sock ET, Le KA, Ith M, Kreis R, Boesch C, Tappy L. Effects of a short-term overfeeding with fructose or glucose in healthy young males. The British Journal of Nutrition. 2010;**103**(7):939-943

[16] Dowman JK, Tomlison JW, and Newsome PN. Pathogenesis of non-alcholic fatty liver disease. 2009;**103**:71-83 QJMed

[17] Jakobsen MU, Berentzen T, Sørensen TI, Overvad K. Abdominal obesity and fatty liver. Epidemiologic Reviews. 2007;**29**:77-87

[18] Chitturi S, Abeygunasekera S, Farrell GC, et al. NASH and insulin resistance: Insulin hypersecretion and specific association with the insulin resistance syndrome. Hepatol. 2002;**35**(2):373-379

[19] Lee JH, Rhee PL, Lee JK, et al. Role of hyperinsulinemia and glucose intolerance in the pathogenesis of nonalcoholic fatty liver in patients with normal body weight. The Korean Journal of Internal Medicine. 1998;**13**(1):12-14

[20] Donnelly KL, Smith CI, Schwarzenberg SJ, Jessurun J, Boldt MD, Parks EJ. Sources of fatty acids stored in liver and secreted via lipoproteins in patients with nonalcoholic fatty liver disease. The Journal of Clinical Investigation. 2005;**115**(5):1343-1351

[21] Kien CL. Dietary interventions for metabolic syndrome: Role of modifying dietary fats. Current Diabetes Reports. 2009;**9**(1):43-50

[22] Spadaro L, Magliocco O, Spampinato D, et al. Effects of n-3 polyunsaturated fatty acids in subjects with nonalcoholic fatty liver disease. Digestive and Liver Disease. 2008;**40**(3):194-199

[23] Tanaka N, Sano K, Horiuchi A, Tanaka E, Kiyosawa K, Aoyama T. Highly purified eicos-
      apentaenoic acid treatment improves nonalcoholic steatohepatitis. Journal of Clinical
      Gastroenterology. 2008;**42**(4):413-418

[24] Solga S, Alkhuraishe AR, Clark JM, et al. Dietary composition and nonalcoholic fatty
      liver disease. Digestive Diseases and Sciences. 2004;**49**(10):1578-1583

[25] Lovejoy JC, Smith SR, Champagne CM, et al. Effects of diets enriched in saturated (pal-
      mitic), monounsaturated (oleic), or trans (elaidic) fatty acids on insulin sensitivity and
      substrate oxidation in healthy adults. Diabetes Care. 2002;**25**(8):1283-1288

[26] Vessby B, Uusitupa M, Hermansen K, et al. Substituting dietary saturated for mono-
      unsaturated fat impairs insulin sensitivity in healthy men and women: The KANWU
      study. Diabetologia. 2001;**44**(3):312-319

[27] Xiao C, Giacca A, Carpentier A, Lewis GF. Differential effects of monounsaturated,
      polyunsaturated and saturated fat ingestion on glucose-stimulated insulin secretion,
      sensitivity and clearance in overweight and obese, non-diabetic humans. Diabetologia.
      2006;**49**(6):1371-1379

[28] Tiikkainen M, Bergholm R, Vehkavaara S, et al. Effects of identical weight loss on body
      composition and features of insulin resistance in obese women with high and low liver
      fat content. Diabetes. 2003;**52**(3):701-707

[29] Vilar L, Oliveira CP, Faintuch J, et al. High-fat diet: A trigger of non-alcoholic steato-
      hepatitis? Preliminary findings in obese subjects. Nutrition. 2008;**24**(11-12):1097-1102

[30] Lefevre M, Champagne CM, Tulley RT, Rood JC. Most MM. Individual variability in car-
      diovascular disease risk factor responses to low-fat and low-saturated-fat diets in men:
      Body mass index, adiposity, and insulin resistance predict changes in LDL cholesterol.
      The American Journal of Clinical Nutrition. 2005;**82**(5):957-963

[31] Utzschneider KM, Bayer-Carter JL, Arbuckle MD, Tidwell JM, Richards TL, Craft S.
      Beneficial effect of a weight-stable, low-fat/low-saturated fat/low-glycaemic index diet to
      reduce liver fat in older subjects. The British Journal of Nutrition. 2013;**109**(6):1096-1104

[32] Eckel RH, Borra S, Lichtenstein AH, Yin-Piazza SY, Trans Fat Conference Planning
      Group. Understanding the complexity of trans fatty acid reduction in the American diet:
      American Heart Association trans fat conference 2006: Report of the trans fat conference
      planning group. Circulation. 2007;**115**(16):2231-2246

[33] Mensink RP, Zock PL, Kester AD, Katan MB. Effects of dietary fatty acids and carbo-
      hydrates on the ratio of serum total to HDL cholesterol and on serum lipids and apo-
      lipoproteins: A meta-analysis of 60 controlled trials. The American Journal of Clinical
      Nutrition. 2003;**77**(5):1146-1155

[34] Dhibi M, Brahmi F, Mnari A, et al. The intake of high fat diet with different trans fatty
      acid levels differentially induces oxidative stress and non alcoholic fatty liver disease
      (NAFLD) in rats. Nutrition & Metabolism (London). 2011;**8**(1):65

[35] Obara N, Fukushima K, Ueno Y, et al. Possible involvement and the mechanisms of excess trans-fatty acid consumption in severe NAFLD in mice. Journal of Hepatology. 2010;**53**(2):326-334

[36] Araya YN, Silvertown J, Gowing DJ, McConway KJ, Peter Linder H, Midgley G. A fundamental, eco-hydrological basis for niche segregation in plant communities. New Phytologist. 2011;**189**:253-258

[37] York LW, Puthalapattu S, Wu GY. Nonalcoholic fatty liver disease and low-carbohydrate diets. Annual Review of Nutrition. 2009;**29**:365-379

[38] Toshimitsu K, Matsuura B, Ohkubo I, et al. Dietary habits and nutrient intake in non-alcoholic steatohepatitis. Nutrition. 2007;**23**(1):46-52

[39] Garg A, Bantle JP, Henry RR, et al. Effects of varying carbohydrate content of diet in patients with non-insulin-dependent diabetes mellitus. Journal of the American Medical Association. 1994;**271**(18):1421-1428

[40] McLaughlin T, Abbasi F, Lamendola C, Yeni-Komshian H, Reaven G. Carbohydrate-induced hypertriglyceridemia: An insight into the link between plasma insulin and triglyceride concentrations. The Journal of Clinical Endocrinology and Metabolism. 2000;**85**(9):3085-3088

[41] Hudgins LC, Hellerstein M, Seidman C, Neese R, Diakun J, Hirsch J. Human fatty acid synthesis is stimulated by a eucaloric low fat, high carbohydrate diet. The Journal of Clinical Investigation. 1996;**97**(9):2081-2091

[42] Nomura K, Yamanouchi T. The role of fructose-enriched diets in mechanisms of nonalcoholic fatty liver disease. The Journal of Nutritional Biochemistry. 2012;**23**(3):203-208

[43] Alisi A, Manco M, Pezzullo M, Nobili V. Fructose at the center of necroinflammation and fibrosis in nonalcoholic steatohepatitis. Hepatology. 2011;**53**(1):372-373

[44] Lim JS, Mietus-Snyder M, Valente A, Schwarz JM, Lustig RH. The role of fructose in the pathogenesis of NAFLD and the metabolic syndrome. Nature Reviews. Gastroenterology & Hepatology. 2010;**7**(5):251-264

[45] Yilmaz Y. Review article: Fructose in non-alcoholic fatty liver disease. Alimentary Pharmacology & Therapeutics. 2012;**35**(10):1135-1144

[46] Huang D, Dhawan T, Young S, Yong WH, Boros LG, Heaney AP. Fructose impairs glucose-induced hepatic triglyceride synthesis. Lipids in Health and Disease. 2011;**10**:20

[47] Koo HY, Wallig MA, Chung BH, Nara TY, Cho BH, Nakamura MT. Dietary fructose induces a wide range of genes with distinct shift in carbohydrate and lipid metabolism in fed and fasted rat liver. Biochimica et Biophysica Acta. 2008;**1782**(5):341-348

[48] Teff KL, Elliott SS, Tschöp M, et al. Dietary fructose reduces circulating insulin and leptin, attenuates postprandial suppression of ghrelin, and increases triglycerides in women. The Journal of Clinical Endocrinology and Metabolism. 2004;**89**(6):2963-2972

[49] Stanhope KL, Havel PJ. Fructose consumption: Considerations for future research on its effects on adipose distribution, lipid metabolism, and insulin sensitivity in humans. The Journal of Nutrition. 2009;**139**(6):1236S-1241S

[50] Assy N, Nasser G, Kamayse I, et al. Soft drink consumption linked with fatty liver in the absence of traditional risk factors. Canadian Journal of Gastroenterology. 2008;**22**(10):811-816

[51] Abid A, Taha O, Nseir W, Farah R, Grosovski M, Assy N. Soft drink consumption is associated with fatty liver disease independent of metabolic syndrome. Journal of Hepatology. 2009;**51**(5):918-924

[52] Thuy S, Ladurner R, Volynets V, et al. Nonalcoholic fatty liver disease in humans is associated with increased plasma endotoxin and plasminogen activator inhibitor 1 concentrations and with fructose intake. The Journal of Nutrition. 2008;**138**(8):1452-1455

[53] Ouyang X, Cirillo P, Sautin Y, et al. Fructose consumption as a risk factor for non-alcoholic fatty liver disease. Journal of Hepatology. 2008;**48**(6):993-999

[54] Abdelmalek MF, Suzuki A, Guy C, et al. Increased fructose consumption is associated with fibrosis severity in patients with nonalcoholic fatty liver disease. Hepatology. 2010;**51**(6):1961-1971

[55] Zelber-Sagi S, Nitzan-Kaluski D, Goldsmith R, et al. Role of leisure-time physical activity in nonalcoholic fatty liver disease: A population-based study. Hepatology. 2008;**48**(6):1791-1798

[56] Krasnoff JB, Painter PL, Wallace JP, Bass NM, Merriman RB. Health-related fitness and physical activity in patients with nonalcoholic fatty liver disease. Hepatology. 2008;**47**(4):1158-1166

[57] Perseghin G, Lattuada G, De Cobelli F, et al. Habitual physical activity is associated with intrahepatic fat content in humans. Diabetes Care. 2007;**30**(3):683-688

[58] Booth FW, Laye MJ, Lees SJ, Rector RS, Thyfault JP. Reduced physical activity and risk of chronic disease: The biology behind the consequences. European Journal of Applied Physiology. 2008;**102**(4):381-390

[59] Helmerhorst HJ, Wijndaele K, Brage S, Wareham NJ, Ekelund U. Objectively measured sedentary time may predict insulin resistance independent of moderate- and vigorous-intensity physical activity. Diabetes. 2009;**58**(8):1776-1779

[60] Harrison SA, Fecht W, Brunt EM, Neuschwander-Tetri BA. Orlistat for overweight subjects with nonalcoholic steatohepatitis: A randomized, prospective trial. Hepatology. 2009;**49**(1):80-86

[61] Shah K, Stufflebam A, Hilton TN, Sinacore DR, Klein S, Villareal DT. Diet and exercise interventions reduce intrahepatic fat content and improve insulin sensitivity in obese older adults. Obesity (Silver Spring). 2009;**17**(12):2162-2168

[62] Promrat K, Kleiner DE, Niemeier HM, et al. Randomized controlled trial testing the effects of weight loss on nonalcoholic steatohepatitis. Hepatology. 2010;**51**(1):121-129

[63] Wong VW, Wong GL, Choi PC, et al. Disease progression of non-alcoholic fatty liver disease: A prospective study with paired liver biopsies at 3 years. Gut. 2010;**59**(7):969-974

[64] Westerbacka J, Lammi K, Häkkinen AM, et al. Dietary fat content modifies liver fat in overweight nondiabetic subjects. The Journal of Clinical Endocrinology and Metabolism. 2005;**90**(5):2804-2809

[65] Petersen KF, Dufour S, Befroy D, Lehrke M, Hendler RE, Shulman GI. Reversal of non-alcoholic hepatic steatosis, hepatic insulin resistance, and hyperglycemia by moderate weight reduction in patients with type 2 diabetes. Diabetes. 2005;**54**(3):603-608

[66] Cowin GJ, Jonsson JR, Bauer JD, et al. Magnetic resonance imaging and spectroscopy for monitoring liver steatosis. Journal of Magnetic Resonance Imaging. 2008;**28**(4):937-945

[67] Sjöström L, Lindroos AK, Peltonen M, et al. Lifestyle, diabetes, and cardiovascular risk factors 10 years after bariatric surgery. The New England Journal of Medicine. 2004;**351**(26):2683-2693

[68] Dixon JB, Bhathal PS, O'Brien PE. Weight loss and non-alcoholic fatty liver disease: Falls in gamma-glutamyl transferase concentrations are associated with histologic improvement. Obesity Surgery. 2006;**16**(10):1278-1286

[69] Silvestre V, Ruano M, Domínguez Y, et al. Morbid obesity and gastric bypass surgery: Biochemical profile. Obesity Surgery. 2004;**14**(9):1227-1232

[70] Stratopoulos C, Papakonstantinou A, Terzis I, et al. Changes in liver histology accompanying massive weight loss after gastroplasty for morbid obesity. Obesity Surgery. 2005;**15**(8):1154-1160

[71] Johansson HE, Haenni A, Ohrvall M, Sundbom M, Zethelius B. Alterations in proinsulin and insulin dynamics, HDL cholesterol and ALT after gastric bypass surgery. A 42-months follow-up study. Obesity Surgery. 2009;**19**(5):601-607

[72] Pontiroli AE, Pizzocri P, Librenti MC, et al. Laparoscopic adjustable gastric banding for the treatment of morbid (grade 3) obesity and its metabolic complications: A three-year study. The Journal of Clinical Endocrinology and Metabolism. 2002;**87**(8):3555-3561

[73] Burza MA, Romeo S, Kotronen A, et al. Long-term effect of bariatric surgery on liver enzymes in the Swedish obese subjects (SOS) study. PLoS One. 2013;**8**(3):e60495

[74] Hafeez S, Ahmed MH. Bariatric surgery as potential treatment for nonalcoholic fatty liver disease: A future treatment by choice or by chance? Journal of Obesity. 2013;**2013**:839275

[75] Mummadi RR, Kasturi KS, Chennareddygari S, Sood GK. Effect of bariatric surgery on nonalcoholic fatty liver disease: Systematic review and meta-analysis. Clinical Gastroenterology and Hepatology. 2008;**6**(12):1396-1402

[76] Estruch R, Ros E, Salas-Salvadó J, et al. Primary prevention of cardiovascular disease with a Mediterranean diet. The New England Journal of Medicine. 2013;368(14):1279-1290

[77] van Herpen NA, Schrauwen-Hinderling VB, Schaart G, Mensink RP, Schrauwen P. Three weeks on a high-fat diet increases intrahepatic lipid accumulation and decreases meta-bolic flexibility in healthy overweight men. The Journal of Clinical Endocrinology and Metabolism. 2011;96(4):E691-E695

[78] Gillingham LG, Harris-Janz S, Jones PJ. Dietary monounsaturated fatty acids are pro-tective against metabolic syndrome and cardiovascular disease risk factors. Lipids. 2011;46(3):209-228

[79] Alonso A, Ruiz-Gutierrez V, Martínez-González MA. Monounsaturated fatty acids, olive oil and blood pressure: Epidemiological, clinical and experimental evidence. Public Health Nutrition. 2006;9(2):251-257

[80] Ryan MC, Itsiopoulos C, Thodis T, et al. The Mediterranean diet improves hepatic steato-sis and insulin sensitivity in individuals with non-alcoholic fatty liver disease. Journal of Hepatology. 2013;59(1):138-143

[81] Bozzetto L, Prinster A, Annuzzi G, et al. Liver fat is reduced by an isoenergetic MUFA diet in a controlled randomized study in type 2 diabetic patients. Diabetes Care. 2012;35(7):1429-1435

[82] Mozaffarian D, Wu JH. Omega-3 fatty acids and cardiovascular disease: Effects on risk factors, molecular pathways, and clinical events. Journal of the American College of Cardiology. 2011;58(20):2047-2067

[83] Grimsgaard S, Bønaa KH, Hansen JB, Myhre ES. Effects of highly purified eicosapen-taenoic acid and docosahexaenoic acid on hemodynamics in humans. The American Journal of Clinical Nutrition. 1998;68(1):52-59

[84] Bucher HC, Hengstler P, Schindler C, Meier G. N-3 polyunsaturated fatty acids in cor-onary heart disease: A meta-analysis of randomized controlled trials. The American Journal of Medicine. 2002;112(4):298-304

[85] Ooi EM, Lichtenstein AH, Millar JS, et al. Effects of therapeutic lifestyle change diets high and low in dietary fish-derived FAs on lipoprotein metabolism in middle-aged and elderly subjects. Journal of Lipid Research. 2012;53(9):1958-1967

[86] Bjermo H, Iggman D, Kullberg J, et al. Effects of n-6 PUFAs compared with SFAs on liver fat, lipoproteins, and inflammation in abdominal obesity: A randomized controlled trial. The American Journal of Clinical Nutrition. 2012;95(5):1003-1012

[87] Khaw KT, Friesen MD, Riboli E, Luben R, Wareham N. Plasma phospholipid fatty acid concentration and incident coronary heart disease in men and women: The EPIC-Norfolk prospective study. PLoS Medicine. 2012;9(7):e1001255

[88]   Ooi EM, Ng TW, Watts GF, Barrett PH. Dietary fatty acids and lipoprotein metabolism: New insights and updates. Current Opinion in Lipidology. 2013;**24**(3):192-197

[89]   McLaughlin T, Carter S, Lamendola C, et al. Effects of moderate variations in macronutrient composition on weight loss and reduction in cardiovascular disease risk in obese, insulin-resistant adults. The American Journal of Clinical Nutrition. 2006;**84**(4):813-821

[90]   Foster GD, Wyatt HR, Hill JO, et al. A randomized trial of a low-carbohydrate diet for obesity. The New England Journal of Medicine. 2003;**348**(21):2082-2090

[91]   Ryan MC, Abbasi F, Lamendola C, Carter S, McLaughlin TL. Serum alanine aminotransferase levels decrease further with carbohydrate than fat restriction in insulin-resistant adults. Diabetes Care. 2007;**30**(5):1075-1080

[92]   Carter P, Khunti K, Davies MJ. Dietary recommendations for the prevention of type 2 diabetes: What are they based on? Journal of Nutrition and Metabolism. 2012;**2012**:847202

[93]   Kim J, Tanabe K, Yokoyama N, Zempo H, Kuno S. Association between physical activity and metabolic syndrome in middle-aged Japanese: A cross-sectional study. BMC Public Health. 2011;**11**:624

[94]   Johnson NA, George J. Fitness versus fatness: Moving beyond weight loss in nonalcoholic fatty liver disease. Hepatology. 2010;**52**(1):370-381

[95]   Carroll JF, Franks SF, Smith AB, Phelps DR. Visceral adipose tissue loss and insulin resistance 6 months after laparoscopic gastric banding surgery: A preliminary study. Obesity Surgery. 2009;**19**(1):47-55

[96]   Rector RS, Thyfault JP, Morris RT, et al. Daily exercise increases hepatic fatty acid oxidation and prevents steatosis in Otsuka long-Evans Tokushima fatty rats. American Journal of Physiology. Gastrointestinal and Liver Physiology. 2008;**294**(3):G619-G626

[97]   Mikus CR, Rector RS, Arce-Esquivel AA, et al. Daily physical activity enhances reactivity to insulin in skeletal muscle arterioles of hyperphagic Otsuka long-Evans Tokushima fatty rats. Journal of Applied Physiology. 2010;**109**(4):1203-1210

[98]   Shojaee-Moradie F, Baynes KC, Pentecost C, et al. Exercise training reduces fatty acid availability and improves the insulin sensitivity of glucose metabolism. Diabetologia. 2007;**50**(2):404-413

[99]   Johnson NA, Sachinwalla T, Walton DW, et al. Aerobic exercise training reduces hepatic and visceral lipids in obese individuals without weight loss. Hepatology. 2009;**50**(4):1105-1112

[100] van der Heijden GJ, Wang ZJ, Chu ZD, et al. A 12-week aerobic exercise program reduces hepatic fat accumulation and insulin resistance in obese, Hispanic adolescents. Obesity (Silver Spring). 2010;**18**(2):384-390

[101] Bonekamp S, Barone BB, Clark J, Stewart KJ. The effect of an exercise training intervention on hepatic steatosis. Hepatology. 2008;**48**(Suppl 1):806a

[102] Know your fats. American Heart Association website. http://www.heart.org/HEARTORG/
       Conditions/Cholesterol/PreventionTreatmentofHighCholesterol/Know-Your-Fats_
       UCM_305628_Article.jsp. [Accessed 06-06-2017]

[103] O'Donovan G, Kearney EM, Nevill AM, Woolf-May K, Bird SR. The effects of 24 weeks
       of moderate- or high-intensity exercise on insulin resistance. European Journal of
       Applied Physiology. 2005;**95**(5-6):522-528

[104] Kistler KD, Brunt EM, Clark JM, et al. Physical activity recommendations, exercise
       intensity, and histological severity of nonalcoholic fatty liver disease. The American
       Journal of Gastroenterology. 2011;**106**(3):460-468

[105] St George A, Bauman A, Johnston A, Farrell G, Chey T, George J. Independent effects
       of physical activity in patients with nonalcoholic fatty liver disease. Hepatology.
       2009;**50**(1):68-76

[106] Chen SM, Liu CY, Li SR, Huang HT, Tsai CY, Jou HJ. Effects of therapeutic lifestyle pro-
       gram on ultrasound-diagnosed nonalcoholic fatty liver disease. Journal of the Chinese
       Medical Association. 2008;**71**(11):551-558

[107] de Mello MT, de Piano A, Carnier J, et al. Long-term effects of aerobic plus resistance
       training on the metabolic syndrome and adiponectinemia in obese adolescents. Journal
       of Clinical Hypertension (Greenwich, Conn.). 2011;**13**(5):343-350

[108] de Piano A, de Mello MT, Sanches LP, et al. Long-term effects of aerobic plus resis-
       tance training on the adipokines and neuropeptides in nonalcoholic fatty liver dis-
       ease obese adolescents. European Journal of Gastroenterology and Hepatology.
       2012;**24**(11):1313-1324

[109] Hallsworth K et al. Resistance exercise reduces liver fat and its mediators in non-alco-
       holic fatty liver disease independent of weight loss. Gut. DOI: 10.1136/gut.2011.242073

[110] Hasegawa T, Yoneda M, et al. Plasma transforming growth factor-beta1 level and effi-
       cacy of alpha-tocopherol in patients with non-alcoholic steatohepatitis: A pilot study.
       Alimentary Pharmacology & Therapeutics. 2001;**15**:1667-1672

[111] Kugelmas M, Hill DB, Vivian B, Marsano L, CJ MC. Cytokines and NASH : A pilot
       study of the effects of lifestyle modification and vitamin E. Hepatology. 2003;**38**:413-419

[112] Sanyal AJ, Chalasini N, Kowdley KV, et al. Pioglitazone, vitamin E, or placebo for non-
       alcoholic steatohepatitis. New England Journal of Medicine. 2010;**362**:16751685. DOI:
       10.1056/NEJMoa0907929

[113] Arendt BM, Allard JP. Effect of atorvastatin, vitamin E and C on nonalcoholic fatty
       liver disease: is the combination required? The American Journal of Gastroenterology.
       2011;**106**:78-80

[114] Sesso HD, Cook NR, Buring JE, Manson JE, Gaziano JM. Alcohol consumption and
       the risk of hypertension in women and men. Hypertension. 2008;**51**:1080-1087. DOI:
       10.1161/HYPERTENSION AHA.107.104968

[115] Bjelakovic G, Nikolova D, Gluud LL, Simonetti RG, Gluud C. Antioxidant supplements for prevention of mortality in healthy participants and patients with various diseases. Cochrane Database of Systematic Reviews. 2012 Mar 14;**3**:CD007176. DOI: 10.1002/14651858.CD007176.pub2. Review

[116] Pittas AG, Harris SS, Stark PC, Dawson-Hughes B. The effects of calcium and vitamin D supplementation on blood glucose and markers of inflammation in non-diabetic adults. Diabetes Care. 2007;**30**:980-986

[117] Kendrick J, Targher G, Smits G, Chonchol M. 25-Hydroxyvitamin D deficiency is independently associated with cardiovascular disease in the third National Health and nutrition examination survey. Atherosclerosis. 2009;**205**:255-260

[118] Musso G, Anty R, Petta S. Antioxidant therapy and drugs interfering with lipid metabolism: could they be effective in NAFLD patients? Current Pharmaceutical Design. 2013;**19**:5297-5313

[119] Di Minno MN, Russolillo A, Lupoli R, Ambrosino P, Di Minno A, et al. Omega-3 fatty acids for the treatment of non-alcoholic fatty liver disease. World Journal of Gastroenterology. 2012;**18**:5839-5847

[120] Compare D, Coccoli P, Rocco A, Nardone OM, De Maria S, Cartenì M, et al. Gut–liver axis: The impact of gut microbiota on non-alcoholic fatty liver disease. Nutrition, Metabolism & Cardiovascular Diseases. 2012;**22**:471-476. DOI: 10.1016/j.numecd.2012.02.007

[121] Loguercio C, DeSimone T, Federico A, Terracciano F, Tuccillo C, DiChicco M, Carteni M. Gut-liver axis: A new point of attack to treat chronic liver damage? The American Journal of Gastroenterology. 2002;**97**:2144-2146

[122] Loguercio C, Federico A, Tuccillo C, Terracciano F, D'Auria MV, et al. Beneficial effects of a probiotic VSL#3 on parameters of liver dysfunction in chronic liver diseases. Journal of Clinical Gastroenterology. 2005;**39**:540-543

[123] Li X, Zhuo R, Tiong S, Di Cara F, King-Jones K, Hughes SC, Campbell SD, Wevrick R. The Smc5/Smc6/MAGE complex confers resistance to caffeine and genotoxic stress in Drosophila melanogaster. PLoS One. 2013;**8**(3):e59866

[124] Aller R, De Luis DA, Izaola O, Conde R, Gonzalez Sagrado M, Primo D, et al. Effect of a probiotic on liver aminotransferases in nonalcoholic fatty liver disease patients: A double blind randomized clinical trial. European Review for Medical and Pharmacological Sciences. 2011;**15**(9):1090e5

[125] Sahebkar A. Potential efficacy of ginger as a natural supplement for nonalcoholic fatty liver disease. World Journal of Gastroenterology. 2011 Jan 14;**17**(2):271-272. DOI: 10.3748/wjg.v17.i2.271

7

Neurocognitive Impairments and Depression and Their Relationship to Hepatitis C Virus Infection

Mihaela Fadgyas Stanculete

Abstract

The hepatitis C virus is a blood-borne virus with a direct cytopathic action. Chronic hepatitis C is a prevalent and costly disease. Studies have shown that it is a significant overlap between hepatitis C virus and mental disorders and that a substantial number of patients infected are suffering from mood disturbances and neurocognitive impairment. Recently, the neurocognitive impairments (attention, memory, and executive function alterations) were recognized as being independent of liver fibrosis and representing the direct effect of hepatitis C virus on neurons. However, until now impairments in neurocognition are not associated with viral replication or overall viral burden. Moreover, interferon alpha is still used to treat patients with hepatitis C. According to various researchers, 30–70% will develop significant psychiatric symptoms, leading to a premature discontinuation of therapy or noncompliance and worsening of quality of life. Several potential mechanisms may be implicated in the onset of a depressive episode following interferon alpha, the most important being the activation of immune-inflammatory pathways. This chapter will present the complex and striking relationships between hepatitis C virus infection and central nervous system symptoms. A variety of approaches, which integrate the extensive research data (including molecular, brain imaging, and neuropsychological findings), will be discussed.

Keywords: hepatitis C, cognitive impairments, psychiatry

1. Introduction

Hepatitis C virus (HCV) infects about 200 million people and is considered a public problem worldwide. Studies suggest that patients with HCV have a high burden of comorbidities such as psychiatric disorders, co-infection with hepatitis B and human immunodeficiency virus

(HIV), atherosclerosis, chronic kidney disease, mixed cryoglobulinemia, insulin resistance, and several cardiovascular diseases [1, 2]. The extrahepatic manifestation is secondary to HCV-related inflammatory responses and autoimmune reactions. According to a recent meta-analysis, the most frequent extrahepatic manifestation occurring in HCV-infected persons is depression, irrespective of alcohol and drug abuse or antiviral treatment [3].

The issue of a direct relationship between hepatitis C virus (HCV) infection and neuropsychiatric symptoms was raised for some years. Initially, the psychiatric and neurocognitive complaints were considered as the results of impairments in liver function. About 50% of the patients complain of chronic fatigue, deficits in attention, memory, learning, and depression [4–8].

Meanwhile, it has been shown that the reduction of global health-related quality of life (HRQoL) and development of psychiatric and neurocognitive impairments are not correlated with the level of hepatic alterations [9, 10].

Data point to an increasing evidence to support central nervous system (CNS) change in HCV patients. Several studies detected HCV in cerebrospinal fluid and brain. Further evidence was provided by studies using imaging techniques like magnetic resonance spectroscopy (MRS), positron emission tomography (PET), and single photon emission computed tomography (SPECT).

The mechanisms through which HCV entries and replicates in the brain are not fully elucidated yet, but evidences point to microstructural changes, and cerebral metabolite abnormalities [11–13].

Historically, the treatment of hepatitis C with interferon (IFN) was burdensome, complicated, and often was associated with neurocognitive abnormalities, depression, anxiety, and psychosis.

This chapter aims to analyze the current data about the relation between chronic HCV infection, depression, and neurocognitive impairments. Also, the effects of pharmacologic viral clearance on cognitive dysfunction and psychiatric features will be discussed.

2. Neurocognitive impairments and hepatitis C virus

The evidence of CNS infection is supported by the detection of replicative intermediate forms of HCV RNA and viral proteins within the CNS. Additional mechanisms, involved in neurological dysfunction, are possibly related to the consequence of circulating inflammatory cytokines and chemokines in the brain tissues through altered sites of the blood–brain barrier [14–17]. HCV ribonucleic acid (RNA) has been detected in peripheral blood mononuclear cells, cerebrospinal fluid (CSF), and the brain of chronically infected patients with neuropathological abnormalities. The majority of reports supporting HCV in the CNS have used PCR-based approaches to detect viral genomes in brain tissue and CSF. The presence of HCV in the brain was demonstrated using immunostaining and Western blot techniques. The presence of RNA negative strand intermediate is considered as a direct evidence of HCV replication. Until now, it is not clear which cells are involved. Some authors demonstrated that HCV infects microglia/macrophages, astrocytes, brain microvascular endothelial cells, neuroepithelioma cells, and neuroblastoma cells. More recent studies showed that CSF was found to be HCV positive in more than 50% of patients with HCV [18–23].

A variety of mechanisms have been hypothesized to explain the biological abnormalities in the brain:

a. direct infection of the brain,

b. chronic neuroinflammatory response,

c. indirect stimulation of neurotoxic cytokine pathways, and

d. toxicity mediated by vascular damage.

2.1. Neuroimaging studies

The imaging techniques that have been used to determine the biological abnormalities in HCV patients were: magnetic resonance spectroscopy, positron emission tomography, single photon computed tomography (SPECT), magnetic resonance-perfusion weighted imaging, and diffusion tensor imaging (DTI).

MRS provides noninvasive measures to evidence the metabolite abnormalities concentration in specific brain regions: myoinositol (mI), choline-containing compounds (Cho), creatine and phosphocreatine (Cr), glutathione, and N-acetyl aspartate (NAA). These metabolites are sensitive to changes in neuronal and glial state and density.

In general, metabolites are reported as a ratio to creatine. The evidence of neuroinflammation in HCV-positive patients is underlined by choline/creatine ratios. The choline-containing compound (Cho) peak is considered a marker for cell turnover and membrane metabolism. They were significantly higher in the basal ganglia (BG) and white matter of HCV positive patients. This data was associated with elevated myoinositol/creatine ratios (a marker of glial density). Myoinositol is a cerebral osmolyte and considered a marker for gliosis. Increases are thought to reflect microglial activation and are associated with CNS inflammation. Choline and myoinositol were significantly higher in the BG. N-acetyl aspartate (NAA) is considered a marker for neurons/axons. NAA and N-acetyl-glutamate were also significantly higher in BG.

Alterations in brain metabolism and neurotransmission are presented in **Table 1**.

In spite of the fact that the results vary greatly in the areas of the brain most affected, HCV positive patients with mild liver disease are characterized on MRS by higher mI (or mI/Cr), higher Cho (or Cho/Cr), and often lower NAA (or NAA/Cr). Those results are considered to represent the results of neuronal dysfunction and immune activation of microglia cells.

The main limitations of these studies are represented by:

• small study sizes,

• heterogeneity and varying selection of patients, and

• differences in data acquisition and data analysis.

Author	Year	Technique	Findings	Journal
Forton et al.	2001	MRS	Elevated choline/creatine (Cho/Cr) ratio in the basal ganglia and frontal white matter	Lancet [24]
Forton et al.	2002	MRS	Higher choline in basal ganglia, white matter	Hepatology [10]
Weissenborn et al	2004	MRS	Decrease of the N-acetyl-aspartate (NAA)/Cr ratio in the frontal gray matter	Journal of Hepatology [12]
			no changes of the Cho/Cr ratio	
Bokemeyer et al.	2011	MRS	Increased Cho and myoinositol concentrations in basal ganglia and white matter	Gut [25]
			Increased Cr, NAA, and N-acetyl-aspartyl-glutamate in basal ganglia	
Nagarajan et al.	2012	Localized two-dimensional correlated spectroscopy (L-COSY)	Increased myoinositol and glutathione	International Journal of Hepatology [26]

Table 1. Neuroimaging findings.

Diffusion tensor imaging (DTI) is a technique of magnetic resonance imaging that provides metrics for the speed and direction of water diffusion along the white matter tracts in the brain. DTI is a sensible method for detecting microscopic differences in tissue properties. The common DTI measures are mean diffusivity (MD), fractional anisotropy (FA), radial diffusivity (Dr), and axial diffusivity (Da). Mean diffusivity (MD) is an averaged measure of speed of diffusion in the three main directions. Fractional anisotropy (FA) measures the degree to which diffusion is faster in one direction than others. FA is used to highlight the microstructural changes, but it seems to be not very specific to the type of changes. Reductions in FA and elevations in MD seem to indicate impaired white matter integrity. Microglial state is also assessed using the positron emission tomography (PET) ligand PK11195, which binds to the mitochondrial membrane translocator protein (TPSO) present in endothelial, astroglial, and microglial cells. It is considered a marker for microglial activation. The most important neuroimaging findings are presented in **Table 2**.

2.2. Cognitive impairments

Approximately more than 50% of patients with chronic HCV infection complain of:

- poor memory,
- impaired attention, and
- fatigue.

Despite its potential clinical significance, cognitive impairments are often missed in patients evaluated for HCV, unless the manifestations are overt or interfere with the functionality, leading to impairments in health-related quality of life. When the symptomatology is very

Author	Year	Technique	Findings	Journal
Bladowska et al.	2013	DTI	Decreased FA in all white matter areas measured	Journal of Hepatology [27]
Thames et al.	2015	DTI	Increased FA in striatum, thalamus, and insula	Neurology Neuroimmunology Neuroinflammation [28]
Grover VPB	2012	PET	Significantly higher binding potential in all subcortical areas assessed (caudate, thalamus, pallidum) but in no cortical areas	Journal of Viral Hepatitis [29]
Pflugrad et al.	2016	PET	No differences between patients with mild HCV and healthy controls	Journal of Viral Hepatitis [30]

Table 2. Neuroimaging findings in HCV patients.

severe, the patients could present word finding difficulties, anomia, and significant deficits in attention performance. In general, constructional abilities and nonverbal recall are intact in these patients. Many studies suggest that approximately 30% of patients with chronic HCV exhibit cognitive dysfunctions even in the absence of cirrhosis. It seems that the cognitive performances are unrelated to viral load or viral genotype. The imaging studies showed significant reduction in striatal and midbrain dopamine availability and reduced metabolism in limbic, frontal, parietal, and temporal cortices. Thus, a crucial role of impaired dopaminergic transmission in causing cognitive impairment in HCV-infected patients was suggested. Moreover, pathologic cerebral serotonin and dopamine transporter binding were observed.

Emerging lines of evidence suggest that the profile of neuropsychological dysfunction in HCV-infected patients is characterized by impairment in:

a. executive function,

b. sustained attention,

c. working memory, and

d. verbal learning and verbal recall.

Several cognitive impairments demonstrated in patient with HCV are presented in **Table 3**.

Author	Year	Domains	Journal
Weissenborn et al.	2004	Impaired executive function	Journal of Hepatology [31]
Karaivazoglou et al.	2007	Impairment of verbal learning and memory	Liver international [32]
Fontana et al.	2007	Impairment in verbal recall and working memory	Hepatology [33]
Lowry et al.	2010	Alterations in memory, sustained attention, and delayed auditory recognition	Journal of Viral Hepatitis [34]
Ibrahim et al.	2016	Worse performance in nonverbal reasoning, attention, spatial orientation, age identification, and working memory	Journal of Clinical and Experimental Neuropsychology [35]

Table 3. Summary of major cognitive dysfunctions observed in patients with chronic hepatitis C virus infection.

There is evidence that cognitive dysfunctions in HCV patients have some impact in the reduction of health-related quality of life, chronic fatigue, and impaired functionality. The literature demonstrates evidence of neurocognitive impairment in patients with chronic HCV infection. However, until now, it is not clear that these dysfunctions can be linked, wholly or in part, to the virus itself. The longitudinal evaluation of the cognitive functioning could provide valuable information regarding the persistence of symptoms after the clearance of virus in the periphery.

3. Depression and hepatitis C virus

Depression has long been recognized and associated with many chronic medical conditions. The occurrence of depression is higher in patients with chronic liver disease than that in the general population. The depression is a very common psychiatric comorbidity in HCV patients. The link between HCV and depression has been the focus of many investigations. Several studies have reported variability in the prevalence of depression among the HCV population. The prevalence of depression in HCV patients has been estimated to be 1.5–4 times higher than in general population. Moreover, the prevalence rate seems to be unrelated to liver disease severity and interferon treatment. However, psychiatric comorbidities are usually underdiagnosed or overlooked when patients seek primary care, even though depression affects overall disease progression in the HCV-infected population [36–40].

Understanding the depressive disorder comorbid with HCV may be critical for developing effective intervention strategies. Most patients with depression will suffer noticeable changes in social and physical activities, a loss of interest in work or leisure activities, or poor academic performance. Another important issue is that HCV infection is often associated with behaviors that are condemned by society (e.g., drug use, alcoholism, and high-risk sexual behaviors), promoting prejudice, discrimination, and abuse against patients. Also, these maladaptive behaviors could further exacerbate the depression.

The high prevalence of psychiatric comorbidities in HCV-infected patients has been typically associated with direct effects of the virus on the central nervous system or adverse effects of hepatitis C treatment. The high prevalence of psychiatric comorbidities in HCV-infected patients has been typically associated with direct effects of the virus on the central nervous system or adverse effects of hepatitis C treatment.

The comorbid depression in HCV patients could be:

a. depression that may be pre-existent,

b. a reactive depression to the diagnosis of HCV,

c. a biological effect of HCV infection, or

d. an α-interferon-induced depression.

Both biological and psychosocial factors are important considerations for the effective clinical management of HCV and the prevention of HCV disease progression.

3.1. Psychosocial factors involved in development of depression

It is very important to distinguish between psychological reactions to the knowledge that one has been infected with HCV and the direct effects of the virus itself. Learning that one has contracted HCV infection represents a significant life stressor and will produce emotional stress in most patients, and psychiatric disorder in many. The psychological reasons for the development of depression are illustrated in **Table 4**. The psychosocial factors involved in the development of depression are illustrated in **Table 4**.

Stigma negatively affects the HRQOL, mental health, and social life of the patients, and leads to difficulties with receiving or accepting treatment. Poor social and work adjustment, lower acceptance of the illness, and higher subjective complaints are other problems associated with stigmatization. Researches showed that women generally are prone to experience more stigmatization. The social stigma may cause some HCV individuals to refuse to disclose their HCV diagnosis. Furthermore, HCV-related stigma is an important stressor that leads to poor treatment adherence. In some cases, HCV-infected individuals tend to isolate themselves to prevent stigma-related negative attitudes. Low income is also a socio-demographic factor significantly associated with the appearance of depressive symptoms [41–46].

The most commonly used coping styles by HCV patients are:

- problem-solving behavior,
- distraction and self-revalorization,
- religiousness and search for meaning,
- cognitive avoidance and dissimulation, and
- depressive coping.

Illness perception
Risk of cirrhosis/cancer and other health-related worries
Fear of transmitting the disease
Concerns about the complications of disease/treatment
Functional disability
Impaired quality of life
Fatigue severity
Personality disorders
Low income
Social stigma
Coping styles
Social support

Table 4. Psychosocial factors associated with the development of depression in HCV patients.

Several studies have reported using inappropriate coping strategies in patients with HCV, which may negatively affect several aspects of their management.

Psychosocial interventions that include cognitive, behavioral and lifestyle strategies may influence the negative impact of HCV symptoms and treatment side effects on HRQOL.

3.2. Biological factors

Biological factors appear to play a significant role as well. Major depressive disorder is associated with the increased production of pro-inflammatory cytokines, such as interleukin-1 (IL-1), IL-6, and interferon gamma (IFN-γ). Chronic HCV infection is also known to increase inflammatory cytokines like IL-1, IL-6, and tumor necrosis factor alpha (TNF-α). The inflammatory model of depression provides a possible link between the HCV infection and major depressive disorder. An increased macrophage migration inhibitory factor was also demonstrated in patients with major depression. Elevated pro-inflammatory cytokines have been found in patients with anxiety and depression symptoms and pharmacological agents who specifically inhibit inflammatory mediators seem to determine a reduction in depression and anxiety symptoms. The rise in cytokine levels is associated with fatigue, malaise, lethargy, and depression. Another effect of pro-inflammatory cytokines is the activation of the hypothalamic–pituitary–adrenal (HPA) axis, which represents the regulator of the stress response.

Many studies suggest that the activation of HPA pathways can modify monoamine expression in the CNS, and as a consequence, leading to symptoms of depression. It was demonstrated that the neurochemical imbalance of serotonin (5-HT), norepinephrine (NE), and dopamine (DA) is linked to the development of depression. Studies in HCV-infected patients demonstrate impaired levels of dopamine and serotonin among distinct brain regions.

Many studies suggest that the activation of HPA pathways can modify monoamine expression in the CNS, and as consequence, leading to symptoms of depression. It was demonstrated that the neurochemical imbalance of serotonin (5-HT), norepinephrine (NE), and dopamine (DA) is linked to the development of depression. Studies in HCV-infected patients demonstrate impaired levels of dopamine and serotonin among distinct brain regions [47–50].

IFN-α-induced depression may increase suicidality, impair quality of life, increase, and lead to noncompliance or even treatment withdrawal among patients with chronic HCV infection. Following IFN treatment of patients with HCV, up to 70% may develop depression. Several mechanisms have been proposed:

a. altered monoamine metabolism,

b. altered hypothalamus–pituitary–adrenal axis function,

c. increased rate of apoptosis, and

d. brain-derived neurotrophic factor (BDNF) reduction.

The predictors of development of depression during antiviral treatment are:

1. history of depressive disorder,

2. sub-threshold depressive symptoms,

3. female gender,

4. low educational level, and

5. high baseline serum interleukin 6 (IL6) concentrations.

Specific risk factors for IFN-induced suicide are still unknown.

Standard treatment for CHC was for a period a combination of pegylated interferon (pegIFN) and ribavirin (RBV), which was known to exacerbate fatigue and depressive symptoms. Interferon-based regimens are related to complicated dosing schedules, weekly administration of subcutaneous injections, and many side effects. Interferon alpha combined with ribavirin has been shown to be more effective than interferon alone on obtaining sustained virologic response. Moreover, it seems that SVR achieved with PEG-IFN-α and RBV combination therapy is durable over time [51].

Until now, we do not have sufficient data whether or not the cognitive impairments are irreversible in patients who have eliminated HCV after successful treatment. A study performed by Byrnes et al. concluded that HCV eradication was associated with an improvement in memory (visual and spatial) and verbal learning [52]. Another survey of 168 HCV patients receiving antiviral therapy with interferon and ribavirin evaluated 12 months after the termination of antiviral treatment concluded that in patients with a sustained viral response a significant improvement was observed in three out five cognitive domains (working memory, vigilance, and shared attention) [53, 54].

3.3. Direct-acting antivirals

Approval of direct-acting antivirals (DAA) against the hepatitis C virus has dramatically changed the management of HCV infection due to high cure rates and a favorable safety profile. It was reported that DAA in certain combinations are curing HCV infection in almost 100% of cases [55]. DAA are taken once-daily in oral combinations. Treatment duration has also been shortened considerably in comparison with interferon therapies, making treatment regimens more tolerable. Patient-reported outcomes (PROs) provide the patient's perspective on the physical, functional, and psychological consequences of treatment and the degree and impact of disease symptoms. Recent regimens are interferon-free, and in many cases, RBV-free, and involve a combination of DAA agents. Many studies showed a consistent improvement in the quality of life, fatigue, and work productivity during treatment in patients receiving IFN and RBV-free strategy. Newly approved oral anti-HCV drugs are very safe and effective, but unfortunately, they are very costly. DAAs do not seem to increase the neuropsychiatric risks to patients undergoing HCV triple therapy [56–60].

In the absence of the neurocognitive side effects of interferon, it should be expected a significant improvement in neurocognitive functioning if, as suggested, the impairments are directly attributable to HCV action on CNS.

3.4. Treatment of depression

Several studies have specifically investigated the treatment of depression in HCV patients. The literature suggests that depression, anxiety symptoms, and cognitive complaints are responsive to selective serotonin reuptake inhibitors (SSRIs) antidepressants. However, the neurovegetative symptoms seem to be less sensitive to SSRIs. Some evidence suggests that dual antidepressants neurovegetative symptoms can be better influenced with serotonin-norepinephrine reuptake inhibitors (SNRIs). Although the data are not strong, it does appear that SSRIs might be the first choice for the treatment of interferon-induced MDD and citalopram is recommended as first-line treatment for IFN-induced depression. Antidepressant medication should be continued for at least 12 weeks following the end of IFN treatment. Antidepressant therapy is also indicated for those patients with baseline depressive symptoms and those with a history of IFN-induced depression. Data showed that antidepressant pre-treatment with SSRIs lowers the incidence and severity of IFN-associated depression in patients with chronic hepatitis C infection. But we need to keep in mind that antidepressants are not recommended for all HCV patients, and the indication should be tailored to each patient [54, 61–65].

4. Conclusions

HCV infection causes multiple provocations to practitioners due to nontreatment and especially treatment-related psychiatric comorbidities. The evidence reviewed in this chapter strongly suggests that HCV patients should be carefully monitored for psychiatric side effects of treatment. The psychiatric comorbidities along with the cognitive dysfunctions affect the patient's care significantly and might influence the course of the disease. The mechanisms involved remain mainly not sufficiently understood. Psychological adjustment to illness is determined by a complex interaction of many factors. Psychosocial factors appear to be of significance, particularly concerning the coping mechanisms and perceived stigma. In the long run, the goal is to offer a multidisciplinary approach for optimal medical and psychosocial management of patients with HCV.

Author details

Mihaela Fadgyas Stanculete

Address all correspondence to: mihaelastanculete@yahoo.com

Department of Neurosciences, Psychiatry, Iuliu Hatieganu University of Medicine and Pharmacy, Cluj Napoca, Romania

References

[1] Louie KS, St Laurent S, Forssen UM, Mundy LM, Pimenta JM. The high comorbidity burden of the hepatitis C virus infected population in the United States. BMC Infectious Diseases. 2012;**12**:86. DOI: 10.1186/1471-2334-12-86

[2] Ferri C, Ramos-Casals M, Zignego AL, Arcaini L, Roccatello D, Antonelli A, Saadoun D, Desbois AC, Sebastiani M, Casato M, Lamprecht P. International diagnostic guidelines for patients with HCV-related extrahepatic manifestations. A multidisciplinary expert statement. Autoimmunity Reviews. 2016;**15**(12):1145-1160. DOI: 10.1016/j.autrev.2016.09.006

[3] Younossi Z, Park H, Henry L, Adeyemi A, Stepanova M. Extrahepatic manifestations of hepatitis C: A meta-analysis of prevalence, quality of life, and economic burden. Gastroenterology. 2016;**150**(7):1599-1608. DOI: 10.1053/j.gastro.2016.02.039

[4] Gill K, Ghazinian H, Manch R, Gish R. Hepatitis C virus as a systemic disease: Reaching beyond the liver. Hepatology International. 2016;**10**(3):415-423. DOI: 10.1007/s12072-015-9684-3

[5] McAndrews MP, Farcnik K, Carlen P, Damyanovich A, Mrkonjic M, Jones S, Heathcote EJ. Prevalence and significance of neurocognitive dysfunction in hepatitis C in the absence of correlated risk factors. Hepatology. 2005;**41**(4):801-808

[6] Mathew S, Faheem M, Ibrahim SM, et al. Hepatitis C virus and neurological damage. World Journal of Hepatology. 2016;**8**:545-556. DOI: 10.4254/wjh.v8.i12.545

[7] Adinolfi LE, Nevola R, Lus G, Restivo L, Guerrera B, Romano C, Zampino R, Rinaldi L, Sellitto A, Giordano M, Marrone A. Chronic hepatitis C virus infection and neurological and psychiatric disorders: An overview. World Journal of Gastroenterology: WJG. 2015;**21**(8):2269. DOI: 10.3748/wjg.v21.i8.2269

[8] Yarlott L, Heald E, Forton D. Hepatitis C virus infection, and neurological and psychiatric disorders–a review. Journal of Advanced Research. 2017;**8**(2):139-148. DOI: 10.1016/j.jare.2016.09.005

[9] Weinstein AA, Price JK, Stepanova M, Poms LW, Fang Y, Moon J, Nader F, Younossi ZM. Depression in patients with nonalcoholic fatty liver disease and chronic viral hepatitis B and C. Psychosomatics. 2011;**52**(2):127-132 doi.org/10.1016/j.psym.2010.12.019

[10] Forton DM, Thomas HC, Murphy CA, Allsop JM, Foster GR, Main J, Wesnes KA, Taylor-Robinson SD. Hepatitis C and cognitive impairment in a cohort of patients with mild liver disease. Hepatology. 2002;**35**:433-439. DOI: 10.1053/jhep.2002.30688

[11] Forton DM, Hamilton G, Allsop JM, Grover VP, Wesnes K, O'Sullivan C, Thomas HC, Taylor-Robinson SD. Cerebral immune activation in chronic hepatitis C infection: A magnetic resonance spectroscopy study. Journal of Hepatology. 2008;**49**(3):316-322. DOI: 10.1016/j.jhep.2008.03.022

[12] Weissenborn K, Krause J, Bokemeyer M, Hecker H, Schüler A, Ennen JC, Ahl B, Manns MP, Böker KW. Hepatitis C virus infection affects the brain—Evidence from psychometric studies and magnetic resonance spectroscopy. Journal of Hepatology. 2004;**41**(5):845-851. DOI: 10.1016/j.jhep.2004.07.022

[13] Vargas HE, Laskus T, Radkowski M, Wilkinson J, Balan V, Douglas DD, Harrison ME, Mulligan DC, Olden K, Adair D, Rakela J. Detection of hepatitis C virus sequences in brain tissue obtained in recurrent hepatitis C after liver transplantation. Liver Transplantation. 2002;**8**(11):1014-1019. DOI: 10.1053/jlts.2002.36393

[14] Revie D, Salahuddin SZ. Human cell types important for hepatitis C virus replication in vivo and in vitro: Old assertions and current evidence. Virology Journal. 2011;**8**:346. DOI: 10.1186/1743-422X-8-346

[15] Monaco S, Ferrari S, Gajofatto A, Zanusso G, Mariotto S. HCV-related nervous system disorders. Clinical & Developmental Immunology. 2012;**2012**:236148. DOI: 10.1155/2012/236148

[16] Fletcher NF, McKeating JA. Hepatitis C virus and the brain. Journal of Viral Hepatitis. 2012;**19**:301-306. DOI: 10.1111/j.1365-2893.2012.01591.x

[17] Fletcher NF, Wilson GK, Murray J, Hu K, Lewis A, Reynolds GM, Stamataki Z, Meredith LW, Rowe IA, Luo G, MA L–R. Hepatitis C virus infects the endothelial cells of the blood-brain barrier. Gastroenterology. 2012 Mar 31;**142**(3):634-643. DOI: 10.1053/j.gastro.2011.11.028

[18] Tully DC, Hjerrild S, Leutscher PD, Renvillard SG, Ogilvie CB, Bean DJ, Videbech P, Allen TM, McKeating JA, Fletcher NF. Deep sequencing of hepatitis C virus reveals genetic compartmentalization in cerebrospinal fluid from cognitively impaired patients. Liver International. 2016 Oct 1;**36**(10):1418-1424. DOI: 10.1111/liv.13134

[19] Martindale SL, Hurley RA, Taber KH. Neurobiology and neuroimaging of chronic hepatitis C virus: Implications for neuropsychiatry. The Journal of Neuropsychiatry and Clinical Neurosciences. 2017 Sep 29;**29**(4):A6-307. DOI: 10.1176/appi.neuropsych.17080163

[20] Da Costa D, Turek M, Felmlee DJ, Girardi E, Pfeffer S, Long G, Bartenschlager R, Zeisel MB, Baumert TF. Reconstitution of the entire hepatitis C virus life cycle in non-hepatic cells. Journal of Virology. 2012;**JVI-01066**. DOI: 10.1128/JVI.01066-12

[21] Fukuhara T, Matsuura Y. Role of miR-122 and lipid metabolism in HCV infection. Journal of Gastroenterology. 2013;**48**(2):169-176. DOI: 10.1007/s00535-012-0661-5

[22] Schaefer M, Capuron L, Friebe A, Diez-Quevedo C, Robaeys G, Neri S, Foster GR, Kautz A, Forton D, Pariante CM. Hepatitis C infection, antiviral treatment and mental health: A European expert consensus statement. Journal of Hepatology. 2012 Dec 31;**57**(6):1379-1390. DOI: 10.1016/j.jhep.2012.07.037

[23] Wilkinson J, Radkowski M, Eschbacher JM, Laskus T. Activation of brain macrophages/microglia cells in hepatitis C infection. Gut. 2010;**59**(10):1394-1400. DOI: 10.1136/gut.2009.199356

[24] Forton DM, Allsop JM, Main J, Foster GR, Thomas HC, Taylor-Robinson SD. Evidence for a cerebral effect of the hepatitis C virus. Lancet. 2001 Jul 7;**358**(9275):38-39. DOI: 10.1016/S0140-6736(00)05270-3

[25] Bokemeyer M, Ding XQ, Goldbecker A, Raab P, Heeren M, Arvanitis D, Tillmann HL, Lanfermann H, Weissenborn K. Evidence for neuroinflammation and neuroprotection in HCV infection-associated encephalopathy. Gut. Mar 2011;**60**(3):370-377. DOI: 10.1136/gut.2010.217976

[26] R N, Sarma MK, Thames AD, Castellon SA, Hinkin CH, Thomas MA. 2D MR spectroscopy combined with prior-knowledge fitting is sensitive to HCV-associated cerebral metabolic abnormalities. International Journal of Hepatology. 2012;**2012**:179365. DOI: 10.1155/2012/179365

[27] Bladowska J, Zimny A, Knysz B, Małyszczak K, Kołtowska A, Szewczyk P, Gąsiorowski J, Furdal M, Sąsiadek MJ. Evaluation of early cerebral metabolic, perfusion and microstructural changes in HCV-positive patients: A pilot study. Journal of Hepatology. Oct 2013;**59**(4):651-657. DOI: 10.1016/j.jhep.2013.05.008

[28] Thames AD, Castellon SA, Singer EJ, Nagarajan R, Sarma MK, Smith J, Thaler NS, Truong JH, Schonfeld D, Thomas MA, Hinkin CH. Neuroimaging abnormalities, neurocognitive function, and fatigue in patients with hepatitis C. Neurology Neuroimmunology and Neuroinflammation. 2015 Jan 14;**2**(1):e59. DOI: 10.1212/NXI.0000000000000059

[29] VP G, Pavese N, Koh SB, Wylezinska M, Saxby BK, Gerhard A, Forton DM, Brooks DJ, Thomas HC, Taylor-Robinson SD. Cerebral microglial activation in patients with hepatitis C: In vivo evidence of neuroinflammation. Journal of Viral Hepatitis. Feb 2012; **19**(2):e89-e96. DOI: 10.1111/j.1365-2893.2011.01510.x

[30] Pflugrad H, Meyer GJ, Dirks M, Raab P, Tryc AB, Goldbecker A, Worthmann H, Wilke F, Boellaard R, Yaqub M, Berding G, Weissenborn K. Cerebral microglia activation in hepatitis C virus infection correlates to cognitive dysfunction. Journal of Viral Hepatitis. May 2016;**23**(5):348-357. DOI: 10.1111/jvh.12496

[31] Weissenborn K, Krause J, Bokemeyer M, Hecker H, Schüler A, Ennen JC, Ahl B, Manns MP, Böker KW. Hepatitis C virus infection affects the brain-evidence from psychometric studies and magnetic resonance spectroscopy. Journal of Hepatology. Nov 2004; **41**(5):845-851

[32] Karaivazoglou K, Assimakopoulos K, Thomopoulos K, Theocharis G, Messinis L, Sakellaropoulos G, Labropoulou-Karatza C. Neuropsychological function in Greek patients with chronic hepatitis C. Liver International. Aug 2007;**27**(6):798-805

[33] Fontana RJ, Bieliauskas LA, Lindsay KL, Back-Madruga C, Wright EC, Snow KK, Lok AS, Kronfol Z, Padmanabhan L. HALT-C trial group. Cognitive function does not worsen during pegylated interferon and ribavirin retreatment of chronic hepatitis C. Hepatology. 2007;**45**(5):1154-1163

[34] Lowry D, Coughlan B, McCarthy O, Crowe J. Investigating health-related quality of life, mood and neuropsychological test performance in a homogeneous cohort of Irish

female hepatitis C patients. Journal of Viral Hepatitis. May 2010;**17**(5):352-359. DOI: 10.1111/j.1365-2893.2009.01188.x

[35] Ibrahim I, Salah H, El Sayed H, Mansour H, Eissa A, Wood J, Fathi W, Tobar S, Gur RC, Gur RE, Dickerson F, Yolken RH, El Bahaey W, Nimgaonkar V. Hepatitis C virus antibody titers associated with cognitive dysfunction in an asymptomatic community-based sample. Journal of Clinical and Experimental Neuropsychology. Oct 2016;**38**(8):861-868. DOI: 10.1080/13803395.2016.1168780

[36] Oxenkrug G, Turski W, Zgrajka W, Weinstock J, Ruthazer R, Summergrad P. Disturbances of tryptophan metabolism and risk of depression in HCV patients treated with IFN-alpha. Journal of Infectious Disease and Therapy. 2014;**2**(2)

[37] Kanwal F, Pyne JM, Tavakoli-Tabasi S, Nicholson S, Dieckgraefe B, Storay E, Goetz MB, Kramer JR, Smith D, Sansgiry S, Tansel A, Gifford AL, Asch SM. A randomized trial of off-site collaborative care for depression in chronic hepatitis C virus. Health Services Research. 2017 Sep 11. DOI: 10.1111/1475-6773.12758

[38] Adinolfi LE, Nevola R, Rinaldi L, Romano C, Giordano M. Chronic hepatitis C virus infection and depression. Clinics in Liver Disease. Aug 2017;**21**(3):517-534. DOI: 10.1016/j.cld.2017.03.007

[39] Machado MO, Oriolo G, Bortolato B, Köhler CA, Maes M, Solmi M, Grande I, Martín-Santos R, Vieta E, Biological CAF. Mechanisms of depression following treatment with interferon for chronic hepatitis C: A critical systematic review. Journal of Affective Disorders. 2016 Nov 27. DOI: 10.1016/j.jad.2016.11.039

[40] Mahajan S, Avasthi A, Grover S, Chawla YK. Role of baseline depressive symptoms in the development of depressive episode in patients receiving antiviral therapy for hepatitis C infection. Journal of Psychosomatic Research. Aug 2014;**77**(2):109-115. DOI: 10.1016/j.jpsychores.2014.05.008

[41] Rogal SS, McCarthy R, Reid A, Rodriguez KL, Calgaro L, Patel K, Daley M, Jonassaint NL, Zickmund SL. Primary care and Hepatology provider-perceived barriers to and facilitators of hepatitis C treatment candidacy and adherence. Digestive Diseases and Sciences. Aug 2017;**62**(8):1933-1943. DOI: 10.1007/s10620-017-4608-9

[42] Schwarzinger M, Baillot S, Yazdanpanah Y, Rehm J, Mallet V. Contribution of alcohol use disorders on the burden of chronic hepatitis C in France, 2008-2013: A nationwide retrospective cohort study. Journal of Hepatology. Sep 2017;**67**(3):454-461. DOI: 10.1016/j.jhep.2017.03.031

[43] Sublette VA, Smith SK, George J, McCaffery K, Douglas MW. The hepatitis C treatment experience: Patients' perceptions of the facilitators of and barriers to uptake, adherence and completion. Psychology & Health. 2015;**30**(8):987-1004. DOI: 10.1080/08870446.2015.1012195

[44] Evon DM, Golin CE, Bonner JE, Grodensky C, Velloza J. Adherence during antiviral treatment regimens for chronic hepatitis C: A qualitative study of patient-reported

facilitators and barriers. Journal of Clinical Gastroenterology. 2015 May-Jun;**49**(5):e41-e50. DOI: 10.1097/MCG.0000000000000151

[45] Cho HJ, Park E. Illness experience of patients with chronic hepatitis C participating in clinical trials. Osong Public Health and Research Perspectives. 2016;**7**(6):394-399. DOI: 10.1016/j.phrp.2016.11.001

[46] Raison CL, Demetrashvili M, Capuron L, Neuropsychiatric MAH. Adverse effects of interferon-alpha: Recognition and management. CNS Drugs. 2005;**19**(2):105-123

[47] Pinto EF, Andrade C. Interferon-related depression: A primer on mechanisms, treatment, and prevention of a common clinical problem. Current Neuropharmacology. 2016; **14**(7):743-748

[48] Keefe B. Interferon-induced depression in hepatitis C: An update. Current Psychiatry Reports. Jun 2007;**9**(3):255-261

[49] Al-Omari A, Cowan J, Turner L, Cooper C. Antidepressant prophylaxis reduces depression risk but does not improve sustained virological response in hepatitis C interferon recipients without depression at baseline: A systematic review and meta-analysis. Canadian Journal of Gastroenterology. Oct 2013;**27**(10):575-581

[50] Sarkar S, Schaefer M. Antidepressant pretreatment for the prevention of interferon alfa-associated depression: A systematic review and meta-analysis. Psychosomatics. 2014; **55**(3):221-234. DOI: 10.1016/j.psym.2013.06.015

[51] Wang X, Gao F, Yuan G, Shi K, Huang Y, Chen Y, Qiu R, Sun L, Liu J, Hu C, Zhou Y. Ten-year follow-up analysis of chronic hepatitis C patients after getting sustained virological response to pegylated interferon-α and ribavirin therapy. Journal of Viral Hepatitis. 2016;**23**(12):971-976. DOI: 10.1111/jvh.12574

[52] Byrnes V, Miller A, Lowry D, Hill E, Weinstein C, Alsop D, Lenkinski R, Afdhal NH. Effects of anti-viral therapy and HCV clearance on cerebral metabolism and cognition. Journal of Hepatology. 2012;**56**(3):549-556. DOI: 10.1016/j.jhep.2011.09.015

[53] Kraus MR, Schäfer A, Teuber G, Porst H, Sprinzl K, Wollschläger S, Keicher C, Scheurlen M. Improvement of neurocognitive function in responders to an antiviral therapy for chronic hepatitis C. Hepatology. 2013;**58**(2):497-504. DOI: 10.1002/hep.26229

[54] Udina M, Hidalgo D, Navinés R, Forns X, Solà R, Farré M, Capuron L, Vieta E, Martín-Santos R. Prophylactic antidepressant treatment of interferon-induced depression in chronic hepatitis C: A systematic review and meta-analysis. The Journal of Clinical Psychiatry. Oct 2014;**75**(10):e1113-e1121. DOI: 10.4088/JCP.13r08800

[55] Saxena V, Koraishy FM, Sise M, Lim JK, Chung RT, Liapakis A, Nelson DR, Schmidt M, Fried MW, Terrault N. LP08: Safety and efficacy of sofosbuvir-containing regimens in hepatitis C infected patients with reduced renal function: Real-world experience from HCV-target. Journal of Hepatology. 2015;**62**:S267. DOI: 10.1111/liv.13102

[56] Flisiak R, Pogorzelska J, Flisiak-Jackiewicz M. Hepatitis C: Efficacy and safety in real life. Liver International. 2017;**37**(S1):26-32. DOI: 10.1111/liv.13293

[57] Younossi Z, Henry L. Systematic review: Patient-reported outcomes in chronic hepatitis C-the impact of liver disease and new treatment regimens. Alimentary Pharmacology & Therapeutics. 2015;**41**(6):497-520. DOI: 10.1111/apt.13090

[58] Moradpour D, Grakoui A, Manns MP. Future landscape of hepatitis C research–basic, translational and clinical perspectives. Journal of Hepatology. 2016 Oct 31;**65**(1):S143-S155. DOI: 10.1016/j.jhep.2016.07.026

[59] Golabi P, Sayiner M, Bush H, Gerber LH, Younossi ZM. Patient-reported outcomes and fatigue in patients with chronic hepatitis C infection. Clinics in Liver Disease. 2017; **21**(3):565-578. DOI: 10.1016/j.cld.2017.03.011

[60] Marcellin F, Roux P, Protopopescu C, Duracinsky M, Spire B, Carrieri MP. Patient-reported outcomes with direct-acting antivirals for the treatment of chronic hepatitis C: Current knowledge and outstanding issues. Expert Review of Gastroenterology & Hepatology. 2017 Mar 4;**11**(3):259-268. DOI: 10.1080/17474124.2017.1285227

[61] Jiang HY, Deng M, Zhang YH, Chen HZ, Chen Q, Ruan B. Specific serotonin reuptake inhibitors prevent interferon-α-induced depression in patients with hepatitis C: A meta-analysis. Clinical Gastroenterology and Hepatology. Sep 2014;**12**(9):1452-60.e3. DOI: 10.1016/j.cgh.2013.04.035

[62] Hou XJ, Xu JH, Wang J, Yu YY. Can antidepressants prevent pegylated interferon-α/ribavirin-associated depression in patients with chronic hepatitis C: Meta-analysis of randomized, double-blind, placebo-controlled trials? PLoS One. 2013 Oct 30;**8**(10):e76799. DOI: 10.1371/journal.pone.0076799

[63] Schäfer A, Wittchen HU, Seufert J, Kraus MR. Methodological approaches in the assessment of interferon-alfa-induced depression in patients with chronic hepatitis C - a critical review. International Journal of Methods in Psychiatric Research. 2007;**16**(4):186-201. DOI: 10.1002/mpr.229

[64] Başterzi AD, Yazici K, Aslan E, Delialioğlu N, Taşdelen B, Tot Acar S, Yazici A. Effects of fluoxetine and venlafaxine on serum brain derived neurotrophic factor levels in depressed patients. Progress in Neuro-Psychopharmacology & Biological Psychiatry. 2009 Mar 17;**33**(2):281-285. DOI: 10.1016/j.pnpbp.2008.11.016

[65] Cooper CM, Godlewska B, Sharpley AL, Barnes E, Cowen PJ, Harmer CJ. Interferon-α induces negative biases in emotional processing in patients with hepatitis C virus infection: A preliminary study. Psychological Medicine. 2017:1-10. DOI: 10.1017/S0033291 717002379

Predictors of 50 Day In-Hospital Mortality in Decompensated Cirrhosis Patients with Spontaneous Bacterial Peritonitis

Chinmaya Kumar Bal, Ripu Daman and
Vikram Bhatia

Abstract

Aim: Predictors of 50 day in-hospital mortality in decompensated cirrhosis patients with spontaneous bacterial peritonitis (SBP).

Methods: 218 SBP patients admitted to intensive care units in a tertiary care hospital were retrospectively analyzed. Student t test, multivariate logistic regression, Cox proportional hazard ratio, receiver operating characteristics curves and Kaplan-Meier survival analysis were utilized for statistical analysis. Predictive powers of the statistical significant variables were compared using the area under receiver operating characteristics curve (AUC). p values <0.05 were considered statistical significant.

Results: SBP related in-hospital mortality rate was 43%. Multivariate regression analysis showed acute kidney injury, hepatic encephalopathy, positive ascitic culture, leucocyte count, bilirubin, serum glutamic oxaloacetic transaminase (SGOT), Child Pugh score, and Model for End stage Liver Disease Sodium (MELD-Na) were significantly associated with 50 day in-hospital mortality. The prognostic accuracy for acute kidney injury, MELD-Na and septic shock was 77, 74 and 71% respectively.

Conclusion: Acute kidney injury, MELD-Na and septic shock were predictors of 50 day in-hospital mortality in decompensated cirrhotic patients with SBP.

Keywords: spontaneous bacterial peritonitis, cirrhosis, acute kidney injury, model for end stage liver disease sodium

1. Introduction

SBP is defined as an ascitic fluid infection without an evident intra-abdominal surgically-treatable source [1]. SBP is a major complication of decompensated cirrhosis with ascites [2]. The diagnosis of SBP is established based on diagnostic paracentesis with an elevated ascitic fluid absolute polymorphonuclear leucocyte (PMN) count ($\geq$250 cells/mm^3) and/or a positive ascitic fluid bacterial culture. The most common pathogens involved are Gram-negative bacteria (60%), usually *Escherichia coli* or *Klebsiella pneumonia* [3]. In about 25% of the cases, Gram-positive bacteria are involved, mainly Streptococcus species and Enterococci [3]. The prevalence of SBP is up to 30% in hospitalized cirrhotic patients with ascites [4]. Despite intensive management, the in-hospital mortality remains between 20 and 40% [5]. MELD scores have clinical utility in terms of predictive ability in SBP patients [6, 7]. Acute kidney injury (AKI) and septic shock are fairly common in patients with decompensated cirrhosis with ascites [8, 9]. Hence our study aimed to have a collective approach to determine common prognostic factors predicting SBP related in-hospital mortality. We also compared the predictive powers of AKI, MELD-Na and septic shock to predict 50 day in-hospital mortality.

2. Materials and methods

2.1. Patients

Retrospective analysis and review of 218 adult patients admitted to hepatology ICU with a diagnosis of SBP was done. The study was approved by the Institutional review Board and was conducted with the provisions of Declaration of Helsinki [10].

The diagnosis of cirrhosis was based on clinical, laboratory and imaging findings. SBP was diagnosed by diagnostic paracentesis in the presence of PMN $\geq$250 cells/mm^3 in the peritoneal fluid with positive culture report and the absence of the features suggestive of secondary bacterial peritonitis [11].

Data from patient's medical records were collected and tabulated. It comprises of demographics, etiology of liver disease, severity of liver disease, laboratory parameters, co-existing medical conditions (diabetes mellitus, hepatocellular carcinoma), previous medication use, organ failure, ascitic fluid analysis results, duration of ICU stay, and patient outcome. In culture-positive cases growth of the organisms and antibiotic sensitivity were recorded.

MELD-Na score was based on laboratory parameters (bilirubin, creatinine levels and INR) collected at admission and determined by using the Internet site MELD calculator [12]. Diagnostic ascitic tapping was done upon admission to ICU in all patients with ascites except in those with severe coagulopathy. Ascitic fluid was sent for differential cell count and culture. Blood sample was also sent for culture at admission in all patients. Antibiotics administered in patients based on previous antibiotic exposure and based on culture and sensitivity.

No patient underwent fluid restriction or hypertonic saline for management of dilution hyponatremia.

AKI was defined by AKIN (acute kidney injury network) criteria [8]. AKI was managed by intravenous vasopressors (terlipressin) and intravenous albumin infusions. The dose was titrated as-per response and tolerance. Intravenous albumin was used in all patients, with a minimal daily dose of 20 g and increased to up to 60 g/d [13], titrated by clinical monitoring and hourly urine output. We did not stratify renal dysfunction into hepatorenal syndrome (HRS) and non-hepatorenal syndrome. Renal replacement therapy (RRT) was used at the bedside to correct fluid overload, ascites, and electrolyte dysfunction. We did not consider advanced liver disease as a contraindication to RRT in our patient cohort.

We defined septic shock according to the American college of chest physicians/society of critical care medicine consensus conference [14].

2.2. Exclusion criteria

Patients with cirrhosis and ascites fluid PMN <250 cells/mm^3. Patients admitted from the community with SBP. Patients presented with ascites unrelated to cirrhosis. Patients with secondary peritonitis, variceal hemorrhage, advanced malignancy and HIV.

2.3. Statistical analysis

All statistical analyses were conducted using Stata version 14 for windows. The continuous clinical and biochemical variables and prognostic scores were expressed as mean ± standard deviation. All the variables were assumed to be normally distributed with equal variance. The means were compared using student's t test. Categorical variables were expressed as proportions and compared with logistics regression. All significant variables were analyzed using multivariate logistics regression. Cox proportional hazard model was used to analyze the hazard ratio of the predictors adjusted by age and gender. Receiver operating characteristics (ROC) curves were plotted for prognostic variables (MELD-Na, AKI and) to measure the predictive accuracy. The best cut-off point for MELD-Na was created using the ROC analysis to determine 50 day in-hospital mortality risk. The sensitivity, specificity, positive predictive values (PPV), negative predictive values (NPV), positive and negative likelihood ratio were calculated for each predictor variable so that patients could be correctly classified for each prognostic model. For all analyses, p value < 0.05 was considered statistically significant. STROBE checklist for retrospective analysis was performed.

3. Results

A total of 218 patients with decompensated cirrhosis with ascites and SBP were included in the study. Patients that were diagnosed with SBP for the first time were 97% (n = 211) with only 0.03% (n = 7) had more than one episode previously. The 50 day in-hospital mortality

Variables	Overall (n = 218)	Survivors (n = 124)	Deaths (n = 94)	P-value
Demographic data				
Age (yrs) mean ± SD	49.90 ± 12.52	49.86 ± 13.37	49.96 ± 11.37	0.950
Male (%)	177 (81.19%)	99 (79.84%)	78 (82.98%)	0.557
Etiology of cirrhosis (%)				
Ethanol	100 (45.87%)	48 (38.71%)	52 (55.32%)	0.689
Crypto/NAFLD	63 (28.90%)	38 (30.65%)	25 (26.60%)	0.104
HCV	23 (10.55%)	16 (12.905)	7 (7.45%)	0.068
Clinical data (%)				
Hepatocellular carcinoma	17 (7.80%)	9 (7.26%)	8 (8.51%)	0.733
Diabetes	47 (21.56%)	27 (21.77%)	20 (21.28%)	0.929
Acute kidney injury	99 (45.41%)	35 (28.23%)	64 (68.09%)	<0.001
Respiratory failure	10 (4.59%)	6 (4.84%)	4 (4.26%)	0.978
Hepatic encephalopathy	109 (50.0%)	50 (40.32%)	59 (62.77%)	0.001
Septic shock	28 (12.84%)	4 (3.23%)	24 (25.53%)	<0.001
Positive culture	48 (22.02%)	21 (16.94%)	27 (28.72%)	0.038
Laboratory data (mean ± SD)*				
Ascitic neutrophil count (cells/mm^3)	3346.07 ± 4700.60	3899.28 ± 5003.75	2616.30 ± 4182.81	0.040
Hemoglobin (g/dl)	9.42 ± 1.88	9.58 ± 1.77	9.21 ± 2.01	0.154
Platelet count (mmol/L)	128.24 ± 102.11	138.43 ± 111.25	115.03 ± 87.69	0.095
Leucocyte count (10^3/μL)	13.30 ± 9.35	11.86 ± 8.65	15.17 ± 9.92	0.009
Sodium (mEq/L)	132.14 ± 7.69	132.50 ± 6.54	131.67 ± 9.01	0.454
Bilirubin (mg/dL)	8.17 ± 8.81	5.85 ± 6.27	11.24 ± 10.61	<0.001
Albumin (g/dL)	2.32 ± 0.50	2.35 ± −0.48	2.28 ± 0.52	0.250
INR	2.31 ± 1.11	2.09 ± 1.08	2.59 ± 1.08	0.001
AST (U/L)	59.66 ± 109.81	79.23 ± 98.71	171.3 ± 321.94	0.003
ALT (U/L)	59.66 ± 109.81	46.49 ± 72.93	77.04 ± 143.41	0.041
Urea (mg/dL)	70.31 ± 52.42	62.24 ± 48.23	80.94 ± 55.98	0.008
Creatinine (mg/dL)	1.67 ± 1.29	1.58 ± 1.39	1.80 ± 1.15	0.217
Scores (mean ± SD)				
CTP (B/C)	10.72 ± 1.82	10.50 ± 1.95	11.02 ± 1.60	0.034

Variables	Overall (n = 218)	Survivors (n = 124)	Deaths (n = 94)	P-value
MELD	24.79 ± 8.28	22.20 ± 7.59	28.20 ± 7.94	<0.001
MELD-Na	27.53 ± 7.57	25.21 ± 7.44	30.59 ± 6.62	<0.001

*Results obtained on the day of diagnosis of SBP.

Table 1. Baseline characteristics of the hospitalized patients with spontaneous bacterial peritonitis in decompensated cirrhosis.

rate was 43.11% (n = 94). Median survival duration for those who died was 9 days. In univariate analysis AKI, hepatic encephalopathy, total leucocyte count, serum bilirubin, INR, SGOT, and MELD-Na are significantly associated with in hospital mortality in patients with SBP (**Table 1**).

The baseline characteristics of the demographics, etiology, clinical and laboratory data shown in **Table 1**. Mean age was 49.90 ± 12.52 years and the male was predominant (83%). Most common etiology of liver cirrhosis was ethanol induced (45.87%) followed by crypto/ NAFLD (28.9%). Liver cirrhosis due to HCV infection constitute only 11% in our study. Total 50.0% patients (n = 109) had hepatic encephalopathy with 62.77% deaths (n = 59, p = 0.001). Overall 45.11% subjects (n = 99) had AKI who were hospitalized, out of which 68.09% (n = 64, $p \leq 0.001$) died. Compared with survivors, the non-survivors had a higher proportion of septic shock (25.53 vs. 3.23%), $p < 0.001$. Mean leucocyte count, bilirubin, INR, AST were significantly higher in the persons who died in comparing to the survivors. Mean MELD-Na score was higher among the non-survivors compared with the survivors (30.59 ± 6.62 vs. 25.21 ± 7.44) ($p < 0.001$). It is surprising to notice that CTP (B/C) score was not different among the survivors and non-survivors. The mean CTP scores were high (10.72 ± 1.82).

On multivariate regression analysis, AKI (p = 0.001), septic shock (p = 0.029), MELD-Na (p<0.001) were found to be independent predictors of 50 day in-hospital mortality in patients with SBP (**Table 2**). Cox proportional hazard model showed the hazard ratio of AKI was 2.16 (95% CI = 1.36–3.42), septic shock (HR 1.73, 95% CI = 1.05–2.83) and MELD-Na (HR 1.1, 95% CI = 1.02–1.21). ROC curve for AKI, septic shock and MELD-Na had better prognostic

Variables	Hazard ratio* (95% CI)	P value
AKI	2.16 (1.36–3.42)	0.001
Septic shock	1.73 (1.05–2.83)	0.029
MELD-Na	1.06 (1.02–1.09)	<0.001

*Hazard ratio adjusted for age and gender.
AKI, acute kidney injury; MELD-Na, model for end-stage liver disease sodium.

Table 2. Cox proportional regression analysis of risk factors for SBP related in-hospital related mortality.

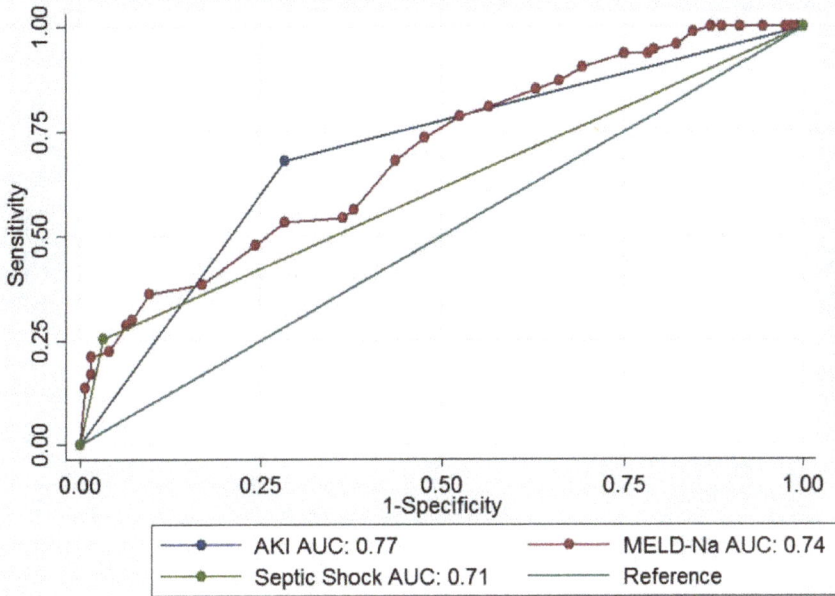

Figure 1. Receiver operator characteristic (ROC) curve for AKI, septic shock and MELD-Na had better prognostic accuracy for 50 day in-hospital mortality in patients with SBP.

Predictors	Sensitivity	Specificity	PPV	NPV	+LR	−LR
AKI	64.6	74.8	68.1	71.8	2.56	0.47
Septic shock	85.7	63.2	25.5	96.8	2.33	0.23
MELD-Na(28)[1]	92.9	60.3	24.5	97.9	2.34	0.12

[1]Cut off score for MELD-Na, PPV: positive predictive value, NPV: negative predictive value, +LR: positive likelihood ratio, −LR: negative likelihood ratio, AKI: acute kidney injury, MELD-Na: model for end stage liver disease sodium.

Table 3. Diagnostic accuracy of prognostic variables to predict SBP related in-hospital mortality.

accuracy for 50 day in-hospital mortality in patients with SBP (**Figure 1**). AKI had highest Area Under Curve (AUC) 0.77, 95% confidence interval (95% CI = 0.71–0.83), followed by MELD-Na (AUC 0.74, 95% CI = 0.69–0.79), septic shock (AUC 0.71, 95% CI = 0.65–0.77). **Table 3** reported the sensitivity, specificity, PPV, NPV, positive likelihood ratio (+LR) and negative likelihood ratio (−LR) for these predictors. The cut off for MELD-Na derived from the ROC with the best ability to predict 50 day in-hospital mortality in decompensated cirrhotic patient with SBP was 28, with sensitivity 92.9%, specificity 60.3%, and NPV of 97.9%. The Kaplan-Meier survival analysis was plotted for the 50 day survival in SBP patients along with individual prognostic variables like AKI, MELD-Na, and septic shock (**Figure 2**).

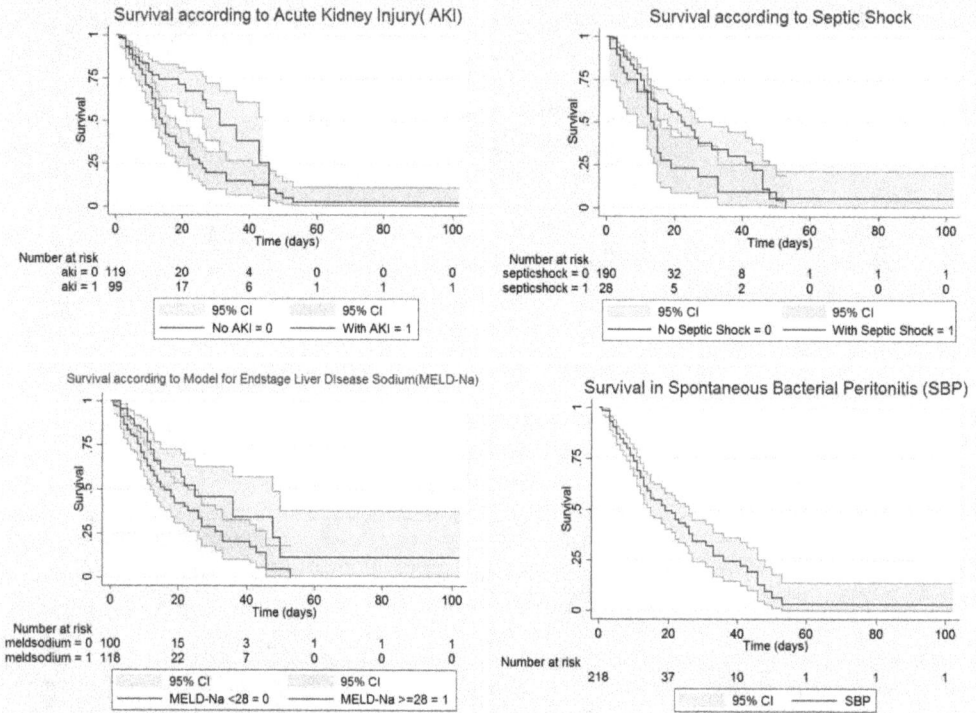

Figure 2. Kaplan-Meier survival analysis was plotted for the 50 day survival in SBP patients along with individual prognostic variables like AKI, MELD-Na, and septic shock.

4. Discussion

The prevalence of SBP in outpatients has been reported to be 1.5–3.5% [15]. The prevalence among in-patients is around 10% [16]. Half of the episodes of SBP are nosocomial related. In our retrospective observational study 43% (n = 93) of the decompensated cirrhotic patients with SBP died within 50 day of hospital admission. Our study considered a variety of prognostic factors that can be used to predict mortality in hospitalized patient with SBP. Our findings support previous study results that variables like hepatic encephalopathy, total leucocyte count, serum bilirubin, SGOT, INR, Child Pugh scores are significantly associated with mortality [5, 6]. The MELD score was found to be an independent predictor of death in cirrhotic patients [7] including those waiting for liver transplantation. MELD-Na is a better prognostic model compared with MELD model [17] for predictive accuracy of mortality in liver cirrhosis. Serum creatinine level measurement for renal dysfunction in decompensated liver cirrhosis is erroneous. It can be due to decrease in creatinine production in liver and associated muscle wasting due to malnutrition [18]. We found that AKI, MELD-Na and septic shock are significant in terms of predicting mortality. We overlooked other predictable variables like total leucocyte count, serum bilirubin, INR to avoid confusion and complexity as those were the components in our predictive model like MELD-Na and septic shock.

Our study demonstrated that AKI has the single best predictive ability (AUC = 0.77) followed by MELD-Na (AUC = 0.74) and septic shock (AUC = 0.71). We set a cut-off value for MELD-Na to be 28. It has sensitivity 92.9% and NPV of 97.9%. AKI has the highest hazards of mortality (HR 2.16, 95% CI 1.36–3.42) followed by septic shock (HR 1.73, 95% CI 1.05–2.83) and MELD-Na (HR 1.06, 95% 1.02–1.09). We plotted graph of Kaplan-Meier survival analysis. The graph illustrated AKI, MELD-Na, and septic shock as predictors for the 50 day in-hospital mortality in decompensated patients with SBP. We hope that these prognostic variables can help in the further improvement of the quality of care of hospitalized SBP patients. The cut-off value 28 for MELD-Na can be utilized to stratify patients diagnosed with SBP into high risk category upon hospital admission.

Diagnosis of SBP is based on the demonstration of an absolute number of polymorphonuclear cells in ascitic fluid equal to or greater than 250/mm^3 with culture positivity. There is a controversy regarding antibiotic therapy in culture positivity with normal ascitic fluid PMN count (bacteriascites). Runyon et al. recommend antibiotic treatment only if the patient shows signs of infection [2]. The first-line of choice antibiotics for treatment of SBP include third generation cephalosporins, amoxicillin-clavulanic acid, ciprofloxacin, and ofloxacin [19]. There is increasing evidence of antibiotic resistance [20].

In our study ascitic fluid culture is positive in 40% of all cases. The most common growth include Gram-negative bacteria (GNB), mostly *Escherichia coli* and Gram-positive cocci (mainly streptococcus species and enterococci) [3]. The epidemiology of bacterial infections differs between community-acquired (in which GNB infections predominate) and nosocomial infections (in which Gram-positive infections predominate) [3]. The infections resistant to first lines of antibiotics are usually caused by *Enterococcus faecium* and extended-spectrum β-lactamase (ESBL) organism like Enterobacteriaceae [21]. There are compelling evidence that nosocomial SBP should be treated with carbapenems or with tigecycline [22].

We included only nosocomial SBP patients in our study because most of the ICU admissions includes referred patients from other hospitals, with a variable but inconsistent antibiotic exposure. Only a minority of our patients are admitted directly from the community, and usually to the wards and not to the ICU. Hospital-acquired infections due to a higher incidence of multidrug resistance (third-generation cephalosporins) were an independent predictor of death [23]. These results are in keeping with recent data showing higher rates of drug resistance in patients with nosocomial SBP and increased rates of and death in patients with multidrug resistance [24].

Dr. Garcia-Tsao recently reviewed 18 studies, and reported that the most common predictors of death were renal dysfunction, lack of SBP resolution, immunosuppressive factors, and hospital-acquired SBP [24]. It identified renal dysfunction and levels of blood urea nitrogen and creatinine as the most important variables. The mortality rate among patients with renal dysfunction was 67%, compared with only 11% of patients who maintained normal renal function. Renal dysfunction was defined somewhat variably in the studies, but most defined it as a creatinine level greater than 1.5 mg/dL.

Our study has certain strengths and limitations. The results clearly show that AKI has greater predictive ability than septic shock and MELD-Na as far as 50 day in-hospital mortality in SBP patient is concerned. Our study did not account for the stages of ascites. We did not stratify our patients according to different stages of AKI as per AKIN criteria. We did not take HRS into account in our study. The standard first line antibiotics were not used in the treatment of SBP. The choice of antibiotics coverage based of culture sensitivity and previous exposure. We did not thoroughly evaluate the antibiotic resistance in SBP patients who are culture positive at the baseline. We included only nosocomial acquired SBP. Most of our patients presented with advanced decompensated liver cirrhosis at the time of SBP diagnosis as it is a tertiary care center. The advanced liver cirrhosis was assessed by lower serum albumin, high serum bilirubin and INR values. As an observational study we were unable to assess the impact of volume expansion and SBP specific therapy on patient outcome. Our study is a single center study, these findings needed to be supplemented by multicenter prospective studies.

Our study findings can guide in advanced liver cirrhosis patients that would benefit them from intensive management where liver transplant is not feasible.

Author details

Chinmaya Kumar Bal*, Ripu Daman and Vikram Bhatia

*Address all correspondence to: chinmaya.bal@gmail.com

Department of Hepatology, Institute of Liver and Biliary Science, New Delhi, India

References

[1] Rimola A, García-Tsao G, Navasa M, Piddock LJ, Planas R, Bernard B, Inadomi JM. Diagnosis treatment and prophylaxis of spontaneous bacterial peritonitis: A consensus document. International Ascites Club. Journal of Hepatology. 2000;**32**:142-153. DOI: 10.1016/S0168-8278(00)80201-9

[2] Such J, Runyon BA. Spontaneous bacterial peritonitis. Clinical Infectious Diseases. 1998;**27**(4):669-674 quiz 675-6

[3] Dever JB, Sheikh MY. Review article: Spontaneous bacterial peritonitis-bacteriology, diagnosis, treatment, risk factors and prevention. Alimentary Pharmacology & Therapeutics. 2015;**41**(11):1116-1131. DOI: 10.1111/apt.13172

[4] Gunjaca I, Francetić I. Prevalence and clinical outcome of spontaneous bacterial peritonitis in hospitalized patients with liver cirrhosis: A prospective observational study in central part of Croatia. Acta Clinica Croatica. 2010;**49**(1):11-18

[5] Thuluvath PJ, Morss S, Thompson R. Spontaneous bacterial peritonitis in-hospital mortality, predictors of survival, and health care costs from 1988 to 1998. The American Journal of Gastroenterology. 2001;**96**:1232-1236. DOI: 10.1111/j.1572-0241.2001.03708.x

[6] Dănulescu RM, Stanciu C, Trifan A. Evaluation of prognostic factors in decompensated liver cirrhosis with ascites and spontaneous bacterial peritonitis. Revista Medico-Chirurgicală a Societăţii de Medici şi Naturalişti din Iaşi. 2015;**119**(4):1018-1024

[7] Nobre SR, Cabral JE, Gomes JJ, Leitão MC. In-hospital mortality in spontaneous bacterial peritonitis: A new predictive model. European Journal of Gastroenterology & Hepatology. 2008;**20**:1176-1181. DOI: 10.1097/MEG.0b013e32830607a2

[8] de Araujo A, Alvares-da-Silva MR. Akin criteria as a predictor of mortality in cirrhotic patients after spontaneous bacterial peritonitis. Annals of Hepatology. 2014;**13**(3):390-395

[9] Moreau R, Hadengue A, Soupison T, Kirstetter P, Mamzer MF, Vanjak D, et al. Septic shock in patients with cirrhosis: Hemodynamic and metabolic characteristics and intensive care unit outcome. Critical Care Medicine. 1992;**20**(6):746-750

[10] WMA declaration of Helsinki-ethical principles for medical research involving human subjects [internet]. 2013. Available from: https://www.wma.net/what-we-do/education/medical-ethics-manual [Accessed: 2018-03-19]

[11] Runyon BA. The evolution of ascitic fluid analysis in the diagnosis of spontaneous bacterial peritonitis. The American Journal of Gastroenterology. 2003;**98**(8):1675-1677

[12] MELDNa/MELD-Na Score for Liver Cirrhosis [Internet]. 2016. Available from: https://www.mdcalc.com/meldna-meld-na-score-liver-cirrhosis [Accessed: 2018-03-19]

[13] de Mattos A. Current indicators for use of albumin in the treatment of cirrhosis. Annals of Hepatology. 2011;**10**(Suppl. 1):S15-S20

[14] Bone RC, Balk RA, Cerra FB, Dellinger RP, Fein AM, Knaus WA, Schein RM, Sibbald WJ. Definitions for sepsis and organ failure and guidelines for the use of innovative therapies in sepsis. The ACCP/SCCM Consensus Conference Committee. American College of Chest Physicians/Society of Critical Care Medicine. 1992. DOI: 10.1378/chest.101.6.1644

[15] Chu CM, Chang KY, Liaw YF. Prevalence and prognostic significance of bacterascites in cirrhosis with ascites. Digestive Diseases and Sciences. 1995;**40**(3):561-565

[16] Terg R, Gadano A, Cartier M et al. Serum creatinine and bilirubin predict renal failure and mortality in patients with spontaneous bacterial peritonitis: A retrospective study. Liver International. 2009;**29**:415-19

[17] Musskopf MI, Fonseca FP, Gass J, de Mattos AZ, John JA, de Mello Brandão AB. Prognostic factors associated with in-hospital mortality in patients with spontaneous bacterial peritonitis. Annals of Hepatology. 2012;**11**(6):915-920

[18] MacAulay J, Thompson K, Kiberd BA, Barnes DC, Peltekian KM. Serum creatinine in patients with advanced liver disease is of limited value for identification of moderate renal dysfunction: Are the equations for estimating renal function better? Canadian Journal of Gastroenterology. 2006;**20**(8):521-526

[19] European Association for the Study of the Liver. EASL clinical practice guidelines on the management of ascites, spontaneous bacterial peritonitis, and hepatorenal syndrome in cirrhosis. Journal of Hepatology. 2010;**53**(3):397-417. DOI: 10.1016/j.jhep.2010.05.004

[20] Cheong HS, Kang CI, Lee JA, et al. Clinical significance and outcome of nosocomial acquisition of spontaneous bacterial peritonitis in patients with liver cirrhosis. Clinical Infectious Diseases. 2009;**48**:1230-1236. DOI: 10.1086/597585

[21] Ariza X, Castellote J, Lora-Tamayo J, Girbau A, Salord S, Rota R, et al. Risk factors for resistance to ceftriaxone and its impact on mortality in community, healthcare and nosocomial spontaneous bacterial peritonitis. Journal of Hepatology. 2012;**56**:825-832. DOI: 10.1016/j.jhep.2011.11.010

[22] Fernández J, Acevedo J, Castro M, Garcia O, de Lope CR, Roca D, Pavesi M, Sola E, Moreira L, Silva A, Seva-Pereira T, Corradi F, Mensa J, Ginès P, Arroyo V. Prevalence and risk factors of infections by multiresistant bacteria in cirrhosis: A prospective study. Hepatology. 2012;**55**:1551-1561. DOI: 10.1002/hep.25532

[23] Umgelter A, Reindl W, Miedaner M, Schmid RM, Huber W. Failure of current antibiotic first-line regimens and mortality in hospitalized patients with spontaneous bacterial peritonitis. Infection. 2009;**37**:2-8. DOI: 10.1007/s15010-008-8060-9

[24] Tandon P, Garcia-Tsao G. Renal dysfunction is the most important independent predictor of mortality in cirrhotic patients with spontaneous bacterial peritonitis. Clinical Gastroenterology and Hepatology. 2011;**9(3)**:260-265. DOI: 10.1016/j.cgh.2010.11.038

9

Noninvasive Evaluation of Fibrosis and Steatosis in Nonalcoholic Fatty Liver Disease by Elastographic Methods

Monica Lupsor-Platon

Abstract

An increasingly common cause of chronic liver disease in adults and children is nonalcoholic fatty liver disease (NAFLD). The diagnosis of NAFLD was traditionally based on the histopathological changes of the liver, evaluated by needle liver biopsy, an invasive method, with potential adverse effects and great inter and intraobserver variability. The noninvasive methods for the assessment of both fibrosis and steatosis in patients with NAFLD have increasingly been studied lately. Of these noninvasive methods, in this chapter, we will focus on the methods assessing the stiffness of liver parenchyma, i.e. elastographic methods, of which, the most widely used are ultrasound elastography techniques. We will discuss the principal elastographic methods of some utility in NAFLD, i.e. shear wdave elastography (SWE) (quantitative elastography), and especially transient elastography, point SWE (acoustic radiation force impulse elastography, ARFI) and two-dimensional real-time SWE (Supersonic). For each method usable in NAFLD cases, we will review the method principle, examination technique and performance in NAFLD evaluation.

Keywords: nonalcoholic fatty liver disease, fibrosis, steatosis, noninvasive, elastography

1. Introduction

An increasingly common cause of chronic liver disease in adults and children is nonalcoholic fatty liver disease (NAFLD) [1]. In adults, the prevalence of NAFLD ranges from 17% to 33% [2], whereas in children, from 2.6% to 9.6%; in obese children, the prevalence is significantly higher: 22.5%–44% [3]. NAFLD may present in various ways: as simple steatosis, nonalcoholic steatohepatitis, liver cirrhosis or even hepatocellular carcinoma (HCC) [2–5].

The diagnosis of NAFLD was traditionally based on the histopathological changes of the liver, evaluated by needle liver biopsy (LB). Unfortunately, this is an invasive method, with potential adverse effects and great inter and intraobserver variability [6–8]. In addition, the interpretation may be erroneous, because of the inhomogeneous distribution of fibrosis. In patients with HCV infection, for instance, differences of at least 1 stage between the right and left lobe in 33% of cases [7] or between 2 samples taken from the same area in even up to 45% of cases have been reported in literature [9]. In patients with nonalcoholic steatohepatitis (NASH), the inhomogeneous distribution of fibrosis appears to be even more pronounced than in HCV patients [10]. Some studies [8] showed that, when taking 2 samples from the right hepatic lobe in each NASH patient, agreement in fibrosis stage was found in only 47% of patients, while differences of at least 1 stage were found in 41% of cases, or 2 stages, in 12% of cases, respectively.

Lately, patients with NASH are increasingly evaluated using rapid, noninvasive methods of assessment of both fibrosis and steatosis. The diagnosis of liver steatosis has several implications in chronic liver diseases [11]. Indeed, in HCV patients, for instance, liver steatosis is associated with fibrosis progression and a decreased rate of sustained viral response [11–13]. Steatosis (which is the primary lesion in nonalcoholic fatty liver disease) may associate graft failure 1 year after liver transplantation, with increased risk of complications after liver resection and, last but not least, increased risk of death [11, 14–16].

The fibrosis may be assessed noninvasively using serum biomarkers (not liver-specific, but proven to correlate with fibrosis), as well as by measuring certain intrinsic physical properties of the liver parenchyma, such as liver stiffness (LS) or shear wave velocity (SWV) within the liver [17]. Of these noninvasive methods, in this chapter, we will focus on the methods assessing the stiffness of liver parenchyma, i.e. elastographic methods, of which, the most widely used are ultrasound (US) elastography techniques.

2. Classification of US-based elastography techniques

Elastography may be considered "a type of remote palpation that allows measurement and display of biomechanical properties associated with the elastic restoring forces in the tissue that act against shear deformation" [18].

In accordance to the European Federation of Societies for Ultrasound in Medicine and Biology (EFSUMB) Guidelines [19, 20], the ultrasound elastographic techniques are either quantitative (shear wave elastography, SWE) or qualitative (strain elastography, real-time elastography). The quantitative techniques are as follows:

- Transient elastography (TE), the only method nonintegrated into a standard ultrasound system.

- Point SWE: Acoustic radiation force impulse elastography (ARFI) or ElastPQ technique.

- Real time SWE: Two-dimensional SWE (2D-SWE) or three-dimensional SWE (3D-SWE)

In the following sections, we will focus on the main quantitative ultrasound elastography techniques, which can help in the noninvasive assessment of nonalcoholic fatty liver disease.

3. Transient elastography (TE)

3.1. Principle

Transient elastography is performed using the Fibroscan® device (Echosens, Paris). The transducer of the device is placed in an intercostal space, above the right lobe, in a point of maximal hepatic dullness (typically the 9–11th intercostal space, on the midaxillary line). A mechanical vibrator is mounted on the axis of the transducer; the vibrator generates a painless vibration, inducing a train of elastic waves, which propagate through the skin and subcutaneous tissue to the liver. In parallel to the vibration, the transducer performs ultrasound acquisitions, at a frequency of 4 kHz. By comparing the ultrasonographic signals thus obtained, tissue deformation records, induced by the propagation of the elastic wave, can be drawn. The time necessary for the train of waves to propagate along the interest area, as well as the velocity of propagation, is recorded [21–25]. The liver stiffness may therefore be calculated using the formula: $E = 3\rho Vs^2$ (E—elasticity modulus; ρ—density, a constant of the material; Vs—the elastic wave propagation velocity within the liver parenchyma). Young's modulus (E) clinically corresponds to the LS and is typically referred to as E or LS. LS values range from 2.5 to 75 kPa. The stiffer the tissue, the higher the train wave propagation velocity [1, 24]. Lower values indicate a more elastic liver.

On the other hand, knowing that fat affects ultrasound propagation, a novel attenuation parameter has been developed to detect and quantify liver steatosis [25]. This parameter, called controlled attenuation parameter (CAP), is based on the ultrasonic properties of the radiofrequency back propagated signals acquired by the Fibroscan® [26]. This ultrasonic attenuation coefficient is an estimate of the total ultrasonic attenuation (go-and-return path) at the central frequency of the regular or M probe of the Fibroscan® probe, i.e. at 3.5 MHz, and is expressed in dB/m and ranges from 100 to 400 dB/m. CAP is evaluated using the same radiofrequency data, and the same region of interest, as the region used to assess the LS [26, 27]. It follows that the equipment can measure the liver stiffness (for the estimation of fibrosis) at the same time with CAP (for the estimation of steatosis) [25].

3.2. Examination technique

The patient is placed in a dorsal decubitus position, with the right arm in maximum abduction, in order to best expose the right quadrant, and the transducer is placed in direct contact with the skin, perpendicularly to the intercostal space, in an area of maximal dullness, free of any large vascular structure. The correct position is ensured either by visualizing the image of the A mode of the system or by using a different ultrasound equipment [22, 24].

When pressing the transducer button, the vibration is generated and transmitted to the liver. The software of the equipment analyses the tissue deformation records and measures the stiffness of the parenchyma. The results are expressed in kiloPascals (kPa) and represent the median value of 10 valid measurements [22, 24]. At the same time, the software can measure the controlled attenuation parameter (CAP), expressed in dB/m.

The monitor of the device will display the instantaneous liver stiffness and CAP values, the median stiffness and CAP values resulting for each of the 10 valid measurements, the measurement success rate as well as the variation of the 10 measurements from the median (IQR).

A necessary condition for a correct assessment is the examination after an overnight fast or at least 2 hours after a meal, because a postprandial examination would increase the stiffness value due to increased hepatic blood flow [28, 29] and would lead to a false interpretation of liver stiffness. The influence of postprandial examination on CAP has not yet been proven.

The measurement can be performed even by a technician after a training period (approximately 100 cases) [30, 31], but the clinical interpretation of results must always be issued by an expert taking into account the demographic data, disease etiology and biochemical profile at the moment of the examination [32].

3.3. Parameters of the examination performance

In accordance to the manufacturer recommendations, the success rate is required to reach at least 60%, and the IQR to be less than 30% of the median (M) liver stiffness [24], although it appears that the best concordance with the biopsy is obtained when its value does not exceed 20% of the median [33].

According to the latest reports, however, the conventional definition of LS measurement accuracy is not relevant. The "success rate $\geq 60\%$" parameter is considered to be no longer necessary, and the examination accuracy depends on the IQR/M ratio, influenced by the median LS value. Three categories of measurement performance are therefore defined [34]:

- "very reliable": IQR/M ≤ 0.10

- "reliable": $0.10 <$ IQR/M ≤ 0.30 or IQR/M > 0.30 and LS <7.1 kPa

- "poorly reliable": IQR/M > 0.30 and LS ≥ 7.1 kPa

3.4. The liver volume examined by TE

The technique can measure the stiffness of a cylinder of parenchyma with a 1 cm diameter and a 4 cm height (the measurement is performed on a distance ranging from 25 and 45 mm from the skin); this represents around 1/500 of the entire liver volume, which is at least 100 times larger than the volume of a biopsy sample [22, 30, 32].

3.5. TE reproducibility

TE has a high degree of reproducibility, with a 0.93–0.98 intraobserver and interobserver correlation coefficient [35, 36]. Interobserver concordance is lower in patients with early stages of fibrosis, in those with $\geq 25\%$ steatosis and in patients with BMI ≥ 25 kg/m^2.

3.6. Normal range of liver stiffness

The mean value of liver stiffness in healthy subjects without any known liver disease and with normal biochemistry and hematology tests is 5.5 ± 1.6 kPa according to some authors [37] and 4.8 ± 1.3 kPa according to others [38]. Age does not appear to influence this value, but stiffness is higher in men than in women. It is very difficult to establish the normal range of liver stiffness without biopsy, but the reverse is not feasible. In a group of HCV patients, without pathological changes on the biopsy sample, the liver stiffness was 4.84 ± 1.49 kPa [39]. In our unit, values of or above 5.3 kPa have a positive predictive value of 90% for the prediction of a fibrosis stage of at least F1.

3.7. Pathological changes influencing liver stiffness in NASH

Our studies performed on a group of biopsied NASH patients proved that LS correlated moderately with fibrosis ($r = 0.661$; $p < 0.0001$) and weakly, but significantly, with hepatocyte ballooning ($r = 0.385$; $p = 0.001$), lobular inflammation ($r = 0.364$; $p = 0.002$) and steatosis ($r = 0.435$; $p < 0.0001$). Of all of these elements, fibrosis was found in a multivariate analysis to be the only factor independently influencing LS in NASH patients [40]. Nevertheless, the correlation between liver stiffness and fibrosis is weaker in NASH ($r = 0.661$) than in hepatitis C ($r = 0.73$–0.79) [41, 42]; this correlation is supported also by the computerized analysis of the biopsy sample that quantifies the amount of fibrosis on the entire sample [43] and is explained by a different distribution pattern of fibrosis in the two conditions [40, 43].

3.8. Diagnostic performance of TE in quantifying fibrosis and steatosis in NASH

Unlike studies performed on diffuse liver diseases of viral etiology, those assessing the role of TE in evaluating NASH patients are rather scarce.

Although liver stiffness is strongly correlated with fibrosis in chronic hepatitis patients, this correlation is weaker in patients with steatohepatitis, because of a different pattern of fibrosis distribution, which, as mentioned earlier, leads to a lower performance of this technique in fibrosis prediction in NASH. Indeed, we observed that liver stiffness in NASH increases alongside the fibrosis stage, but there appears to be an apparent overlap of LS values, especially for the F1-F2 patients [40].

In a meta-analysis including 854 NASH patients [44], TE was found to have a very good performance in diagnosing stages $F \geq 3$ (Se 82%, Sp 82%) and F4 (Se 92%, Sp 92%), but only moderate in diagnosing significant fibrosis $F \geq 2$ (Se 79%, Sp 75%).

The cut-off values for the prediction of fibrosis resulting from various studies differ considerably in NAFLD patients, due to the different prevalence of fibrosis stages in the analyzed groups, as well as to the aim of the analysis (sensibility >90% or specificity >90% or a maximal diagnostic accuracy). Therefore, the proposed cut-offs range between 5.3 and 7 kPa (for $F \geq 1$), with 61.7–93.48% sensitivity and 68–100% specificity (**Table 1**); 5.8–11 kPa (for $F \geq 2$), with 52.5–91.1% sensitivity and 50.3–91.7% specificity (**Table 2**); 7.8–12 kPa (for $F \geq 3$), with 75–100% sensitivity and 78–96.87% specificity (**Table 3**) and between 10.2 and 20 kPa

≥F1	Cut-off (kPa)	AUROC	Se (%)	Sp (%)	PPV (%)	NPV (%)
Yoneda et al. [45]	5.9	0,93	86.1	88.9	97.1	59.3
Lupsor et al. [40]	5.3	0.879	93.48	78.26	89.6	85.7
Kumar et al. [46]	6.1	0.82	78	68	87	53
Imajo et al. [47]	7	0.78	61.7	100	100	86.6

Table 1. Performance of liver stiffness measurement compared with liver biopsy in the detection of fibrosis ≥F1 in nonalcoholic fatty liver disease patients.

(for the prediction of cirrhosis), with 70–100% sensitivity and 68–96.6% specificity (**Table 4**) [40, 45–50]. The studies have shown that TE performance is better for cirrhosis than for significant fibrosis [51, 52].

The available data indicate that, in patients with NAFLD, TE is a highly accurate, noninvasive method for the exclusion of advanced fibrosis and a moderately accurate method for the exclusion of significant fibrosis. According to the EFSUMB and EASL Guidelines and Recommendations on the Clinical Use of Liver Ultrasound Elastography, TE can be used in NAFLD patients to confidently exclude severe fibrosis and especially cirrhosis, with a high negative predictive value (around 90%) [17, 18].

The major challenge for the use of transient elastography in patients with NAFLD in clinical practice is the high rate of failure (no valid shot) or unreliable results (not meeting the manufacturer's first recommendations). In these patients, the failure rate varies between 3.8 and 50% [40, 45, 48, 51, 53–56] and appears to be correlated mainly with obesity [57]. In fact, different studies report increased failure rates owing to increased body mass index (BMI > 30 kg/m²) or waist circumference, which may interfere with the transmission of the push impulses and the tracking ultrasound, thus preventing a correct estimation of liver stiffness [17]. Apart from

≥F2	Cut-off (kPa)	AUROC	Se (%)	Sp (%)	PPV (%)	NPV (%)
Yoneda et al. [45]	6.65	0.865	88.2	73.9	78.9	85
Lupsor et al. [40]	6.8	0.789	66.67	84.31	60	87.8
Wong et al. [48]	5.8 (Sn > 90%)	0.84	91.1	50.3	56.1	89.0
	7 (max DA)		79.2	75.9	69.6	84.0
	9 (Sp > 90%)		52.5	91.7	81.5	73.5
Kumar et al. [46]	7	0.85	77	78	75	81
Pathik et al. [49]	9.1	—	—	—	—	—
Imajo et al. [47]	11	0.82	65.2	88.7	88.2	66.2
Cassinotto et al. [50]	8.5	0.82	72	79	—	—

Table 2. Performance of liver stiffness measurement compared with liver biopsy in the detection of fibrosis ≥F2 in nonalcoholic fatty liver disease patients.

≥F3	Cut-off (kPa)	AUROC	Se (%)	Sp (%)	PPV (%)	NPV (%)
Yoneda et al. [45]	9.8	0.904	85.2	81.4	63.9	93
Lupsor et al. [40]	10.2	0.978	100	96.87	71.4	100
Wong et al. [48]	7.9 (Sn > 90%)	0.93	91.1	75.3	52.0	96.6
	8.7 (max DA)		83.9	83.2	59.5	94.6
	9.6 (Sp > 90%)		75.0	91.6	72.4	92.6
Kumar et al. [46]	9 (Se + Sp max)	0.94	85	88	68	95
	7.8 (Sn > 90%)		96	78	43	98
	11.2 (Sp > 90%)		71	93	57	91
Pathik et al. [49]	12	–	90	80	–	–
Cassinotto et al. [50]	9.3	0.86	82	75	NR	NR
Imajo et al. [47]	11.4	0.88	85.7	83.8	75	91.9

Table 3. Performance of liver stiffness measurement compared with liver biopsy in the detection of fibrosis ≥F3 in nonalcoholic fatty liver disease patients.

obesity, measurement failure correlates also with more general features of the metabolic syndrome, as well as with limited operator experience [57].

A new transient elastography probe (XL) has been proposed to overcome these limitations for patients who are overweight or obese [54, 55, 58–60]. While the M probe, with a transducer central frequency of 3.5 MHz, can be used when the skin-to-liver capsule distance <2.5 cm (measurement depth 2.5–6.5 cm), the XL probe has a transducer central frequency of 2.5 MHz, so that the LS measurement can be made at a depth of 3.5–7.5 cm and, therefore, can be used

F4	Cut-off (kPa)	AUROC	Se (%)	Sp (%)	PPV (%)	NPV (%)
Yoneda et al. [45]	17.5	0.991	100	96.6	75	100
Wong et al. [48]	10.3 (Sn > 90%)	0.95	92.0	87.8	46.0	99.0
	10.3 (max DA)		92.0	87.8	46.0	99.0
	11.5 (Sp > 90%)		76.0	91.0	48.7	97.1
Kumar et al. [46]	11.8 (Se + Sp max)	0.96	90	88	41	98
	10.6 (Sn > 90%)		100	82	33	100
	19.4 (Sp > 90%)		70	98	78	97
Pathik et al. [49]	20	NR	90	80	NR	NR
Imajo et al. [47]	14	0.92	100	75.9	73	100
Cassinotto et al. [50]	10.2	0.87	89	68	NR	NR

Table 4. Performance of liver stiffness measurement compared with liver biopsy in the detection of cirrhosis in nonalcoholic fatty liver disease patients.

when the skin-to-liver capsule distance ranges between 2.5 and 3.5 cm. The measurement failure is significantly less frequent when using the XL probe than the standard M probe (1.1% versus 16%; p < 0.00005) [54]. Unreliable results were still observed with the XL probe, but only in 25%, as opposed to 50% of cases with the M probe ($p < 0.00005$) [57]. The main limiting factors for the XL probe are a skin-to-liver capsule distance >3.4 cm and extreme obesity (BMI > 40 kg/m^2) [54].

It is worth mentioning that, when measured with the XL probe, the median LS is significantly lower than that measured with the M probe (6.9 kPa vs. 8.4 kPa, respectively) [55, 58]. In accordance to the existing literature, the LS cut-off values should be approximately 1.5–2 kPa lower for the same stage of fibrosis when the XL probe is used rather than the M probe [1]. As a result, the cut-off values defined for the M probe cannot be applied to the XL probe, as well.

3.9. Follow-up of patients

Monitoring the progression of fibrosis is also necessary in the follow-up of these patients. European Association for Study of Liver and Asociacion Latinoamericana para el Estudio del Higado [17] and some authors [61] have shown that, indeed, LS measurement may be used to monitor hepatic fibrosis severity in patients with NAFLD, but additional prospective studies are necessary [1]. According to the existing guidelines, follow-up assessment by either serum biomarkers or TE for the progression of liver fibrosis should be performed among NAFLD patients at 3-year interval [17].

3.10. Errors of interpretation of LS values

The liver is an organ wrapped in a distensible but nonelastic envelope (Glisson's capsula). As a result, additional tissue abnormalities (edema, inflammation, cholestasis, congestion), may interfere with LS measurements, independently of fibrosis: increased cytolysis [62–64], extrahepatic cholestasis [65], congestive heart failure [66] and food intake [28, 29]. These error factors should be taken into consideration whenever interpreting LS values since they may overestimate the fibrosis stage [57]. The influence of steatosis on liver stiffness is still rather controversial; some studies indicate that steatosis may lead to higher liver stiffness, independently of fibrosis [53, 67], whereas others did not find the same effect [48]. It follows that more studies are needed to clarify this aspect, especially in NAFLD patients examined with both the M and the XL probe.

3.11. Prediction of steatosis in NAFLD patients using CAP measurements

The new parameter, which can be measured using the Fibroscan® equipment, the controlled attenuation parameter (CAP), has proven, in our and other authors' experience, to correlate significantly only with steatosis, not with other pathological anomalies encountered in patients with diffuse liver diseases (inflammation, ballooning or fibrosis) [26, 47, 54, 68–75].

An increase of the CAP value can be seen alongside the increase in steatosis grade, but there is some degree of overlap between adjacent grades, especially between moderate and severe steatosis [68].

The studies on the assessment of CAP performance in grading steatosis were predominantly aimed at groups of patients with various diffuse liver diseases, not only NAFLD. For the prediction of steatosis >10%, the CAP cut-off values vary in different studies between 214 dB/m and 289 dB/m, with a 64–91% sensitivity range and a 64–94% specificity range and the AUROC between 0.68 and 0.91. For the prediction of steatosis >33%, the cut-offs range between 259 dB/m and 311 dB/m, with a 57–89% sensitivity range and a 62–94% specificity range and the AUROC between 0.73 and 0.95. For the prediction of severe steatosis (>66%), the cut-offs range between 281 dB/m and 318 dB/m, with a 71–100% sensitivity range and a 47–82.5% specificity range and the AUROC between 0.70 and 0.93 [26, 47, 68–76]. According to these studies, CAP is useful in the detection of $S \geq 10\%$, $S \geq 33\%$ and $S \geq 66\%$, as a result of its good sensitivity and specificity; however, the exact cut-off values remain to be defined [1].

A recent meta-analysis including 2735 patients, 20% having NAFLD [77], has established the optimal CAP cut-offs for the prediction of mild, moderate and severe steatosis as, respectively, 248 dB/m, 268 dB/m, and 280 dB/m, with 66.8%, 77.3%, respectively 88.2% sensibility, and 82.2%, 81.2%, respectively 77.6% specificity (**Table 5**). According to this meta-analysis [77], covariates such as etiology, BMI and diabetes should be taken into account when interpreting CAP, but sex, age and fibrosis play a much smaller role. The authors recommend using the cut-offs established here, but deducting 10 dB/m from the CAP value for NAFLD/NASH patients, 10 dB/m for diabetes patients and deducting or adding 4.4 dB/m for each unit of BMI above or below 25 kg/m² over the range of 20–30 kg/m² [77].

In conclusion, CAP is a noninvasive method for the assessment of steatosis in chronic liver disease patients, including NASH, with a diagnosis accuracy of 76.11–82.06% [68], which is independently influenced only by the amount of steatosis. Due to its negative predictive value of 93.5–98.7%, CAP could become a useful clinical tool especially in excluding significant steatosis grades [68]. Large studies are required in order to develop new cut-off values for liver

	S0 vs. S1–S3	S0–S1 vs. S2–S3	S0–S2 vs. S3
Optimal cut off, dB/m	248 (237–261)	268 (257–284)	280 (268–294)
AUC	0.823 (0.809–0.837)	0.865 (0.850–0.880)	0.882 (0.858–0.906)
Sensitivity	0.688 (0.600–0.750)	0.773 (0.690–0.838)	0.882 (0.765–0.956)
False negative rate	0.312 (0.250–0.400)	0.227 (0.162–0.310)	0.118 (0.044–0.235)
Specificity	0.822 (0.761–0.897)	0.812 (0.749–0.879)	0.776 (0.720–0.821)
False positive rate	0.178 (0.103–0.239)	0.188 (0.121–0.251)	0.224 (0.179–0.280)

Table 5. Optimal CAP cut-off values, based on the maximal sum of sensitivity and specificity (Youden index) in predicting steatosis (modified after Karlas et al. [77]).

fibrosis staging using the XL probe and to investigate the differences between the CAP cut-off values used for the M and XL probes [1].

3.12. Advantages of transient elastography with controlled attenuation parameter

TE, the most widely used and validated noninvasive technique, offers several advantages [1, 26, 57, 68, 71]: it is user-friendly, machine-independent and painless, has a short duration of examination and does not require corrections to be made for gain, frequency, focusing or beam diffraction. This technique is highly reproducible, has well-defined quality criteria and allows the simultaneous assessment of liver stiffness (for fibrosis) and CAP (for steatosis) in the same region of the liver. Compared to liver biopsy, the technique is less prone to sampling errors as it explores a liver volume about 100 times larger. Furthermore, the method also has several clinical applications for patients with NAFLD.

3.13. Limitations of transient elastography with controlled attenuation parameter

TE does have some limitations [1], which may lead to measurement failure: ascites (the vibrations do not propagate through liquids), obesity (especially at BMI > 30 kg/m^2) and narrow intercostal spaces. On the other hand, however, some of these limitations may be overcome by using the XL probe (for obese patients) and the S probe (for children). Another limitation of the technique is the overestimation of fibrosis because of increased liver stiffness due to high cytolysis, extrahepatic cholestasis and congestive heart failure.

3.14. Conclusion about the use of TE in NAFLD

In conclusion, TE may prove useful to NAFLD patients especially for the exclusion of significant fibrosis and cirrhosis. However, we must consider the rather high rate of measurement failure in these patients. The XL probe may overcome this problem in obese patients, but new cut-offs should be defined for the prediction of fibrosis, since the ones of the M probe are not applicable for the XL one [1, 57]. Follow-up assessment by TE for the progression of liver fibrosis should be performed among NAFLD patients at 3-year interval [17].

On the other hand, CAP provides a standardized noninvasive measure of hepatic steatosis. According to the latest and most comprehensive meta-analysis [77], the optimal cut-offs for the prediction of mild, moderate and severe steatosis are 248, 268, and 280 dB/m, respectively. Some authors recommend using the cut-offs established here, but deducting 10 dB/m from the CAP value for NAFLD/NASH patients, 10 dB/m for diabetes patients and deducting or adding 4.4 dB/m for each unit of BMI above or below 25 kg/m^2 over the range of 20–30 kg/m^2 [77]. Longitudinal data are needed to demonstrate how CAP relates to clinical outcomes.

4. Acoustic radiation force impulse elastography (ARFI)

Of the "Point SWE" techniques, we will review some features of the ARFI technique (acoustic radiation force impulse elastography), the only technique in this category whose role in the assessment of NAFLD patients has, albeit insufficiently, been analyzed.

4.1. Principle

The ARFI imaging technology involves the mechanical excitation of tissue using short-duration acoustic pulses (push pulses) in a region of interest chosen by the examiner, producing shear waves that spread away from the region of interest, perpendicularly to the acoustic push pulse, generating localized, micron-scale displacements in the tissue [78–80]. Simultaneously, detection waves of lower intensity than that of the push pulse are generated. The shear wave velocity—SWV (m/s) can be calculated taking into account the place and moment of interaction between the shear waves and the detection waves [80–83]. The stiffer the tissue, the higher the shear wave velocity [80–83]. The shear wave velocity is measured in a smaller volume than in transient elastography (10 mm long and 6 mm wide), but, unlike TE, it can be chosen by the operator under B-mode visualization [57], since ARFI is implemented on some ultrasound equipments, alongside the B-mode, color Doppler and contrast modes [17, 80, 84].

4.2. Examination technique

The patient is placed in a dorsal decubitus position, with the right arm in maximum abduction. The transducer is placed in an intercostal space, and the region of interest (10/5 mm) is chosen in an area of the right liver parenchyma (segments 5 or 8), 1–2 cm below the liver capsule; the measurement is performed after asking the patient to hold his/her breath after an expiration to prevent breathing movements [85]. In general, the median value of 10 valid measurements of the shear wave is taken into consideration; sometimes, no valid measurement can be obtained. When taking into account the manufacturer recommendations, we can identify some possible causes, which, alone or in combination, may lead to this situation:

- excessive movements of the liver tissue—for instance, cardiac pulsations transmitted to the liver parenchyma (impaired estimation of shear wave velocity);

- marked signal attenuation in obese patients (impaired identification of the shear wave by the system);

- marked tissue stiffness (impaired estimation of shear wave velocity—shear wave outside of the confidence interval).

On the whole, however, the failure rate of ARFI is significantly lower than that of TE (2.9% vs. 6.4%, $p < 0.001$), especially in patients with ascites or obesity [86].

Ten valid measurements are performed in the right liver lobe, a median value is calculated and the result is expressed in meters/second.

pSWE measurements using Virtual Touch Quantification (VTQ®) in healthy populations range between 1.01 and 1.59 m/s, but in most studies the range is 1.07–1.16 m/s [87–89].

4.3. Errors of interpretation of LS values using the ARFI technique

Like TE, ARFI results are influenced by food intake [90] as well as necroinflammatory activity and aminotransferase levels [91], all of which lead to an overestimation of liver fibrosis and have to be taken into account when interpreting the results [17].

LS values obtained with ARFI, in contrast to TE values, have a narrow range (0.5–4.4 m/s). Defining cut-off values for discriminating certain fibrosis stages is therefore restricted, as well as making management decisions.

4.4. Diagnostic performance of ARFI in NASH

There are few studies assessing the performance of ARFI in NAFLD. The majority of studies included patients with diffuse liver diseases, with only a fraction of NAFLD patients. In most studies, the cut-offs for the prediction of F1 vary between 1.105–1.34 m/s, with 76.7% sensibility and 71.4% specificity; for F $\geq$ 2, between 1.137–1.179 m/s, with Se 71–97% and Sp 67–92%; for F $\geq$ 3, between 1.45–2.20 m/s, with Se 75–100% and Sp 68–95.2%, and for the prediction of cirrhosis, between 1.61–2.90 m/s, with Se 74–100% and Sp 67–96% [92–98].

ARFI performs better in severe fibrosis and cirrhosis than in significant fibrosis, with AUROCs ranging from 0.91 to 0.98 and from 0.66 to 0.86, respectively [97].

A systematic review of seven studies with a total of 723 patients who underwent shear wave velocity measurements with VTQ® technique to evaluate the diagnostic efficacy of pSWE in patients with NAFLD showed that the summary Se and Sp of ARFI in detecting significant fibrosis were 80.2 and 85.2% [99], which is not an appropriate endpoint [17].

In conclusion, ARFI elastography appears to be modestly accurate in detecting significant fibrosis, but performs well in predicting severe fibrosis and cirrhosis in NAFLD patients. As for its use in the follow-up of patients, no data are available for this technique for the moment.

5. Two-dimensional SWE (2D-SWE)

5.1. Principle

2D-SWE is based on the combination of a radiation force induced in tissues by focused ultrasonic beams and a very high frame rate ultrasound imaging sequence capable of catching in real time the transient propagation of resulting shear waves [17, 19, 100]. The shear wave speed is estimated by a Doppler-like acquisition over a region of interest (ROI) and it is used to calculate the tissue stiffness. The relationship between Young's modulus (E) and the shear wave (c) is $E = 3\rho c^2$ (ρ = tissue density) [19, 20, 100, 101].

The elasticity is displayed using a color-coded image superimposed on a B-mode image: stiffer tissues in red and softer tissues in blue [19, 20, 100, 101]. In addition, a quantitative measurement of the liver stiffness in the chosen region of interest is performed. The equipment allows the visualization of results both in kPa and in m/s, with a maximum value reaching 300 kPa (10 m/s) [102, 103].

Almost all 2D-SWE studies for liver applications have been carried out using Supersonic Imagine equipments (Aixplorer, Supersonic Imagine, Aix en Provence, France), because other companies have only recently introduced 2D-SWE products [17].

5.2. The examination technique

The examination is performed after an overnight fast, with the patient placed in a dorsal decubitus position, with the right arm in maximum abduction, in order to enlarge the intercostal spaces and ensure the best access to the right liver lobe parenchyma [103]. The region of interest (ROI) for the elastography examination is placed in the center of the screen, choosing an homogeneous area of parenchyma, free of any large vascular structure and at least 2 cm below the liver capsule, to prevent any risk of overestimation of fibrosis due to the higher capsular and subcapsular fibrosis content. The ROI with color-coded elastographic information is displayed overlapped on the 2D image; its size can be adjusted up to 3×3 cm, and the depth, although adjustable, should be kept within 8 cm [102].

There is no consensus on the *number of measurements* required for a good quality assessment [20]: some studies recommend 3 [104–106], 4 [107] or 5 [108–110].

Similar to pSWE/ARFI, *quality criteria* for 2D-SWE remain to be defined. Until now, such criteria have only been proposed in a study on patients with portal hypertension, but they still require validation on prospective studies on large groups of biopsied patients [106]: "highly reliable" (when the ratio between standard deviation/median LS ≤0.10 and measurement depth < 5.6 cm); "reliable" (when standard deviation/median LS >0.10 or measurement depth ≥ 5.6 cm); respectively "unreliable" (when standard deviation/median LS >0.10 and measurement depth ≥ 5.6 cm). The "highly reliable" and "reliable" measurements are considered acceptable; only the "unreliable" ones are considered unacceptable for evaluation and should be rejected [106].

5.3. Technique failure

The liver stiffness cannot be assessed by 2D-SWE in around 10.4% of cases, more frequently in obese patients or in patients with a thoracic wall thicker than 25 mm in the intercostal spaces [111]. Generally speaking, the following factors may be associated with a higher rate of invalid measurements: narrow intercostal spaces [107], high BMI and thoracic wall thicker than 25 mm in the intercostal spaces [111].

5.4. Normal range of liver stiffness as evaluated by 2D-SWE

Studies performed on subjects with healthy livers, pathologically confirmed potential donors, yielded a mean normal value of liver stiffness in 2D-SWE of 4.4–4.9 kPa (range 2.2–6.2 kPa), not correlated significantly with age, BMI or steatosis [100, 105, 107, 109].

5.5. Performance of 2D-SWE in assessing nonalcoholic steatohepatitis

Some studies on the performance of this method in diffuse liver diseases of various etiologies included a certain proportion of NASH patients. The resulting cut-offs varied between 6.2–7.8 kPa for ≥F1, 7.1–10.49 kPa for ≥F2, 8.7–11.5 kPa for ≥F3 and 9.59–18.1 kPa for F4 [112]. 2D-SWE performance for the prediction of each fibrosis stage seems to be similar when including all patients, regardless of etiology, as well as when including only viral hepatic diseases, with AUROCs between 0.80 and 0.82 [103]. In two meta-analyses, with a total of 2303 and 934 patients, respectively, the summary area under the curve (AUC) was 0.85 for ≥F1, 0.87–0.88 for ≥F2, 0.93–0.94 for ≥F3 and 0.92–0.94 for F4 [112, 113].

In a study performed on 291 NAFLD patients, the chosen cut-offs for the prediction of ≥F2 were 6.3 kPa (Se 90%, Sp 50%) and 8.7 kPa (Se 71%, Sp 90%), with AUROC 0.86; for the prediction of fibrosis ≥F3, 8.3 kPa (Se 91%, Sp 71%) and 10.7 kPa (Se 71%, Sp 90%), with AUROC 0.89 and for the prediction of cirrhosis, 10.5 kPa (Se 90%, Sp 72%) and 14.4 kPa (Se 58%, Sp 90%), with AUROC 0.88 [50].

6. Conclusions: SSI, Fibroscan® or ARFI?

After comparing the performance in the assessment of NAFLD of the three elastographic methods discussed above, we can conclude, on the preliminary results, that the diagnostic performance according to the AUROC values for the diagnosis of significant fibrosis, severe fibrosis and cirrhosis is good for SSI (0.86–0.89); good for Fibroscan® (0.82–0.87) and fair or good for ARFI (0.77–0.84) [50]. The AUROC values for diagnosing severe fibrosis or cirrhosis are particularly good for SSI or Fibroscan® (0.86 and 0.89) [50].

The prediction of steatosis, however, can at this moment only be made using the controlled attenuation parameter measured with Fibroscan®.

As for the causes of measurement failure or unreliable results, we mention clinical factors related to obesity (BMI > 30 kg/m^2, waist circumference ≥ 102 cm or increased wall thickness), which are associated with liver stiffness measurement failures when using SSI or Fibroscan® and with unreliable results when using ARFI [50].

In conclusion, SSI, Fibroscan® and ARFI are valuable diagnostic tools for the staging of liver fibrosis in NAFLD patients. However, the diagnostic accuracy of SSI appears to be superior to that of ARFI for the diagnosis of F2 or above [50]. Most of the cut-off values for SSI for the diagnosis of different stages of liver disease are quite similar to those of Fibroscan®; this is an issue of great importance for the applicability of this technique and its wide dissemination among radiologists and hepatologists in their daily practice. However, as for the M probe of Fibroscan®, the SSI technique remains limited by a high failure rate in cases of obesity, whereas ARFI has a high rate of unreliable results [50].

Acknowledgements

This work was supported by a grant of the Romanian National Authority for Scientific Research and Innovation, CNCS – UEFISCDI, project number PN-II-RU-TE-2014-4-2023.

Author details

Monica Lupsor-Platon

Address all correspondence to: monica.lupsor@umfcluj.ro

Department of Medical Imaging, Iuliu Hatieganu University of Medicine and Pharmacy, Regional Institute of Gastroenterology and Hepatology "Prof. Dr. Octavian Fodor", Cluj-Napoca, Romania

References

[1] Mikolasevic I, Orlic L, Franjic N, Hauser G, Stimac D, Milic S. Transient elastography (FibroScan(®)) with controlled attenuation parameter in the assessment of liver steatosis and fibrosis in patients with nonalcoholic fatty liver disease—Where do we stand? World Journal of Gastroenterology. 2016;**22**(32):7236-7251. DOI: 10.3748/wjg.v22.i32.7236

[2] Bang KB, Cho YK. Comorbidities and metabolic derangement of NAFLD. Journal of Lifestyle Medicine. 2015;**5**(1):7-13. DOI: 10.15280/jlm.2015.5.1.7

[3] Cho Y, Tokuhara D, Morikawa H, Kuwae Y, Hayashi E, Hirose M, et al. Transient elastography-based liver profiles in a hospital-based pediatric population in Japan. PLoS One. 2015;**10**(9):e0137239. DOI: 10.1371/journal.pone.0137239

[4] Byrne CD, Targher GNAFLD. A multisystem disease. Journal of Hepatology. 2015;**62** (1 Suppl):S47-S64. DOI: 10.1016/j.jhep.2014.12.012

[5] Smits MM, Ioannou GN, Boyko EJ, Utzschneider KM. Non-alcoholic fatty liver disease as an independent manifestation of the metabolic syndrome: Results of a US national survey in three ethnic groups. Journal of Gastroenterology and Hepatology. 2013;**28**(4):664-670. DOI: 10.1111/jgh.12106

[6] Bedossa P, Dargère D, Paradis V. Sampling variability of liver fibrosis in chronic hepatitis C. Hepatology. 2003;**38**(6):1449-1457. DOI: 10.1016/j.hep.2003.09.022

[7] Regev A, Berho M, Jeffers LJ, Milikowski C, Molina EG, Pyrsopoulos NT, et al. Sampling error and intraobserver variation in liver biopsy in patients with chronic HCV infection. The American Journal of Gastroenterology. 2002;**97**(10):2614-2618. DOI: 10.1111/j.1572-0241.2002.06038.x

[8] Ratziu V, Charlotte F, Heurtier A, Gombert S, Giral P, Bruckert E, et al. Sampling variability of liver biopsy in nonalcoholic fatty liver disease. Gastroenterology. 2005;**128**(7):1898-1906. DOI: http://dx.doi.org/10.1053/j.gastro.2005.03.084

[9] Siddique I, El-Naga HA, Madda JP, Memon A, Hasan F. Sampling variability on percutaneous liver biopsy in patients with chronic hepatitis C virus infection. Scandinavian Journal of Gastroenterology. 2003;**38**(4):427-432

[10] Goldstein NS, Hastah F, Galan MV, Gordon SC. Fibrosis heterogeneity in nonalcoholic steatohepatitis and hepatitis C virus needle core biopsy specimens. American Journal of Clinical Pathology. 2005;123(3):382-387. DOI: 10.1309/EY72-F1EN-9XCB-1KXX

[11] Boursier J, Calès P. Controlled attenuation parameter (CAP): A new device for fast evaluation of liver fat? Liver International. 2012;32(6):875-877. DOI: 10.1111/j.1478-3231.2012.02824.x

[12] Leandro G, Mangia A, Hui J, Fabris P, Rubbia-Brandt L, Colloredo G, et al. HCV Meta-Analysis (on) Individual Patients' Data Study Group. Relationship between steatosis, inflammation, and fibrosis in chronic hepatitis C: A meta-analysis of individual patient data. Gastroenterology. 2006;130:1636-1642. DOI: http://dx.doi.org/10.1053/j.gastro.2006.03.014

[13] Poynard T, Ratziu V, McHutchison J, Manns M, Goodman Z, Zeuzem S, et al. Effect of treatment with peginterferon or interferon alfa-2b and ribavirin on steatosis in patients infected with hepatitis C. Hepatology. 2003;38(1):75-85. DOI: 10.1053/jhep.2003.50267

[14] Spitzer AL, Lao OB, Dick AA, Bakthavatsalam R, Halldorson JB, Yeh MM, Upton MP, Reyes JD, Perkins JD. The biopsied donor liver: Incorporating macrosteatosis into high-risk donor assessment. Liver Transplantation. 2010;16:874-884. DOI: 10.1002/lt.22085

[15] de Meijer VE, Kalish BT, Puder M, Ijzermans JN. Systematic review and meta-analysis of steatosis as a risk factor in major hepatic resection. The British Journal of Surgery. 2010;97:1331-1339. DOI: 10.1002/bjs.7194

[16] Younossi ZM, Stepanova M, Afendy M, Fang Y, Younossi Y, Mir H, et al. Changes in the prevalence of the most common causes of chronic liver diseases in the United States from 1988 to 2008. Clinical Gastroenterology and Hepatology. 2011;9:524-530. DOI: 10.1016/j.cgh.2011.03.020

[17] European Association for Study of Liver; Asociacion Latinoamericana para el Estudio del Higado. EASL-ALEH clinical practice guidelines: Non-invasive tests for evaluation of liver disease severity and prognosis. Journal of Hepatology. 2015;63(1):237-264. DOI: 10.1016/j.jhep.2015.04.006

[18] Dietrich CF, Bamber J, Berzigotti A, Bota S, Cantisani V, Castera L, et al. EFSUMB guidelines and recommendations on the clinical use of liver ultrasound elastography, update 2017 (long version). Ultraschall Med. 2017:38(4):e16-e47. DOI: 10.1055/s-0043-103952

[19] Bamber J, Cosgrove D, Dietrich CF, Fromageau J, Bojunga J, Calliada F, et al. EFSUMB guidelines and recommendations on the clinical use of ultrasound elastography. Part 1: Basic principles and technology. Ultraschall in der Medizin. 2013;34(2):169-184. DOI: 10.1055/s-0033-1335205

[20] Sporea I, Bota S, Săftoiu A, Şirli R, Gradinăru-Taşcău O, Popescu A, et al. Romanian national guidelines and practical recommendations on liver elastography. Medical Ultrasonography. 2014;16(2):123-138. DOI: 10.11152/mu.2013.2066.162.is1sb2

[21] Lupşor M, Badea R. Elastografia unidimensională tranzitorie. In Badea R, Dudea S, Mircea PM. Stamate M. Tratat de Ultrasonografie clinică, Vol III. Bucuresti: Ed Medicala; 2008. pp. 675-685

[22] Lupşor M, Badea R, Stefănescu H. Evaluarea neinvazivă a fibrozei hepatice. In: Pascu O, Grigorescu M, Acalovschi M, Andreica V, editors. Gastroenterologie. Hepatologie – Bazele practicii clinice. Cluj Napoca: Ed. Medicală Universitară Iuliu Haţieganu; 2010. pp. 402-408

[23] Yeh WC, Li PC, Jeng YM, Hsu HC, Kuo PL, Li ML, et al. Elastic modulus measurements of human liver and correlation with pathology. Ultrasound in Medicine & Biology. 2002;**28**(4):467-474

[24] Sandrin L, Fourquet B, Hasquenoph JM, Yon S, Fournier C, Mal F, et al. Transient elastography: A new noninvasive method for assessment of hepatic fibrosis. Ultrasound in Medicine & Biology. 2003;**29**(12):1705-1713. DOI: http://dx.doi.org/10.1016/j.ultrasmedbio.2003.07.001

[25] Lupsor M, Stefanescu H, Feier D, Badea R. Non-invasive evaluation of liver steatosis, fibrosis and cirrhosis in hepatitis C virus infected patients using unidimensional transient elastography (Fibroscan®). In: Tagaya N, editor. Liver Biopsy—Indications, Procedures, Results. Croatia: Intech; 2012. pp. 209-234. DOI: 10.5772/52621

[26] Sasso M, Beaugrand M, de Ledinghen V, Douvin C, Marcellin P, Poupon R, et al. Controlled attenuation parameter (CAP): A novel VCTE™ guided ultrasonic attenuation measurement for the evaluation of hepatic steatosis: Preliminary study and validation in a cohort of patients with chronic liver disease from various causes. Ultrasound in Medicine & Biology. 2010;**36**(11):1825-1835. DOI: 10.1016/j.ultrasmedbio.2010.07.005

[27] Sasso M, Miette V, Sandrin L, Beaugrand M. The controlled attenuation parameter (CAP): A novel tool for the non-invasive evaluation of steatosis using Fibroscan. Clinics and Research in Hepatology and Gastroenterology. 2012;**36**(1):13-20. DOI: 10.1016/j.clinre.2011.08.001

[28] Mederacke I, Wursthorn K, Kirschner J, Rifai K, Manns MP, Wedemeyer H, et al. Food intake increases liver stiffness in patients with chronic or resolved hepatitis C virus infection. Liver International. 2009;**29**(10):1500-1506. DOI: 10.1111/j.1478-3231.2009.02100.x

[29] Arena U, Lupsor Platon M, Stasi C, Moscarella S, Assarat A, Bedogni G, et al. Liver stiffness is influenced by a standardized meal in patients with chronic hcv hepatitis at different stages of fibrotic evolution. Hepatology. 2013;**58**(1):65-72. DOI: 10.1002/hep.26343

[30] Kettaneh A, Marcellin P, Douvin C, Poupon R, Ziol M, Beaugrand M, et al. Features associated with success rate and performance of FibroScan measurements for the diagnosis of cirrhosis in HCV patients: A prospective study of 935 patients. Journal of Hepatology. 2007;**46**(4):628-634. DOI: http://dx.doi.org/10.1016/j.jhep.2006.11.010

[31] Boursier J, Konate A, Guilluy M, Gorea G, Sawadogo A, Quemener E, et al. Learning curve and interobserver reproducibility evaluation of liver stiffness measurement by transient

elastography. European Journal of Gastroenterology & Hepatology. 2008;**20**(7):693-701. DOI: 10.1097/MEG.0b013e3282f51992

[32] Castera L, Forns X, Alberti A. Non-invasive evaluation of liver fibrosis using transient elastography. Journal of Hepatology. 2008;**48**(5):835-847. DOI: 10.1016/j.jhep.2008.02.008

[33] Lucidarme D, Foucher J, Le Bail B, Vergniol J, Castera L, Duburque C, et al. Factors of accuracy of transient elastography (fibroscan) for the diagnosis of liver fibrosis in chronic hepatitis C. Hepatology. 2008;**49**(4):1083-1089. DOI: 10.1002/hep.22748

[34] Boursier J, Zarski JP, de Ledinghen V, Rousselet MC, Sturm N, Lebail B, et al. Determination of reliability criteria for liver stiffness evaluation by transient elastography. Hepatology. 2013;**57**(3):1182-1191. DOI: 10.1002/hep.25993

[35] Fraquelli M, Rigamonti C, Casazza G, Conte D, Donato MF, Ronchi G, et al. Reproducibility of transient elastography in the evaluation of liver fibrosis in patients with chronic liver disease. Gut. 2007;**56**(7):968-973. DOI: 10.1136/gut.2006.111302

[36] Boursier J, Konaté A, Gorea G, Reaud S, Quemener E, Oberti F, et al. Reproducibility of liver stiffness measurement by ultrasonographic elastometry. Clinical Gastroenterology and Hepatology. 2008;**6**(11):1263-1269. DOI: 10.1016/j.cgh.2008.07.006

[37] Roulot D, Czernichow S, Le Clésiau H, Costes JL, Vergnaud AC, Beaugrand M. Liver stiffness values in apparently healthy subjects: Influence of gender and metabolic syndrome. Journal of Hepatology. 2008;**48**(4):606-613. DOI: 10.1016/j.jhep.2007.11.020

[38] Sirli R, Sporea I, Tudora A, Deleanu A, Popescu A. Transient elastographic evaluation of subjects without known hepatic pathology: Does age change the liver stiffness? Journal of Gastrointestinal and Liver Diseases. 2009;**18**(1):57-60

[39] Lupsor Platon M, Stefanescu H, Feier D, Maniu A, Badea R. Performance of unidimensional transient elastography in staging chronic hepatitis C. Results from a cohort of 1,202 biopsied patients from one single center. Journal of Gastrointestinal and Liver Diseases. 2013;**22**(2):157-166

[40] Lupsor M, Badea R, Stefanescu H, Grigorescu M, Serban A, Radu C. Performance of unidimensional transient elastography in staging non-alcoholic steatohepatitis. Journal of Gastrointestinal and Liver Diseases. 2010;**19**(1):53-60

[41] Lupşor M, Badea R, Stefănescu H, Grigorescu M, Sparchez Z, Serban A, et al. Analysis of histopathological changes that influence liver stiffness in chronic hepatitis C. Results from a cohort of 324 patients. Journal of Gastrointestinal and Liver Diseases. 2008;**17**:155-163

[42] Foucher J, Chanteloup E, Vergniol J, Castéra L, Le Bail B, Adhoute X, et al. Diagnosis of cirrhosis by transient elastography (FibroScan): A prospective study. Gut. 2006;**55**:403-408. DOI: 10.1136/gut.2005.069153

[43] Ziol M, Kettaneh A, Ganne-Carrié N, Barget N, Tengher-Barna I, Beaugrand M. Relationships between fibrosis amounts assessed by morphometry and liver stiffness measurements in

chronic hepatitis or steatohepatitis. European Journal of Gastroenterology & Hepatology. 2009;**21**:1261-1268. DOI: 10.1097/MEG.0b013e32832a20f5

[44] Kwok R, Tse YK, Wong GL, Ha Y, Lee AU, Ngu MC, et al. Systematic review with meta-analysis: Non-invasive assessment of non-alcoholic fatty liver disease—The role of transient elastography and plasma cytokeratin-18 fragments. Alimentary Pharmacology & Therapeutics. 2014;**39**(3):254-269. DOI: 10.1111/apt.12569

[45] Yoneda M, Yoneda M, Mawatari H, Fujita K, Endo H, Iida H, et al. Noninvasive assessment of liver fibrosis by measurement of stiffness in patients with nonalcoholic fatty liver disease (NAFLD). Digestive and Liver Disease. 2008;**40**(5):371-378. DOI: http://dx.doi.org/10.1016/j.dld.2007.10.019

[46] Kumar R, Rastogi A, Sharma MK, Bhatia V, Tyagi P, Sharma P, et al. Liver stiffness measurements in patients with different stages of nonalcoholic fatty liver disease: Diagnostic performance and clinicopathological correlation. Digestive Diseases and Sciences. 2013;**58**(1):265-274. DOI: 10.1007/s10620-012-2306-1

[47] Imajo K, Kessoku T, Honda Y, Tomeno W, Ogawa Y, Mawatari H, et al. Magnetic resonance imaging more accurately classifies steatosis and fibrosis in patients with nonalcoholic fatty liver disease than transient elastography. Gastroenterology. 2016;**150**:626-637. DOI: 10.1053/j.gastro.2015.11.048

[48] Wong VW, Vergniol J, Wong GL, Foucher J, Chan HL, Le Bail B, et al. Diagnosis of fibrosis and cirrhosis using liver stiffness measurement in nonalcoholic fatty liver disease. Hepatology. 2010;**51**(2):454-462. DOI: 10.1002/hep.23312

[49] Pathik P, Ravindra S, Ajay C, Prasad B, Jatin P, Prabha S. Fibroscan versus simple noninvasive screening tools in predicting fibrosis in high-risk nonalcoholic fatty liver disease patients from western India. Annals of Gastroenterology. 2015;**28**(2):281-286

[50] Cassinotto C, Boursier J, de Lédinghen V, Lebigot J, Lapuyade B, Cales P, et al. Liver stiffness in nonalcoholic fatty liver disease: A comparison of supersonic shear imaging, FibroScan, and ARFI with liver biopsy. Hepatology. 2016;**63**(6):1817-1827. DOI: 10.1002/hep.28394

[51] Petta S, Vanni E, Bugianesi E, Di Marco V, Cammà C, Cabibi D, et al. The combination of liver stiffness measurement and NAFLD fibrosis score improves the noninvasive diagnostic accuracy for severe liver fibrosis in patients with nonalcoholic fatty liver disease. Liver International. 2015;**35**:1566-1573. DOI: 10.1111/liv.12584

[52] Naveau S, Lamouri K, Pourcher G, Njiké-Nakseu M, Ferretti S, Courie R, et al. The diagnostic accuracy of transient elastography for the diagnosis of liver fibrosis in bariatric surgery candidates with suspected NAFLD. Obesity Surgery. 2014;**24**:1693-1701. DOI: 10.1007/s11695-014-1235-9

[53] Gaia S, Carenzi S, Barilli AL, Bugianesi E, Smedile A, Brunello F, et al. Reliability of transient elastography for the detection of fibrosis in non-alcoholic fatty liver disease

and chronic viral hepatitis. Journal of Hepatology. 2011;**54**(1):64-71. DOI: 10.1016/j. jhep.2010.06.022

[54] Myers RP, Pomier-Layrargues G, Kirsch R, Pollett A, Duarte-Rojo A, Wong D, et al. Feasibility and diagnostic performance of the FibroScan XL probe for liver stiffness measurement in overweight and obese patients. Hepatology. 2012;**55**(1):199-208. DOI: 10.1002/hep.24624

[55] Wong VW, Vergniol J, Wong GL, Foucher J, Chan AW, Chermak F, et al. Liver stiffness measurement using XL probe in patients with nonalcoholic fatty liver disease. The American Journal of Gastroenterology. 2012;**107**(12):1862-1871. DOI: 10.1038/ ajg.2012.331

[56] Petta S, Di Marco V, Cammà C, Butera G, Cabibi D, Craxì A. Reliability of liver stiffness measurement in non-alcoholic fatty liver disease: The effects of body mass index. Alimentary Pharmacology & Therapeutics. 2011;**33**(12):1350-1360. DOI: 10.1111/ j.1365-2036.2011. 04668.x

[57] Castera L, Vilgrain V, Angulo P. Noninvasive evaluation of NAFLD. Nature Reviews. Gastroenterology & Hepatology. 2013;**10**(11):666-675. DOI: 10.1038/nrgastro.2013

[58] Friedrich-Rust M, Hadji-Hosseini H, Kriener S, Herrmann E, Sircar I, Kau A, et al. Transient elastography with a new probe for obese patients for non-invasive staging of non-alcoholic steatohepatitis. European Radiology. 2010;**20**(10):2390-2396. DOI: 10.1007/ s00330-010-1820-9

[59] de Lédinghen V, Vergniol J, Foucher J, El-Hajbi F, Merrouche W, Rigalleau V. Feasibility of liver transient elastography with FibroScan using a new probe for obese patients. Liver International. 2010;**30**(7):1043-1048. DOI: 10.1111/j.1478-3231.2010.02258.x

[60] de Lédinghen V, Wong VW, Vergniol J, Wong GL, Foucher J, Chu SH, et al. Diagnosis of liver fibrosis and cirrhosis using liver stiffness measurement: Comparison between M and XL probe of FibroScan®. Journal of Hepatology. 2012;**56**(4):833-839. DOI: 10.1016/j. jhep.2011.10.017

[61] Suzuki K, Yoneda M, Imajo K, Kirikoshi H, Nakajima A, Maeda S, et al. Transient elastography for monitoring the fibrosis of non-alcoholic fatty liver disease for 4 years. Hepatology Research. 2013;**43**:979-983. DOI: 10.1111/hepr.12039

[62] Coco B, Oliveri F, Maina AM, Ciccorossi P, Sacco R, Colombatto P, et al. Transient elastography: A new surrogate marker of liver fibrosis influenced by major changes of transaminases. Journal of Viral Hepatitis. 2007;**14**(5):360-369. DOI: 10.1111/j.1365-2893.2006. 00811.x

[63] Sagir A, Erhardt A, Schmitt M, Häussinger D. Transient elastography is unreliable for detection of cirrhosis in patients with acute liver damage. Hepatology. 2008;**47**(2):592-595. DOI: 10.1002/hep.22056

[64] Arena U, Vizzutti F, Corti G, Ambu S, Stasi C, Bresci S, et al. Acute viral hepatitis increases liver stiffness values measured by transient elastography. Hepatology. 2008;47(2): 380-384. DOI: 10.1002/hep.22007

[65] Millonig G, Reimann FM, Friedrich S, Fonouni H, Mehrabi A, Büchler MW, et al. Extrahepatic cholestasis increases liver stiffness (FibroScan) irrespective of fibrosis. Hepatology. 2008;48(5):1718-1723. DOI: 10.1002/hep.22577

[66] Millonig G, Friedrich S, Adolf S, Fonouni H, Golriz M, Mehrabi A, et al. Liver stiffness is directly influenced by central venous pressure. Journal of Hepatology. 2010;52(2): 206-210. DOI: 10.1016/j.jhep.2009.11.018

[67] Petta S, Maida M, Macaluso FS, Di Marco V, Cammà C, Cabibi D, et al. The severity of steatosis influences liver stiffness measurement in patients with nonalcoholic fatty liver disease. Hepatology. 2015;62(4):1101-1110. DOI: 10.1002/hep.27844

[68] Lupşor-Platon M, Feier D, Stefănescu H, Tamas A, Botan E, Sparchez Z, et al. Diagnostic accuracy of controlled attenuation parameter measured by transient elastography for the non-invasive assessment of liver steatosis: A prospective study. Journal of Gastrointestinal and Liver Diseases. 2015;24:35-42. DOI: 10.15403/jgld.2014.1121.mlp

[69] Wang Y, Fan Q, Wang T, Wen J, Wang H, Zhang T. Controlled attenuation parameter for assessment of hepatic steatosis grades: A diagnostic meta-analysis. International Journal of Clinical and Experimental Medicine 2015;8(10):17654-17663. eCollection 2015

[70] Shi KQ, Tang JZ, Zhu XL, Ying L, Li DW, Gao J, et al. Controlled attenuation parameter for the detection of steatosis severity in chronic liver disease: A meta-analysis of diagnostic accuracy. Journal of Gastroenterology and Hepatology. 2014;29:1149-1158. DOI: 10.1111/jgh.12519

[71] de Lédinghen V, Vergniol J, Foucher J, Merrouche W, le Bail B. Non-invasive diagnosis of liver steatosis using controlled attenuation parameter (CAP) and transient elastography. Liver International. 2012;32:911-918. DOI: 10.1111/j.1478-3231.2012.02820.x

[72] Kumar M, Rastogi A, Singh T, Behari C, Gupta E, Garg H, et al. Controlled attenuation parameter for noninvasive assessment of hepatic steatosis: Does etiology affect performance? Journal of Gastroenterology and Hepatology. 2013;28:1194-1201. DOI: 10.1111/jgh.12134

[73] Shen F, Zheng RD, Mi YQ, Wang XY, Pan Q, Chen GY, et al. Controlled attenuation parameter for non-invasive assessment of hepatic steatosis in Chinese patients. World Journal of Gastroenterology. 2014;20:4702-4711. DOI: 10.3748/wjg.v20.i16.4702

[74] Chan WK, Nik Mustapha NR, Mahadeva S. Controlled attenuation parameter for the detection and quantification of hepatic steatosis in nonalcoholic fatty liver disease. Journal of Gastroenterology and Hepatology. 2014;29:1470-1476. DOI: 10.1111/jgh.12557

[75] de Lédinghen V, Vergniol J, Capdepont M, Chermak F, Hiriart JB, Cassinotto C, et al. Controlled attenuation parameter (CAP) for the diagnosis of steatosis: A prospective

study of 5323 examinations. Journal of Hepatology. 2014;**60**:1026-1031. DOI: 10.1016/j. jhep.2013.12.018

[76] Myers RP, Pollett A, Kirsch R, Pomier-Layrargues G, Beaton M, Levstik M, et al. Controlled attenuation parameter (CAP): A noninvasive method for the detection of hepatic steatosis based on transient elastography. Liver International. 2012;**32**:902-910. DOI: 10.1111/j.1478-3231.2012.02781.x

[77] Karlas T, Petroff D, Sasso M, Fan JG, Mi YQ, de Lédinghen V, et al. Individual patient data meta-analysis of controlled attenuation parameter (CAP) technology for assessing steatosis. Journal of Hepatology. 2017;**66**(5):1022-1030. DOI: 10.1016/j.jhep.2016.12.022

[78] Madsen EL, Sathoff HJ, Zagzebski JA. Ultrasonic shear wave properties of soft tissues and tissuelike materials. The Journal of the Acoustical Society of America. 1983;**74**:1346-1355

[79] Frizzell LA, Carstensen EL. Shear properties of mammalian tissues at low megahertz frequencies. The Journal of the Acoustical Society of America. 1976;**60**:1409-1411

[80] Lupsor M, Badea R, Stefanescu H, Sparchez Z, Branda H, Serban A, et al. Performance of a new elastographic method (ARFI technology) compared to unidimensional transient elastography in the noninvasive assessment of chronic hepatitis C. Preliminary results. Journal of Gastrointestinal and Liver Diseases. 2009;**18**(3):303-310

[81] Zhai L, Palmeri ML, Bouchard RR, Nightingale RW, Nightingale KR. An integrated indenter-ARFI imaging system for tissue stiffness quantification. Ultrasonic Imaging. 2008;**30**:95-111. DOI: 10.1177/016173460803000203

[82] Nightingale K, Soo MS, Nightingale R, Trahey G. Acoustic radiation force impulse imaging: In vivo demonstration of clinical feasibility. Ultrasound in Medicine & Biology. 2002;**28**:227-235. DOI: http://dx.doi.org/10.1016/S0301-5629(01)00499-9

[83] Mauldin FW Jr, Zhu HT, Behler RH, Nichols TC, Gallippi CM. Robust principal component analysis and clustering methods for automated classification of tissue response to ARFI excitation. Ultrasound in Medicine & Biology. 2008;**34**:309-325. DOI: 10.1016/j. ultrasmedbio.2007.07.019

[84] Fahey BJ, Nightingale KR, Nelson RC, Palmeri ML, Trahey GE. Acoustic radiation force impulse imaging of the abdomen: Demonstration of feasibility and utility. Ultrasound in Medicine & Biology. 2005;**31**:1185-1198. DOI: http://dx.doi.org/10.1016/j. ultrasmedbio.2005.05.004

[85] Bota S, Mare R, Sporea I. Point shear wave elastography. In: Sporea I, Sirli R, editors. Hepatic Elastography Using Ultrasound Waves. Revised edition of volume 1. Sharjah, UAE: Bentham Science Publishers; 2016. pp. 44-87. DOI: 10.2174/97816080546331120101

[86] Bota S, Herkner H, Sporea I, Salzl P, Sirli R, Neghina AM, et al. Meta-analysis: ARFI elastography versus transient elastography for the evaluation of liver fibrosis. Liver International. 2013;**33**(8):1138-1147. DOI: 10.1111/liv.12240

[87] Popescu A, Sporea I, Sirli R, Bota S, Focşa M, Dănilă M, et al. The mean values of liver stiffness assessed by acoustic radiation force impulse elastography in normal subjects. Medical Ultrasonography. 2011;13(1):33-37

[88] Son CY, Kim SU, Han WK, Choi GH, Park H, Yang SC, et al. Normal liver elasticity values using acoustic radiation force impulse imaging: A prospective study in healthy living liver and kidney donors. Journal of Gastroenterology and Hepatology. 2012;27(1): 130-136. DOI: 10.1111/j.1440-1746.2011.06814.x

[89] Madhok R, Tapasvi C, Prasad U, Gupta AK, Aggarwal A. Acoustic radiation force impulse imaging of the liver: Measurement of the normal mean values of the shearing wave velocity in a healthy liver. Journal of Clinical and Diagnostic Research. 2013;7(1): 39-42. DOI: 10.7860/JCDR/2012/5070.2665

[90] Popescu A, Bota S, Sporea I, Sirli R, Danila M, Racean S, et al. The influence of food intake on liver stiffness values assessed by acoustic radiation force impulse elastography-preliminary results. Ultrasound in Medicine & Biology. 2013;39(4):579-584. DOI: 10.1016/j.ultrasmedbio.2012.11.013

[91] Bota S, Sporea I, Peck-Radosavljevic M, Sirli R, Tanaka H, Iijima H, et al. The influence of aminotransferase levels on liver stiffness assessed by acoustic radiation force impulse elastography: A retrospective multicentre study. Digestive and Liver Disease. 2013;45(9):762-768. DOI: 10.1016/j.dld.2013.02.008

[92] Fierbinteanu Braticevici C, Sporea I, Panaitescu E, Tribus L. Value of acoustic radiation force impulse imaging elastography for non-invasive evaluation of patients with non-alcoholic fatty liver disease. Ultrasound in Medicine & Biology. 2013;39(11):1942-1950. DOI: 10.1016/j.ultrasmedbio.2013.04.019

[93] Cassinotto C, Lapuyade B, Aït-Ali A, Vergniol J, Gaye D, Foucher J, et al. Liver fibrosis: Noninvasive assessment with acoustic radiation force impulse elastography— Comparison with FibroScan M and XL probes and FibroTest in patients with chronic liver disease. Radiology. 2013;269(1):283-292. DOI: 10.1148/radiol.13122208

[94] Friedrich-Rust M, Romen D, Vermehren J, Kriener S, Sadet D, Herrmann E, et al. Acoustic radiation force impulse-imaging and transient elastography for non-invasive assessment of liver fibrosis and steatosis in NAFLD. European Journal of Radiology. 2012;81(3):e325-ee31. DOI: 10.1016/j.ejrad.2011.10.029

[95] Guzmán-Aroca F, Frutos-Bernal M, Bas A, Luján-Mompeán J, Reus M, de Dios Berná-Serna J, et al. Detection of non-alcoholic steatohepatitis in patients with morbid obesity before bariatric surgery: Preliminary evaluation with acoustic radiation force impulse imaging. European Radiology. 2012;22(11):2525-2532. DOI: 10.1007/s00330-012-2505-3

[96] Osaki A, Kubota T, Suda T, Igarashi M, Nagasaki K, Tsuchiya A, et al. Shear wave velocity is a useful marker for managing nonalcoholic steatohepatitis. World Journal of Gastroenterology. 2010;16(23):2918-2925. DOI: 10.3748/wjg.v16.i23.2918

[97]   Palmeri ML, Wang MH, Rouze NC, Abdelmalek MF, Guy CD, Moser B, et al. Noninvasive evaluation of hepatic fibrosis using acoustic radiation force-based shear stiffness in patients with nonalcoholic fatty liver disease. Journal of Hepatology. 2011;**55**(3):666-672. DOI: 10.1016/j.jhep.2010.12.019

[98]   Yoneda M, Suzuki K, Kato S, Fujita K, Nozaki Y, Hosono K, et al. Nonalcoholic fatty liver disease: US-based acoustic radiation force impulse elastography. Radiology. 2010;**256**(2):640-647. DOI: 10.1148/radiol.10091662

[99]   Liu H, Fu J, Hong R, Liu L, Li F. Acoustic radiation force impulse elastography for the non-invasive evaluation of hepatic fibrosis in non-alcoholic fatty liver disease patients: A systematic review & meta-analysis. PLoS One. 2015;**10**(7):e0127782. DOI: 10.1371/journal.pone.0127782. eCollection 2015

[100] Muller M, Gennisson JL, Deffieux T, Tanter M, Fink M. Quantitative viscoelasticity mapping of human liver using supersonic shear imaging: Preliminary in vivo feasibility study. Ultrasound in Medicine & Biology. 2009;**35**(2):219-229. DOI: 10.1016/j.ultrasmedbio.2008.08.018

[101] Ferraioli G, Tinelli C, Zicchetti M, Above E, Poma G, Di Gregorio M, et al. Reproducibility of real-time shear wave elastography in the evaluation of liver elasticity. European Journal of Radiology. 2012;**81**:3102-3106. DOI: 10.1016/j.ejrad.2012.05.030

[102] Kudo M, Shiina T, Moriyasu F, Iijima H, Tateishi R, Yada N, et al. JSUM ultrasound elastography practice guidelines: Liver. Journal of Medical Ultrasonics. 2013;**40**:325-357. DOI: 10.1007/s10396-013-0460-5

[103] Lupşor-Platon M, Badea R, Gersak M, Maniu A, Rusu I, Suciu A, et al. Noninvasive assessment of liver diseases using 2D shear wave elastography. Journal of Gastrointestinal and Liver Diseases. 2016;**25**(4):525-532. DOI: http://dx.doi.org/10.15403/jgld.2014.1121.254.lup

[104] Leung VY, Shen J, Wong VW, Abrigo J, Wong GL, Chim AM, et al. Quantitative elastography of liver fibrosis and spleen stiffness in chronic hepatitis B carriers: Comparison of shear-wave elastography and transient elastography with liver biopsy correlation. Radiology. 2013 Dec;**269**(3):910-918. DOI: 10.1148/radiol.13130128

[105] Suh CH, Kim SY, Kim KW, Lim YS, Lee SJ, Lee MG, et al. Determination of normal hepatic elasticity by using real-time shear-wave elastography. Radiology. 2014;**271**(3):895-900. DOI: 10.1148/radiol.14131251

[106] Procopet B, Berzigotti A, Abraldes JG, Turon F, Hernandez-Gea V, García-Pagán JC, et al. Real-time shear-wave elastography: Applicability, reliability and accuracy for clinically significant portal hypertension. Journal of Hepatology. 2015;**62**:1068-1075. DOI: 10.1016/j.jhep.2014.12.007

[107] Ferraioli G, Tinelli C, Dal Bello B, Zicchetti M, Filice G, Filice C, Liver Fibrosis Study Group. Accuracy of real-time shear wave elastography for assessing liver fibrosis in chronic hepatitis C: A pilot study. Hepatology. 2012;**56**:2125-2133. DOI: 10.1002/hep.25936

[108] Bavu E, Gennisson JL, Couade M, Bercoff J, Mallet V, Fink M, et al. Noninvasive in vivo liver fibrosis evaluation using supersonic shear imaging: A clinical study on 113 hepatitis C virus patients. Ultrasound in Medicine & Biology. 2011;**37**(9):1361-1373. DOI: 10.1016/j.ultrasmedbio.2011.05.016

[109] Yoon JH, Lee JY, Woo HS, Yu MH, Lee ES, Joo I, et al. Shear wave elastography in the evaluation of rejection or recurrent hepatitis after liver transplantation. European Radiology. 2013;**23**(6):1729-1737. DOI: 10.1007/s00330-012-2748-z

[110] Sporea I, Bota S, Jurchis A, Sirli R, Grădinaru-Tascău O, Popescu A, et al. Acoustic radiation force impulse and supersonic shear imaging versus transient elastography for liver fibrosis assessment. Ultrasound in Medicine & Biology. 2013;**39**(11):1933-1941. DOI: 10.1016/j.ultrasmedbio.2013.05.003

[111] Cassinotto C, Lapuyade B, Mouries A, Hiriart JB, Vergniol J, Gaye D, et al. Non-invasive assessment of liver fibrosis with impulse elastography: Comparison of supersonic shear imaging with ARFI and FibroScan®. Journal of Hepatology. 2014;**61**:550-557. DOI: 10.1016/j.jhep.2014.04.044

[112] Jiang T, Tian G, Zhao Q, Kong D, Cheng C, Zhong L, et al. Diagnostic accuracy of 2D-shear wave elastography for liver fibrosis severity: A meta-analysis. PLoS One. 2016;**11**:e0157219. DOI: 10.1371/journal.pone.0157219

[113] Li C, Zhang C, Li J, Huo H, Song D. Diagnostic accuracy of real-time shear wave elastography for staging of liver fibrosis: A meta-analysis. Medical Science Monitor. 2016;**22**:1349-1359. DOI: 10.12659/MSM.895662

10

Non-Alcoholic Fatty Liver Disease, Diabetes Mellitus, and Zinc/Zinc Transporters: Is there a Connection?

Kurt Grüngreiff

Abstract

Immune response and metabolic regulation are closely connected with each other in such a way that dysfunction could lead to a variety of metabolic diseases such as obesity, diabetes mellitus (Dm), lipid metabolism disorders, and fatty liver disorders. Combined with uncritical "sugar-based" overeating and malnutrition, these multisystem metabolic diseases expand into a global epidemic. There are correlations between a fatty liver disease and diabetic metabolism state. A fatty liver leads to insulin resistance and thus to the development of a type 2 Dm; insulin resistance in turn augments the fatty liver. Zinc is a trace element of fundamental importance for a variety of biological processes. The liver is the main organ of the zinc metabolism. Metallothionein and zinc transporters are the key regulators of cellular zinc homeostasis. Molecular studies support the assumption of a correlation between zinc and Dm. Zinc is essential for the synthesis, secretion, and storage of insulin. ZnT8 is a significant autoantigen for type 1 Dm. Genetic polymorphisms in the ZnT8 gene are associated with an increased risk of developing type 2 Dm. Cellular zinc restriction induces the release of stress, particularly in the endoplasmic reticulum (ER). ER stress alone or coupled with cellular stress, as well as chronic inflammation, are central to the development of insulin resistance and type 2 Dm. The present insights into the context of a non-alcoholic fatty liver disease (NAFLD) and a type 2 Dm indicate that zinc and zinc transporters at the cellular level in various forms and in interactions with other mediators both in the regulation of physiological processes and in the formation of pathological processes, such as the cellular and ER stress, as well as chronic inflammation, and the development of metabolic disorders are involved.

Keywords: NAFLD, HCC, insulin resistance, diabetes mellitus, zinc, zinc transporter

1. Main text

Non-alcoholic fatty liver diseases (NAFLD) comprise a broad spectrum of liver diseases that go from non-alcoholic fatty liver (NAFL) to non-alcoholic fatty liver hepatitis (NASH), secondary fatty liver to fatty liver cirrhosis [1–4]. NAFLD represent 11–46% of all chronic liver diseases in the world [1]. NAFLD-induced liver changes look similar to those of alcoholic liver damage [4]. The accumulation of triglycerides and free fatty acids in the hepatocytes and an increased lipogenesis are typical features of an NAFLD. NAFLD is in part also causally associated with other diseases (e.g., metabolic multisystemic diseases such as obesity, type 2 diabetes mellitus (Dm), dyslipidemia, and hypertension [5, 6]. These diseases show a strongly increasing prevalence in particular in the Western and Asian industrialized states [4]. Due to the central role of the liver in the glucose metabolism, fatty acids and amino acids, there is a close interaction between the fatty liver and development of a diabetic metabolic state. On the one hand, the fatty liver will lead to insulin resistance and development of type 2 Dm; on the other hand, insulin resistance compounds the fatty liver [1, 7, 8]. Insulin resistance results in a reduction of glucose intake of the liver and other organs at concurrently increased hepatic glucose production. For this reason, modulation of the hepatic glucose metabolism is a target for antidiabetic treatment [9]. It is not clear yet whether the fatty liver is a cause or consequence of insulin resistance [8]. To differentiate NAFLD from alcoholic fatty liver disease or a mixed form, a daily alcohol limit of 10 g/day in women and 20 g/day in men is assumed. NASH, which can occur in up to 30% of the patients with NAFLD, is characterized by the presence of a mixed-cell infiltration in the hepatic lobules and a cell swelling of the hepatocytes (ballooning). NASH has a multifactorial genesis where genetic as well as environmental factors (e.g., excessive fat accumulation, mitochondrial dysfunction, influence of endotoxins and proinflammatory cytokines) contribute to chronic inflammation of the hepatocytes [1, 5, 6]. NASH as such is deemed a risk factor for the development of cirrhosis and hepatocellular carcinoma (HCC) [1, 4, 10]. Liver biopsy with subsequent histopathological evaluation is the diagnostic gold standard for differentiation between NASH and NAFLD [2, 6, 11]. At this time, NASH is the second most frequent underlying liver disease in the USA in patients to receive a liver transplant for HCC [12]. In a large, population-based study, Younoussi et al. [11] examined the prevalence and incidence of HCC in 2004–2009. Chronic hepatitis C-infection, at 54.9%, was the most frequent cause, and NAFLD was the third most frequent one at 14.1%. The authors explain the annual increase of the HCC incidence around the world with increased HCC screening, as well as with the increase of NAFLD [4, 11]. It is forecast that NAFLD will be the main cause of HCC development in approximately 20 years, after successful eradication of chronic hepatitis C infection, reduction of hepatitis B infection, and concurrent global increase of overnutrition [11, 13]. In particular, type 2 Dm is considered an independent risk factor of HCC [14]. Although liver cirrhosis is a precancerous condition and more than 90% of liver carcinomas develop based on cirrhosis, HCC can, similar to hepatitis B, develop without cirrhotic changes to the liver in NASH as well [15–17].

Zinc is an essential trace element that can be found in all tissues and that is of fundamental relevance for many biological processes, including the division, growth, and differentiation of cells [18–20]. Regulation of zinc homeostasis involves many proteins such as metallothioneins, zinc transporters, and specific permeable channels [21, 22]. Metallothioneins are important for the resorption and storage of zinc.

There are two major protein families that mammalian zinc transporters belong to [23, 24]. The first group of transporters are ZIP (Zrt/-like proteins), which are responsible for transporting zinc into the cytosol from either extracellular space or from intracellular compartments. There are 14 ZIP transporters, designated as solute family SLC39A1-A14 [23, 24]. The second group of 10 transporters are ZnT (zinc transporters), which designated as SLC30A1-A10 [23, 24]. They generally transport zinc out the cytosol into extracellular space or intracellular organelles such as zincosomes. Zincosomes are vesicles that can sequester high levels of zinc [25].

The liver is essential for zinc homeostasis, with zinc deficits leading to the impairment of many hepatic functions. On the other hand, liver diseases are often associated with zinc deficits [26, 27]. The scope of zinc deficit is not determined as much by the genesis (alcohol, viruses, etc.), but rather by the severity of liver damage, fibrosis or cirrhosis, with or without metabolic and/or portal decompensation, or the presence of a HCC [28]. Although a connection between zinc and the development of Dm has been discussed for years, only molecular studies of the last few years have supported this hypothesis [29]. Zinc increases the insulin effect in peripheral tissues and is indispensable for synthesis, secretion, and storage of insulin in the pancreatic ß-cells. It stabilizes the insulin structure, protects against insulin degradation, and is secreted together with insulin, proinsulin, and C-peptide in the early phase of glucose-stimulated insulin secretion; it has an insulin mimetic effect [30]. Type 2 Dm is usually associated with decreased plasma or serum zinc concentrations, whereas type 1 Dm plasma or serum zinc mostly elevates [30]. This is interpreted that at the beginning of type 1 Dm, a destruction of ß-cells takes places, and with decreased zinc concentration later, when the hyperzincuria outweighs the zinc release from ß-cells [30]. **Table 1** shows the causes of zinc deficiency in liver cirrhosis and diabetes mellitus.

Liver cirrhosis [28]	Diabetes mellitus [30]
Inadequate intake	Inadequate intake
Changes in protein and amino	Polyuria, hyperzincuria
acid metabolism	Osmotic diuresis
Diminished hepatic extraction	Increased intestinal secretion
Portosystemic shunts	Decreased intestinal absorption
Alcohol-induced impaired absorption	
Cytokines, IL-1, IL-6	Inflammation, cytokines, IL-1, IL-6
Endotoxins	Acidosis
Catabolism	

Table 1. Causes of zinc deficiency in liver cirrhosis and diabetes mellitus.

Current studies on the function of zinc transporters show that genetic variations of ZIP or ZnT genes, as well as changes to the expression and activity of the zinc transporters, are involved in the pathogenesis of various diseases [31–33]. Pancreatic ß-cells express various zinc transporters (e.g., ZnT3, ZnT5, ZnT8), which are required to ensure zinc homeostasis [29, 34, 35]. Examinations by Yi et al. [32] show that reduced expression of ZnT8 impairs biosynthesis and release of insulin and ß-cell functions. For example, hypoglycemia releases glucagon from pancreatic a-cells as regulated by the activity of ZnT8 [36]. Impaired ß-cell function leads to an absolute or relative deficit of insulin, which subsequently causes type 1 or type 2 Dm. The functional relevance of the ZnT8-function for glucose regulation is supported by association of the auto-antibodies against ZnT8 (ZnT8A) with diabetes; these auto-antibodies have an increased prevalence (in type 1: 60%, type 2: 6–24%) as compared to healthy persons (8%; [33]). Genetic polymorphisms in the SLC30A81 ZnT8-gene are associated with an increased risk of developing Dm type 2 [29, 37–40]. Genetic variants of the ZnT8 protein (e.g., rs13266634) lead to different hepatic insulin "clearance" rates that regulate the peripheral insulin concentration [41]. Individuals with the above risk allele have an impaired insulin metabolization and storage. This is also associated with reduced effectiveness of zinc substitution [33]. Reduced function of ZnT8 and the resulting reduced zinc content in islet cells are a genetic predisposition of such persons for an impaired glucose regulation and type 2 Dm [40, 42]. Predictive examinations of these gene versions that are sensible for clinical relevance in the meaning of diagnostic risk stratification (e.g., at positive family history for Dm, metabolic syndrome, NAFLD) will require further studies [43]. Modulation of ZnT8 activities also provides a new potential therapeutic point of attack for Dm and NAFLD [38]. In addition to ZnT8, the "influx transporter" ZIP14 plays a functionally relevant role in hepatic zinc regulation [24, 44]. According to the examinations by Aydemir et al. [9], ZIP14-mediated zinc transport is involved in regulation of the insulin receptor activity and maintenance of the glucose homeostasis in the hepatocyte. They also observed that there was an increase of ZIP14 and an increase of controlled zinc transport during glucose absorption on the cell surface. In the course of this, zinc is relocated to various locations in the hepatocyte through sequential translocations, from the membrane surface to the earlier and late endosomes. The authors conclude from this that ZIP14 may have a relevance analogue to that of ZnT8 regarding the diagnosis and treatment of type 2 Dm and NAFLD. Current findings by Kim et al. [45] showed the relevance of zinc trafficking and the functional ZIP14 activity for adaptation to endoplasmic reticulum (ER) stress connected to metabolic diseases. According to Zhang [46], zinc restriction in the cells triggers ER stress, which highlights the relevance of zinc for maintaining a normal ER function. There are epidemiological, clinical, and experimental indications that cellular stress (impaired biological processes in the cell) and excessive inflammation are causatively connected to various metabolic conditions, for example, obesity, type 1 and 2 Dm and arteriosclerosis [47–49]. Öczan et al. [50] found that ER stress plays a central role in peripheral insulin resistance and type 2 Dm on a molecular, cellular, and organismal level. The conditions triggering ER include glucose and food withdrawal, viral infections, lipids, increased synthesis of secretory proteins as well as mutated or incorrectly designed proteins [50].

In an excellent review for expression of ZIP 9 transporters in ß-cells of the pancreas, Lawson et al. [51] showed how complex, overlapping, and interlocking zinc transporters work. They identified ZIP6, ZIP7, ZIP9, ZIP13, and ZIP14 in humans and rodents and ZIP1 in rodents as potentially biologically relevant for the zinc effects in the ß-cells of the pancreas.

Inflammation is the first reaction of the immune system to infection or other damage to cells and tissues to protect the human or animal organism. Prolonged or chronic inflammations are harmful and release inflammatory substrates such as pro-inflammatory cytokines (IL-1, IL-6, TNF-alpha), free radicals, hormones and other small molecules, leading to impairment and damage of the physiological cellular processes [47]. Zinc and zinc transporters are involved in the development of ER stress and impairment of the protein synthesis, the unfold protein response (UPR; 45). UPR could be triggered in yeasts and in some mammals by zinc restriction UPR [45, 52, 53]. In the liver, impaired apoptosis leads to dysregulation of the lipid metabolism, causing hepatic steatosis [54]. Kim et al. [45] were able to show that the ZIP14-mediated zinc transport is critical for the prevention of prolonged apoptotic cell death and steatosis during ER stress, that is, for hepatocellular adaptation to ER stress.

Hashimoto et al. [55] found in patients with chronic hepatitis C that zinc deficiency promotes the insulin resistance by exacerbating iron overload in the liver and induces hepatic steatosis by facilitating lipid peroxidation.

Both type 2 Dm and NAFLD are consequences of chronic inflammation and cellular and ER stress. Although the processes that occur during this have not been fully determined yet, it seems highly likely that zinc and zinc transporters play an essential role in the pathogenesis of such diseases.

Zinc supplementation has been investigated as a potential adjunct therapy in the management of Dm; however, the outcomes of such interventions are conflicting [56, 57]. Capdor et al. [57] found a modest reduction in glucose concentration and tendency for a decrease in HbA1c following zinc supplementation and suggested that zinc may contribute to the management of hyperglycemia in individuals with chronic metabolic disease. Ruz et al. [58] remarked that studies available to date on zinc supplementation in type 2 Dm suggest that zinc supplementation is only effective in patients with initially reduced zinc concentrations.

Pia et al. [59] studied the protective effects of zinc supplementation on diabetic liver injury in a rat model of type 2 Dm. They found that zinc supplementation improved liver conditions in type 2 Dm rat models through multiple pathways, in which GRP78 linked ER stress and LC3-II-linked autophagy are ameliorated to some degree. The results of a systematic review by Barbosa de Carvalho et al. [60] about the role of zinc in patients with type 2 Dm confirming the role of zinc in controlling circulating glucose concentration through maintenance of insulin homeostasis. Based on these positive findings, the authors concluded that adequate dietetic ingestion and/or zinc supplementation are essential in the control of type 2 Dm. Lastly, Islam et al. [61] reported in a double-blind randomized placebo controlled pilot study an improving of glucose handling in pre-diabetes by zinc supplementation.

According to the long-term experiences with zinc supplementation in patients with chronic liver diseases, in particular in case of decompensated liver cirrhosis, administration of zinc leads to an increase and often normalization of the zinc levels, with the duration depending on the scope of zinc deficit in the serum [28]. Zinc supplementation improved in patients with liver cirrhosis and hepatic encephalopathy with and without Dm neurologic symptoms and signs of malnutrition [62–64]. Zinc administration increased glucose disposal entirely due to noninsulin-mediated glucose uptake without any systematic effect on insulin secretion and sensitivity [65]. Ruz et al. [58] recommended to further determine the role of zinc in type 2 Dm and therapeutic effectiveness of supplementation by long-term studies under observation of factors such as stage of disease, comorbidities, that is, also NAFLD, duration and type of medication (zinc preparation), and, finally, also examining the genetic variations in SLC30A8 as well due to the heterogeneity and complexity with multiple influences on the disease (**Figure 1**).

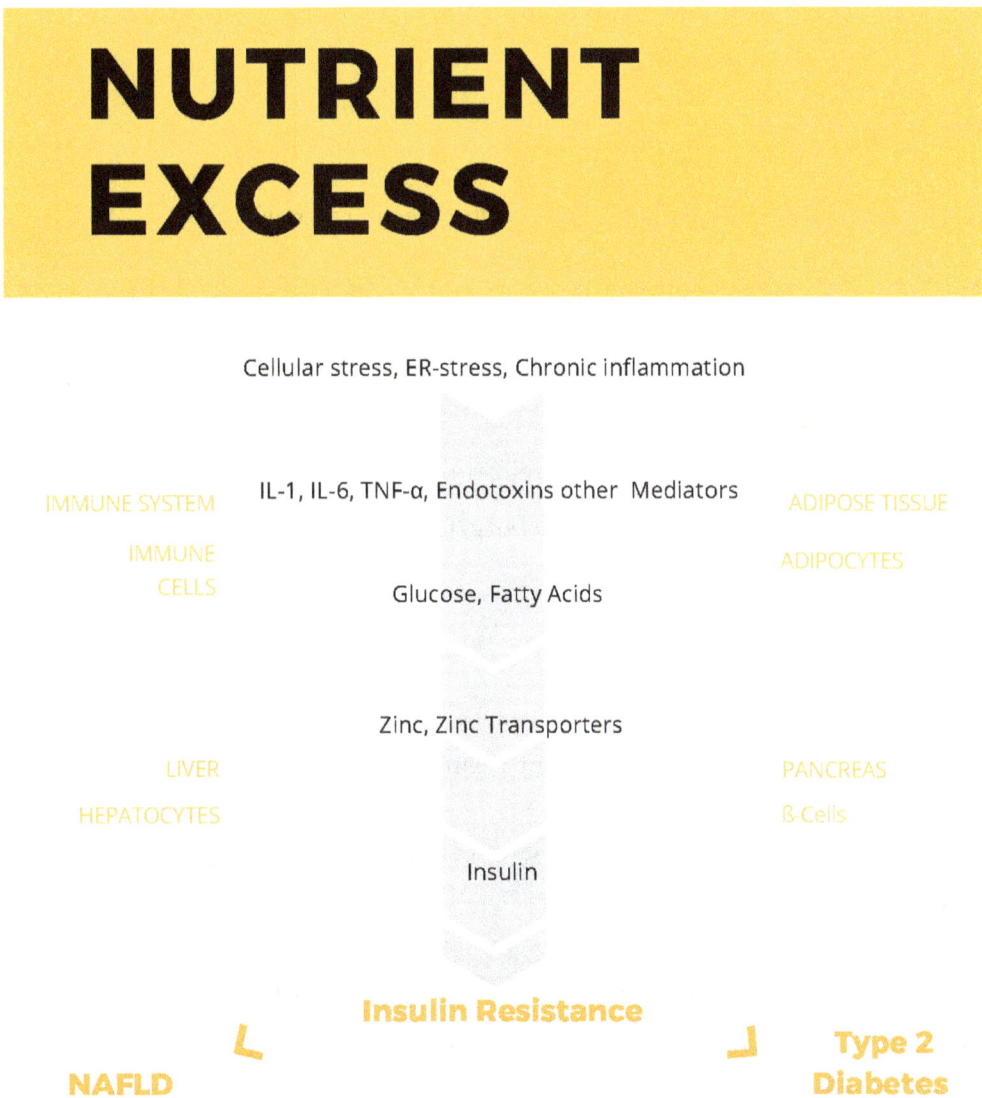

Figure 1. Schematic illustration of the organs, cells, substrates and main mediators involved in the development of insulin resistance linking NAFLD and type 2 Dm.

2. Concluding remarks

The data and findings that are available to date, and certainly not comprehensive, on the interrelation of fatty liver disease and type 2 diabetes mellitus show that zinc and zinc transporters on a cellular level are involved in the regulation of physiological processes as well as the development of pathological processes such as cellular stress, ER stress and not least chronic inflammation in diverse manners and interactions with other mediators, and therefore also in the development of such metabolic diseases.

Due to high complexity of the diseases, there are no simple solutions, that is, normalization of one "pathway" is not enough to recover functional homeostasis (controlling the diseases, health) of the integrated processes. Sole zinc substitution is surely ineffective in most cases, but may promise success in combination with other substrates.

Acknowledgements

I thank Anne Grüngreiff, my daughter, for excellent technical assistance.

Author details

Kurt Grüngreiff

Address all correspondence to: dr.kgruengreiff@t-online.de

Clinic of Gastroenterology Klinikum Magdeburg, Germany

References

[1] Banini BA, Sanyal AJ. Nonalcoholic fatty liver disease: Epidemiology, pathogenesis, natural history, diagnosis, and current treatment options. Clinical Medicine Insights: Therapeutics. 2016;**8**:75-84

[2] Roeb E, Steffen HM, Bantel H, et al. S2 k-Leitlinie nicht alkoholische Fettlebererkrankungen. Zeitschrift für Gastroenterologie. 2015;**53**:668-723

[3] Roeb E, Steffen MH, Bojunga J. S2 k-Leitlinie Nicht-alkoholische Fettlebererkrankungen—Was gibt's Neues? Deutsche Medizinische Wochenschrift. 2016;**141**:494-496

[4] Michelotti GA, Machado MV, Diehl AM. NAFLD, NASH and liver cancer. Nature Reviews. Gastroenterology & Hepatology. 2013;**10**(11):656-665

[5] Tilg H, Moschen AR. Evolution of inflammation in non-alcoholic-fatty liver disease: the multiple parallel hits hypothesis. Hepatology. 2010;**52**:1836-1846

[6] Rotman Y, Sanyal S. Current and upcoming pharmacotherapy for non-alcoholic fatty liver disease. Gut. 2017;**66**:180-190

[7] DÀdamo E, Cali AMG, Weiss R, et al. Central role of fatty liver in the pathogenesis of insulin resistance in obese adolescents. Diabetes Care. 2010;**33**:1817-1822

[8] Cali AMG, De Oliveira AM, Kim H, et al. Glucose dysregulation and hepatic steatosis in obese adolescents: Is there a link? Hepatology. 2009;**49**:1896-1903

[9] Aydemir TB, Troche C, Kim M-H, Cousins RJ. Hepatic ZIP14-mediated zinc transport contributes to endosomal insulin receptor trafficking and glucose metabolism. The Journal of Biological Chemistry. 2016;**291**:23,939-23,951

[10] Wu R, Nakatsu G, Yu J. Pathophysiological mechanisms and therapeutic potentials of macrophages in non-alcoholic steatohepatitis. Expert Opinion on Therapeutic Targets. 2016;**20**:615-626

[11] Younoussi ZM, Otgonsuren M, Venkatesan C, et al. Association of nonalcoholic fatty liver disease (NAFLD) with hepatocellular carcinoma (HCC) in United States from 2004 to 2009. Hepatology. 2015;**62**:1723-1730

[12] Wong RJ, Ahmed A. Obesity and none-alcoholic fatty liver disease: Disparate association among Asian populations. World Journal of Hepatology. 2014;**6**:263-273

[13] Llovet JM, Zucman-Rossi J, Pikarski E, et al. Hepatocellular carcinoma. Nature Reviews. 2016;**2**:1-23

[14] Chen HF, Chen P, Li CY. Risk of malignant neoplasms and biliary tract in diabetic patients with different age and sex stratifications. Hepatology. 2010;**55**:155-163

[15] Hashimoto E, Tokushige K. Hepatocellular carcinoma in non-alcoholic steatohepatitis: Growing evidence of an epidemic? Hepatology Research. 2012;**42**:1-14

[16] Grüngreiff K. Die Leberzirrhose als Präkanzerose. Verdauungskrankheiten. 2003;**21**: 129-134

[17] Ertle J, Dechene A, Sowa JP, et al. Nonalcoholic fatty liver disease progresses to hepatocellular carcinoma in the absence of apparent cirrhosis. International Journal of Cancer. 2011;**128**:2436-2443

[18] Leoni G, Rosato A, Perozzi. Zinc proteome interaction network as a model to identify nutrient-affected pathways in human pathologies. Genes & Nutrition. 2014;**9**:436

[19] Grüngreiff K, Reinhold D. Zink: Bedeutung in der ärztlichen Praxis. J. Hartmann Verlag, Heßdorf-Klebheim; 2007

[20] Maret W. Human zinc biochemistry. In: Rink L, editor. Zinc in Human Health. 1st ed. Amsterdam: IOS Press; 2011. pp. 45-62

[21] Lindenmayer GW, Stoltzfus RJ, Prendergast AJ. Interactions between zinc deficiency and environmental enteropathy in developing countries. Advances in Nutrition. 2014;**5**:16

[22] Fukada T, Yamasaki S, Nishida K, Murakami M, Hirano T. Zinc homeostasis and signaling in health and diseases. Journal of Biological Inorganic Chemistry. 2011;**16**(7):1123-1134

[23] Cousins RJ, Lichten LA. Zinc transporters. In: Rink L, editor. Zinc in Human Health. 1st ed. Amsterdam: IOS Press; 2011. pp. 136-162

[24] Luizzi JP, Cousins RJ. Mammalian zinc transporters. Annual Review of Nutrition. 2004;**24**:151-172

[25] Gammoh NZ, Rink L. Zinc in infection and inflammation. Nutrients. 2017;**9**:624. DOI: 10.3390/nu9060624

[26] Grüngreiff K, Reinhold D. Zinc and liver. In: Rink L, editor. Zinc in Human Health. 1st ed. Amsterdam: IOS Press; 2011. pp. 473-492

[27] Bartholomay AF, Robin ED, Vallee RL, et al. Zinc metabolism in hepatic dysfunction. Serum zinc concentrations in Laennec's cirrhosis and their validation by sequential analysis. The New England Journal of Medicine. 1956;**255**(9):403-408

[28] Grüngreiff K, Reinhold D, Wedemeyer H. The role of zinc in liver cirrhosis. Annals of Hepatology. 2016;**15**(1):7-16

[29] Maret W. Zinc in human disease. Metal Ions in Life Sciences. 2013;**123**:389-414

[30] Jansen J, Karges W, Rink L. Zinc and diabetes—Clinical links and molecular mechanisms. The Journal of Nutritional Biochemistry. 2009;**20**:399-417

[31] Kambe T, Hashimoto A, Fujimoto S. Current understanding of ZIP and ZnT zinc transporters in human health and diseases. Cellular and Molecular Life Sciences. 2014;**71**:3281-3295

[32] Yi B, Zhou Z. Different role of zinc transporter 8 between type 1 diabetes and type 2 diabetes mellitus. Journal of Diabetes Investigation. 2016;**7**:459-465

[33] Hogstrand C, Maret W. Genetics of human zinc deficiencies. In: Encyclopedia of Life Sciences. Chichester: John Wiley & Sons, Ltd. DOI: 10.1002/9780470015902.a0026346

[34] Wijesekara N, Chimienti F, Wheeler MB. Zinc, a regulator of islet function and glucose homeostasis. Diabetes, Obesity & Metabolism. 2009;**11**(Suppl 4):202-214

[35] Chimienti F. Zinc, pancreatic islet cell function and diabetes: New insights into an old story. Nutrition Research Reviews. 2013;**26**:1-11

[36] Solomou A, Philippe E, Chabosseau P, et al. Over-expression of Slc30ab/ZnT8 selectively in the mouse a cell impairs glucagon release and responses to hypoglycemia. Nutrition and Metabolism. 2016;**13**:46

[37] Maruthur NM, Mitchell BD. Zinc-rs 13,266,634 and the arrival of diabetes pharmacogenetics: The "zinc mystique". Diabetes. 2014;**63**:1463-1464

[38] Rutter GA, Chabosseau, Bellomo E, et al. Intracellular zinc in insulin secretion and action: A determinant of diabetes risk? In: The Proceedings of the Nutrition Society. 2016. pp. 61-72. DOI: 10.1017/S0029665115003237

[39] Pearson E. Zinc transport and diabetes risk. Nature Genetics. 2014;**46**(4):323-324

[40] Rutter GA. Think zinc. New roles for zinc in the control of insulin secretion. Islets. 2014;**2**: 49-50

[41] Tamaki M, Fujitani Y, Hara A, et al. The diabetes-susceptible gene SLC30A8/ZnT8 regulates hepatic insulin clearance. The Journal of Clinical Investigation. 2013;**123**:4513-4524

[42] Shan Z, Bao W, Rong Y, et al. Interactions between zinc transporter-8 gene (SLC30AB) and plasma zinc concentrations for impaired glucose regulation and type 2 diabetes. Diabetes. 2014;**63**:1796-1803

[43] Ziegler A-G, Bonifacio E, Powers AC, et al. Type 1 diabetes prevention: A goal dependent on accepting a diagnosis of an asymptomatic disease. Diabetes. 2016;**65**(11):3233-3239. DOI: 10.2337/db16-0687

[44] Franklin RB, Levy BA, Zou J, et al. ZIP14 zinc transporter downregulating and zinc depletion in the development and progression of hepatocellular cancer. Journal of Gastrointestinal Cancer. 2012;**43**(2):249-257

[45] Kim M-H, Aydemir TB, Kim J, Cousins RJ. Hepatic ZIP14-mediated zinc transport is required for adaptation to endoplasmic reticulum stress. PNAS. 2017. DOI: 10.1073/ pnas.1704012114. Published online july 3

[46] Zhang K. Integration of ER stress, oxidative stress and the inflammatory response in heath and disease. International Journal of Clinical and Experimental Medicine. 2010; **3**(1):33-40

[47] Zhang K, Kaufman RJ. From endoplasmic-reticulum stress to the inflammatory response. Nature. 2008;**454**:455-462

[48] Hotamisligil GS. Inflammation and metabolic disorders. Nature. 2006;**444**:860-867

[49] Hanson GK, Libby P. The immune response in atherosclerosis: A double-edged sword. Nature Reviews. Immunology. 2006;**6**:508-519

[50] Öscan U, Cao Q, Vilmaz E, Lee A-H, Iwakoshi NN, et al. Endoplasmic reticulum stress links obesity, insulin action, and type 2 diabetes. Science. 2004;**306**:457-461

[51] Lawson R, Maret W, Hogstrand C. Expression of the ZIP/SLC349A transporters in ß-cells: A systematic review and integration of multiple datasets. BMC Genomics. 2017;**18**:719. DOI: 10.1186/s12864-017-4119-2

[52] Ellis CD et al. Zinc and the Msc2 zinc transporter protein are required for endoplasmic reticulum function. The Journal of Cell Biology. 2004;**166**:325-335

[53] Homma K et al. SOD1 as a molecular switch for initiating homeostatic ER stress response under zinc deficiency. Molecular Cell. 2013;**52**:75-86

[54] Rutkowski DT et al. URP pathways combine to prevent hepatic steatosis caused by ER stress-mediated suppression of transcriptional master regulators. Developmental Cell. 2008;**15**:829-840

[55] Himoto Z, Nomura T, Tani J, Mioyoshi H, et al. Exacerbation of insulin resistance and hepatic steatosis deriving from zinc deficiency in patients with HCV-related chronic liver disease. Biological Trace Element Research. 2015;**163**:81-88

[56] Zampelas A. Zinc supplementation: Another myth or we are heading towards a new era in the treatment of diabetes? Arteriosclerosis. 2011;**219**:22-23

[57] Capdor J, Foster M, Samman S. Zinc and glycemic control: A meta-analysis of randomized placebo controlled supplementation trials in humans. Journal of Trace Elements in Medicine and Biology. 2013;**27**:137-142

[58] Ruz M, Carrasco F, Sanchez A, Perez A, Rojas P. Does zinc really "metal" with diabetes? The epidemiologic evidence. Current Diabetes Reports. 2016;**16**:111. DOI: 10.1007/s11892-016-0803-x

[59] Pia M, Liu Y, Yu T, Lu Y. Zinc supplementation ameliorates ER stress and autophagy in liver in a rat model of type 2 diabetes mellitus. Biomedical Research. 2016;**27**:1075-1081

[60] Barbosa de Carvalho G, Nascimento Brandao-Lima P, Costa Maia CS, Ferreira Barbosa KB, et al. Zinc's role in the glycemic control of patients with type 2 diabetes: A systematic review. Biometals. 2017;**30**:151-162

[61] Islam MR, Attia J, Ali L, McEvoy M, et al. Zinc supplementation for improving glucose handling in pre-diabetes: A double blind randomized placebo controlled pilot study. Diabetes Research and Clinical Practice. 2016;**115**:39-46

[62] Bianchi GP, Marchesini G, Brizi M, Rossi M, et al. Nutritional effects of zinc supplementation in cirrhosis. Nutrition Research. 2000;**20**:1079-1089

[63] Grüngreiff K, Grüngreiff S, Reinhold D. Zinc deficiency and hepatic encephalopathy. Results of a long-term zinc supplementation. Journal of Trace Elements in Experimental Medicine. 2000;**13**:12-31

[64] Marchesini G, Fabri A, Bianchi G, Brizi M, Zoli M. Zinc supplementation and amino acid-nitrogen metabolism in patients with advanced cirrhosis. Hepatology. 1996;**23**:1084-1092

[65] Marchesini G, Bugianesi F, Ronchi M, Flamia R, et al. Zinc supplementation improves glucose disposal in patients with cirrhosis. Metabolism. 1998;**8**:792-798

11

Molecular Basis for Pathogenesis of Steatohepatitis: Contemporary Understanding and New Insights

Om Parkash and Subha Saeed

Abstract

Nonalcoholic fatty liver disease (NAFLD) is characterized by a broad spectrum of clinical and histological presentations, ranging anywhere from simple steatosis to steatohepatitis. Of the patients with NAFLD, only a small fraction goes on to develop inflammation and fibrosis (i.e. NASH). Hence, understanding the underlying molecular mechanisms, which play part in progression of NAFLD and determine the disease severity, is extremely important. Almost two decades ago, Day and colleagues first described the "two-hit hypothesis" to explain progression of NAFLD. However, since then, the advances in field of molecular research have identified that NAFLD development and progression involves complex interplay of numerous determinants, including gut-derived signals, endoplasmic reticulum stress, adipose-derived adipokines, nutritional factors, hormonal imbalances and components of innate immunity which act in concert on genetically predisposed individuals to induce liver inflammation. This chapter reviews the different players of this "multiple-hit model".

Keywords: NAFLD, NASH, molecular basis, "multiple-hit model", steatohepatitis

1. Introduction

Nonalcoholic fatty liver disease (NAFLD) encompasses a broad spectrum of clinical and histo-pathological presentations, ranging from simple steatosis to nonalcoholic steatohepatitis (NASH), the latter being characterized by inflammation, macrovesicular steatosis and apoptosis, with or without fibrosis. NAFLD can further progress to liver fibrosis, cirrhosis and hepatocellular carcinoma (HCC) [1]. The prevalence of NAFLD in Western countries ranges from 30–46% [2], whereas in Asian populations, it is about 15% [3]. About 30% of patients with NAFLD may have NASH [4].

Regarding progression of NASH to cirrhosis, estimated 10% of patients with NASH can progress to decompensated liver disease over 10 years and about 25% of patients develop cirrhosis over a span of 9 years [5]. It is very important to understand and uncover the underlying molecular mechanisms which explain the variable incidence and severity of steatohepatitis in only few patients with NAFLD, while most patients with steatosis never progress to steatohepatitis [6]. After Day and Colleagues first described "two-hit" model for pathogenesis of steatohepatitis in 1998, wherein steatosis ("first hit") progresses to steatohepatitis due to rampant lipid peroxidation in liver ("second hit") [7], recent advances in field of molecular research have identified numerous other culprits, collectively summed up in "multiple-hit" hypothesis [8]. The "multiple-hit" hypothesis examines multiple insults which act collectively and in-parallel on genetically predisposed individuals to induce development of NAFLD and expedite progression to further adverse pathologies. This chapter provides a review of literature for multiple culprits identified in development of NAFLD and NASH.

2. Development of hepatic steatosis

Several mechanisms are involved in development of hepatic steatosis [9–11], including increased fatty acid supply due to increased lipogenesis from both visceral and subcutaneous adipose tissue, increased dietary intake of fats, increased de novo hepatic lipogenesis, decreased free fatty acid oxidation, and decreased secretion of VLDL from liver. Increased free fatty acid delivery to liver and elevated *de novo* lipogenesis are major contributors to fatty acid accumulation in NAFLD.

Elevated hepatic *de novo* lipogenesis may be due to activation by transcription factors such as *SREBP-1*(activated by Insulin, regulated via *Insulin Receptor Substrate* (IRS) and maintains cellular cholesterol homeostasis), *ChREBP* (activated by glucose and increased hepatic *de novo* lipogenesis) and *PPAR-γ*. Studies have demonstrated that *de novo* lipogenesis in liver is elevated in insulin-resistant state and NAFLD [12, 13].

2.1. Lipoapoptosis: free fatty acids and cholesterol

Free fatty acid and Cholesterol are considered main players in lipotoxicity. Increased concentration of serum free fatty acids (16 Carbons and more; saturated or unsaturated) are seen in patients with NAFLD [14]. Apoptosis of hepatocytes, which is morphologic and pathologic feature of human NASH, is partly due to free fatty acids, as explained below.

Hepatocytes can undergo apoptosis via extrinsic pathway (activated by FAS ligand and tumor necrosis factor related apoptosis-inducing ligands) or intrinsic pathway (activated by intracellular stress of membrane-bound organelle, such as mitochondria, endoplasmic reticulum and mitochondria) [15]. Free fatty acids can induce apoptosis via following mechanisms, as demonstrated in **Figure 1**:

- *Mitochondrial pathway* [16] (palmitic acid and stearic acid activate intrinsic apoptotic pathway via C-jun N-terminal kinase and Bim, leading to Bax activation, mitochondrial permeabilization, release of cytochrome c, and activation of Caspase 3 and 7),

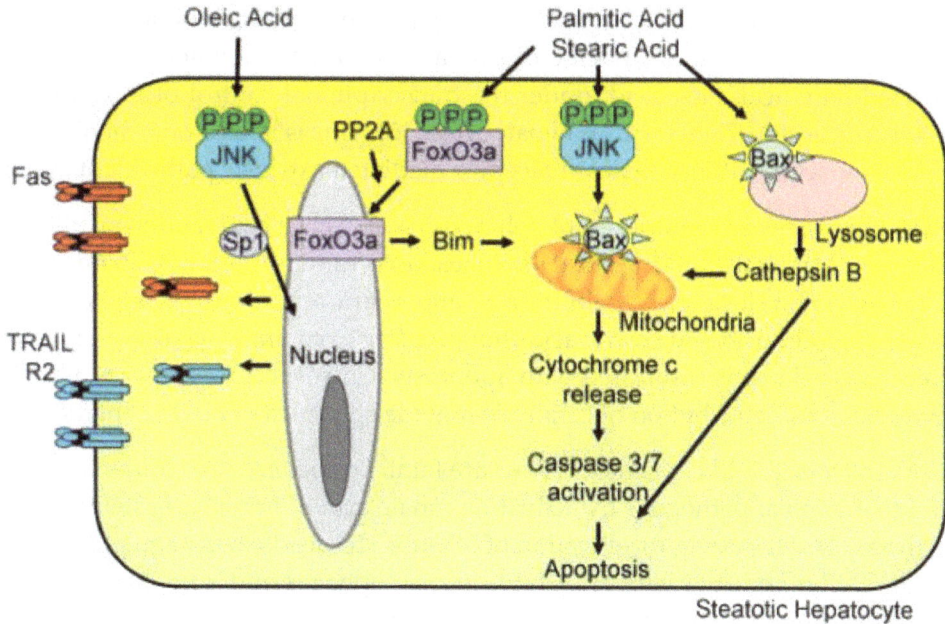

Figure 1. The figure demonstrates different mechanisms by which fatty acids impart lipotoxicity to hepatocytes.

- *Induction of Bim expression* [17] (palmitic acid and stearic acid can activate transcription factor FoxO3a, which further induces expression of pro-apoptotic protein Bim),

- *Lysosomal pathway* [18, 19]: Oleic acid and palmitic acid activate Bax which trans-locates to lysosomes, increases the permeability of lysosomes and causes release of cathepsin B, which further increase permeability of mitochondria and activates Caspases. Furthermore, Lysosomal permeabilization is also associated with activation of NF-κB, which results in generation of tumor necrosis factor-α (TNF-α) in hepatocytes,

- *Endoplasmic Reticulum* [20]:Palmitic acid and stearic acid lead to activation of Endoplasmic reticulum (ER) stress pathway, which can lead to apoptosis, as explained later,

- *C-Jun N-Terminal Kinase:* JNK belongs to family of intracellular mitogen-activated protein (MAP). The murine dietary models of obesity were associated with increased activation of JNK in liver [21]. JNK leads to activation of pro-apoptotic protein Bax [22] while it inactivates anti-apoptotic protein, Bcl-2 [23]

- *Death Receptors*: Tumor Necrosis Factor Receptors, TNFR-1 and TNFR-2, and Fas are implicated in pathogenesis of steatohepatitis [24]. Obesity, being a chronic inflammatory state [25], is characterized by infiltration of adipose tissue by macrophages which release of inflammatory mediators, including TNF-α [26], with increased levels of TNF-α being observed in obesity. Upon activation by TNF-α, TNFR-1 activates NF-κB which leads to activation of pro-inflammatory genes and further apoptosis, if NF-κB mediated survival signals are inhibited. TNF-α can also lead to JNK activation, which can also lead to apoptosis if its activation is sustained [15].

Fas is expressed on hepatocytes and upon binding by Fas ligand, it signals apoptotic cell death [15]. In dietary murine models, such as methionine and choline-deficient diet and high sucrose diet, steatosis is accompanied by increased expression of hepatic Fas [27], and increase in Fas expression confers increased Fas ligand-mediated apoptosis. Also, Mono-unsaturated fatty acid, oleic acid, under the transcriptional control of JNK, increases the expression of Fas and TRAIL-R2 on hepatocytes [15]. This is another mechanism by which fatty acids impart sensitivity to death receptor mediated extrinsic pathway of apoptosis,

- *Ceramide*: Ceramides are composed of sphingosine and fatty acid, and availability of long chain fatty acids is a rate limiting step in synthesis of ceramide in ER [28]. In nutritional obesity with associated elevation of palmitic acid and stearic acid, excess synthesis of ceramide is possible. Palmitic acid and stearic acid-induced *de novo* ceramide synthesis in hematopoietic precursor cell line is associated with apoptosis. However, more studies are needed to highlight the exact contribution of ceramide to wide spectrum of NAFLD pathologies [29]

- *Toll-Like Receptors*: toll-like receptors (TLR) are family of pattern recognition receptors that respond to microbial pathogens by activating innate arm of immune system [15]. Palmitic acid activates TLR4, leading to activation of NK-κB. This leads to upregulation of its target genes- i.e. TNF-α and Interleukin-6 (IL-6)- in macrophages and adipocytes [30]. When a high-fat diet is fed to mice lacking TLR4, there is a lack of inflammatory gene expression induction by high-fat diet, pointing towards the role of TLR4 in hepatic inflammation seen in NASH [31].

- *Oxidative Stress*: Enhanced mitochondrial and microsomal fatty acid β oxidation and cytochrome P450 (CYP2E1) induction can lead to oxidative stress via generation of Reactive Oxygen species (ROS), as observed in human models of steatohepatitis [15, 32]. 4-hydroxy-2-noneal (HNE) and Thiobarbituric acid reacting substrate (TBARS), both markers of lipid peroxidation, are increased in patients with NAFLD and NASH [33, 34]. Thus, oxidative stress may contribute towards development of steatosis and steatohepatitis.

- *Long chain poly unsaturated fatty acids (LCPUFA)*: Oxidative stress leads to depletion of n-3 LCPUFA (e.g Eicosapentaenoic acid, *EPA*, and docosahexaenoic Acid, *DHA*) due to increased peroxidation or defective desaturation processes. Depletion of n-3 LCPUFA leads to upregulation of lipogenic and glycogenic effects from SREBP-1c and down-regulation of fatty acid oxidation effects from peroxisome proliferator activated receptor-α (PPAR-α), ultimately promoting hepatic steatosis [35]. In addition, depletion of LCPUFA can also lead to insulin resistance due to disturbance in membrane mediated processes such as insulin signaling [36]. From dietary prospective, a study aimed at assessing the influence of high-fat diet on Δ5 and Δ6 desaturase enzymes involved in LCPUFA formation, found that HFD lead to enhanced oxidative stress and macrovesicular steatosis, with diminution in desaturase activity and hence, depletion of LCPUFA [37].

The role of cholesterol in lipoapoptosis requires special mention. In an analysis conducted on human liver samples, subjects with NAFLD and NASH exhibited almost a 2-fold increase in free cholesterol, as compared to controls [38]. Furthermore, in a study to evaluate the effect of dietary free cholesterol loading in rodents, rats fed high cholesterol diet developed microvesicular steatosis and were sensitized to apoptotic effect of TNF-α, which may explain the lipoapoptosis due to cholesterol [39].

2.2. Triglycerides

Triglycerides are the main lipids stored in liver of patients with hepatic steatosis and recent studies suggest that triglycerides may in fact have protective functions. Diacylglycerol acyl-transferase 1 and 2 (DGAT) catalyze final step in triglyceride synthesis. In a model of diet-induced obesity, mice with over-expression of DGAT1 in adipocytes and macrophages were protected from macrophage activation and accumulation in white adipose tissue, and from systemic inflammation and insulin resistance [9, 40]. In another study, DGAT2 antisense oli-gonucleotides lead to inhibition of triglycerides synthesis which improved liver steatosis but worsened liver damage, further strengthening the notion that liver triglycerides are protective in nature [41]. Thus, in summary, accumulation of triglycerides in liver might not actually be a pathology but in fact, an adaptive, beneficial response in situations where hepatocytes are exposed to toxic triglyceride metabolites and fatty acid excess due to increased caloric consumption [9, 42].

2.3. Inflammation leads to Steatosis or vice versa: chicken or the egg?

- Treatment with anti-TNF antibody and metformin (an anti-diabetic drug that inhibits he-patic TNFα expression) in ob/ob mice (the laboratory model of nonalcoholic fatty liver disease) showed marked improvement in hepatic steatosis [43, 44].

- In patients with alcoholic steatosis, treatment with anti-TNF antibody can improve hepatic steatosis [45].

- Similarly, loss of Kupffer cells lead to decreased production of anti-inflammatory cytokine (IL-10), which lead to hepatic steatosis [46].

The above examples support the notion that Inflammation activates stress response in hepa-tocytes, which leads to lipid accumulation. In fact, hepatic steatosis may be considered a *"bystander phenomenon"* following inflammatory attacks. It may be a possibility that inflam-mation proceeds steatosis in NASH and, benign and non-progressive simple steatosis and NASH are different disease entities altogether [9].

2.4. Insulin resistance in NAFLD

NAFLD is strongly associated with hepatic and adipose tissue insulin resistance, as well as reduced whole body insulin sensitivity [47]. Different underlying molecular mechanisms have been identified which account for insulin resistance [8]:

1. Serine phosphorylation of insulin receptor substrate (IRS) by inflammatory signals, such *as c-jun N-terminal protein kinase 1* (JNK) or *inhibitor of nuclear factor-jB kinase-b* (IKKb) [48]

2. *Activation of nuclear factor kappa B* (NF-κB) and *Suppressors of cytokine signaling* (SOCS) [49]

Insulin Resistance would mean that ability of Insulin to suppress lipolysis has been supressed, leading to increased delivery of free fatty acids to liver [50]. The free fatty acid can further exacerbate hepatic insulin resistance by causing translocation of PKC-γ isoform from cytosol to the membrane where it impairs hepatic *insulin receptor substrate* (IRS)-associated phosphatidylinositol activity [51].

2.4.1. Oxidative stress and insulin resistance

Prolonged excess oxidative load in steatosis, due to carbohydrates and lipids, leads to redox disequilibrium characterized by lower than normal hepatic anti-oxidative potential, for example, decreased hepatic glutathione (GSH) and reduced superoxide dismutase (SOD) activity, which further triggers insulin resistance (IR) [52]. This is validated by a data from study where increased reactive oxygen species (ROS) in 3T3-L1 cultured pre-adipocytes preceded the onset of Insulin resistance [53], by molecular mechanisms listed above. The insulin resistance due to exacerbated hepatic oxidative stress can in turn lead to upregulation of pro-oxidative CYP2E1 expression, the response which is normally attenuated by repressive effects of Insulin on CYP2E1 expression [54]. Thus, there is increasing evidence for positive reinforcement and interdependency between oxidative stress and insulin resistance in patients with Hepatic steatosis [52].

Thus, due to impairment in IRS activity and further down-regulation of IRS due to insulin resistance, SREBP is unregulated and over-expressed, leading to increased hepatic *de novo* lipogenesis [55]. Insulin Resistance, due to its ability to induce lipotoxicity, oxidative stress and inflammatory cascade, may be one of the "multiple hit" in pathogenesis of NAFLD and progression towards NASH [8, 56].

3. The gut-derived factors

The gut microbiota is implicated in the pathogenesis and progression of NAFLD, through so-called gut-liver axis [8]. A study aimed at analyzing human gut microbiome recognized different "enterotypes" [57] and "obese microbiome", which has an ability to harvest increased amount of energy from diet, has been demonstrated in obese mice [58]. In fact, colonization of germ-free mice with "obese microbiome" leads to greater increase in total body fat as compared to colonization with "lean microbiome" [58]. The **Figure 2** summarizes the role of gut-liver axis and adipose tissue in pathogenesis of NAFLD.

The liver receives more than 50% of its blood supply from splanchnic circulation [8], and hence, it is always exposed to gut-derived toxins. The ability of gut-derived factors like lipopolysaccharide (LPS) to flow in portal vein requires intestinal permeability, which in NAFLD is due to disrupted intercellular tight junctions in the intestine [59]. In Murine models of NAFLD, intestinal mucosa has bacterial overgrowth with increased intestinal permeability and concurrent reduction in expression of tight junction proteins [60]. Consequentially, plasma endotoxin levels are significantly high in patients with NAFLD and NASH [61], and high-fat diet is associated with 2–3 fold increase in plasma LPS levels [62]. LPS may act as a ligand for TLR with consequent activation of inflammatory cascade, including stress- and mitogen-activated protein kinases-JNK (explained later), p38, Interferon regulatory factors 3 and nuclear factor-jB – each having

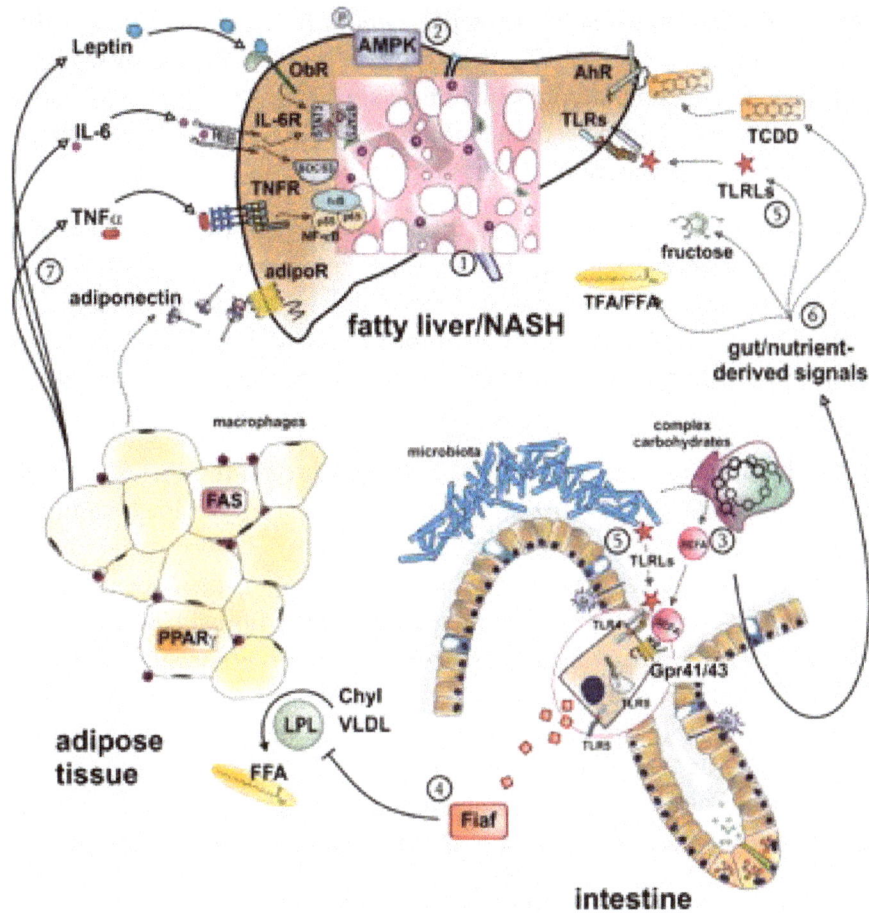

Figure 2. "The multiple parallel hits model. Lipotoxicity: (1) a liver loaded with lipids consisting primarily of trigylcerides might reflect a benign process because triglycerides might exert mostly protective effects. Furthermore, hyperleptinemia leads to oxidation of hepatic lipids, thereby also protecting this organ from lipotoxicity. When the capacity of peripheral and central organs of detoxifying "aggressive lipids" fails, lipotoxic attack of the liver might begin. Inflammation may precede steatosis in NASH. Gut-derived signals: Many signals beyond endotoxin might affect hepatic steatosis and inflammation. Several pathways have been identified how the gut microbiota might influence host energy metabolism: (2) Absence of the microbiota in germ-free mice correlates with increased activity of phosphorylated AMPK in the liver and the muscle (not shown). (3) Some of the breakdown products of polysaccharides are metabolized to SCFAs. SCFAs such as propionate and acetate are ligands for the G protein-coupled receptors Gpr41 and Gpr43. Shortage of SCFAs might allow the evolution of systemic inflammatory events. Such mechanisms elegantly combine diet, microbiota, and the epithelial cell as "nutrient sensor." (4) The microbiota decreases epithelial expression of fasting-induced adipocyte factor (Fiaf), which functions as a circulating lipoprotein lipase (LPL) inhibitor and therefore is an important regulator of peripheral fat storage. (5) Several TLRs, such as TLR5 or TLR9, are not only able to affect microbiota but also to regulate metabolism, systemic inflammation, and insulin resistance, thus highlighting the role of the innate immune system in metabolic inflammation as observed in NASH. (6) Various nutrients such as trans fatty acids (TFAs), fructose or aryl hydrocarbon receptor (AhR) ligands such as 2,3,7,8-tetrachlorodibenzodioxin (TCDD) may directly lead to steatosis/liver inflammation. Adipose tissue-derived signals: Signals derived from the adipose tissue beyond toxic lipids might play a central role in NAFLD/NASH. (7) here, adipocytokines such as adiponectin and leptin, certain pro-inflammatory cytokines such as TNFα or IL-6, and others (the death receptor Fas, PPARγ) are of key relevance. The cytokine/adipocytokine milieu might be critical because ob/ob-adiponectin tg mice, although becoming severely obese, are not insulin-resistant. This suggests that in the hierarchy of processes soluble mediators play the central role. Adipose-derived mediators might indeed affect target organs such as the liver, because JNK1 adipose-deficient mice are protected from diet-induced obesity, and experiments have demonstrated that this effect is mediated mainly by IL-6 (a cytokine), which is of key importance in human obesity." [9] (figure and associated caption used after permission from "John Wiley and Sons" [9]).

significant contribution towards insulin resistance, hepatic fat accumulation, obesity and NASH development and progression [63, 64]. Evidently, a continuous infusion of LPS for 4 weeks in mice mimicked high-fat diet phenotype, with noticeable increase in insulin resistance, increased liver triglyceride content and adipose tissue inflammation [62]. Similarly, the use of antibiotics reduced the intensity of inflammation in high-fat diet and ob/ob mice [65].

Another mechanism for gut microbiota to influence the host immune system is via their capacity to digest dietary fibers, such as resistant starch and nonstarch polysaccharide, to short chain fatty acids (SCFAs, mainly propionate, butyrate and acetate), which are absorbed by intestinal epithelium [66]. SCFAs, via their interactions with G protein-coupled receptor 43 (Gpr43), have anti-inflammatory function in various models of human ulcerative colitis [67, 68].

Enteric bacteria also suppress the synthesis of fasting-induced adipocyte factor (Fiaf), resulting in increased lipoprotein lipase activity and increased triglyceride accumulation in the liver [8, 9]. Gut microbiota also produce enzymes which cause the conversion of dietary choline to toxic compounds, particularly methylamines which, in the liver, are transformed to trimethylamine-N-oxide and induce inflammation and liver fibrosis [69]. Intestinal microbiome is a major source for production of hepatotoxic compounds such as alcohol, phenols and ammonia which are delivered to the liver by portal circulation. These compounds activate kupffer cells and stimulate the production of nitric oxide and other inflammatory cytokines [70]. Patients with NASH show abundance of alcohol-producing bacteria as compared to healthy children and children with simple steatosis [71]. This endogenous production of alcohol has a well-established role in generation of ROS and liver inflammation [72].

Furthermore, NLRP6 and NLRP3 inflammasomes, through their production of IL-18, play an important role in modulation of gut microbiota. In different mouse models, inflammasomes deficiency is associated with modifications in configuration of gut microbiota, and exacerbation of hepatic steatosis and inflammation. This is due to increased influx of TLR4 and TLR9 ligands into the portal circulation, leading to enhanced tumor necrosis factor-α (TNF-α) production in liver which leads to NASH progression [73].

3.1. Bile acids

The primary bile acids cholic acid and chenodeoxycholic acid are conjugated to glycine and taken up in distal ileum for transport to the liver [74]. By binding to cellular receptor farnesoid X receptor (FXR) in various organs of the body, bile acids act as signaling molecules to control overall metabolism of the host [75]. Upon activation of FXR by primary bile acids, downstream signals are generated which lead to inhibition of hepatic *de novo* lipogenesis, increased insulin sensitivity and protection of hepatocytes from bile acid-induced cytotoxicity [76]. However, the gut microbiota in distal ileum can deconjugate the bile acids and can further metabolize them to secondary bile acids, and thus, contribute towards obesity by altering lipid metabolism, through changes in bile acid pools and modulation of FXR signaling [74].

3.2. Dietary factors

The recent decades saw a dramatic increase in consumption of trans-fatty acids, and as evident from studies on mice, trans-fatty acids consumption leads to larger liver with NASH-like lesions and Insulin resistance [77]. Similarly, Fructose is a lipogenic, pro-inflammatory dietary factor associated with oxidative stress and upregulation of TNF-α [78], and daily fructose consumption is associated with liver inflammation and fibrosis [79]. Fructose diet can induce oxidative stress and hepatocellular damage by different mechanisms, including induction of protein fructosylation which activates SREBP and generates reactive oxygen species (ROS) [80]. Also fructose phosphorylation leads to depletion of ATP, which stimulates increased uric acid synthesis which in turn stimulates production of ROS [81]. Lastly fructose can induce mitochondrial disturbance which lead to disequilibrium between *De novo Lipogenesis* and VLDL, which promotes alteration of respiratory chain and uncoupling of oxidative phosphorylation with excess ROS production [82, 83].

Another receptor, aryl hydrocarbon receptor (AhR), is a ligand activated transcription factor which is activated by many constituents of our diet such as indolo-(3,2-b)-carbazole and 3,3'-diindolyl-methane (metabolized from indole 2-carbinol), or flavonoids, and this pathway plays an important role in inflammation [84]. This is evident in transgenic mice with constitutively activated AhR as they develop spontaneous hepatic steatosis and increased hepatic oxidative stress [85].

Studies show that Low-Calorie, Low-carbohydrate soy-containing diet and Mediterranean diet rich in antioxidants and polyunsaturated fatty acids of n-3 series are known to be protective in reducing hepatic steatosis [86].

4. Adipose tissue-derived signal

Adipose tissue, with its ability to generate cytokines and adipocytokines, can be classified as a complex endocrine and immune organ which mediates different metabolic, immunological and inflammatory responses.

4.1. Adiponectin

Adiponectin is an anti-inflammatory cytokine with anti-lipogenic effects which protect non-adipocyte tissue, such as liver, from lipid accumulation [87]. Reduced levels of adiponectin are seen in conditions associated with development of NAFLD, namely obesity [88] and insulin resistance [89]. Hence, adiponectin levels are inversely related to visceral obesity and insulin resistance, and weight loss is an inducer of adiponectin synthesis [90]. The levels of adiponectin are significantly reduced in patients with NASH as compared to simple steatosis [91]. Thus adiponectin protects the liver against steatosis.

By activating cyclic-AMP dependent protein kinase (AMPK), adiponectin opposes fatty acid synthesis and promotes mitochondrial β-oxidation [92]. The anti-inflammatory effects of adiponectin are due to its ability to block activation of NF-κB which inhibits the release of pro-inflammatory cytokines such as TNFα and IL-6 [93]. The anti-inflammatory and hepatic lipid modulating effects of adiponectin may also be due to activation of peroxisome proliferator activated receptor-α (PPAR-α), as pharmacological treatment with PPAR-α agonist reverses experimental steatohepatitis [94]. Furthermore, PPAR-γ agonist, such as thiazolidinedione, stimulate adiponectin synthesis, and latter activates PPAR-α [95].

4.2. Leptin

Leptin is a gene product of *ob* gene and is produced by visceral adipocytes [96]. The levels of leptin directly correlate with body fat mass and adipocyte size [97]. Leptin has a potential dual action on NAFLD experimental models, exerting anti-steatotic, and pro-inflammatory/pro-fibrogenic actions [98]. In non-adipose tissue, such as liver, it prevents lipid accumulation by decreasing the expression of SREBP-1. Leptin exerts pro-fibrogenic effects by activating stellate cell in liver through hedgehock [99], mTOR [100] or kupffer cell-mediated TGF-β1 secretion which then activates stellate cell [101]. In mice models of NASH, gut-derived endo-toxins can induce hyper-responsiveness to leptin, with subsequent upregulation of CD14 and accelerated fibrosis [102]. Experimental studies have demonstrated that leptin deficiency in mice may lead to hepatic steatosis which can be reversed by leptin replacement. On the other hand, excess leptin contributes towards hepatic inflammation and fibrosis [98]. It may be a possibility that anti-steatosis effects of leptin may predominate in initial stages of NAFLD while pro-inflammatory and pro-fibrotic effects might take over during disease progression phase [103]. However, the exact magnitude of contribution by Leptin towards NAFLD remains to be elucidated.

4.3. IL-6 and TNFα

In severe obesity, adipocytes are major source of IL-6 production, as evident by a study results where IL-6 expression was 100-fold elevated in adipose tissue as compared to liver in obese patients [9]. Similarly, elevated TNF-α production has been observed in cultures of peripheral blood cells collected from obese patients with NASH [104]. These two important pro-inflammatory cytokines are found to be elevated in obese patients and weight loss is associated with dramatic decrease in serum levels of these cytokines [105, 106].

The liver is the target organ for adipose tissue-derived 1 L-6 and TNFα. It is known that high-fat diet, also called "inflammatory diet", stimulates *JNK1* (mitogen-activated protein kinase, associated with apoptosis) signaling in adipocytes, which leads to IL-6 secretion by adipocytes. IL-6 further acts on hepatic cell, leading to hepatic steatosis and hepatic insulin resistance [48]. Continuous exposure to elevated levels of IL-6/TNF-α leads to many of the histological features of NASH such as hepatocyte necrosis and apoptosis, neutrophil chemotaxis and activation of hepatic stellate cells [107]. Also, they caused insulin resistance by upregulating hepatic suppressor of cytokine signaling 3 (SOCS3) [108].

Transcription factor *nuclear factor-jB kinase b* (NF-κB) and its IKK2 subunits is also important mediators of chronic inflammatory states. Persistent activation of NF-κB has been shown in animal models of NAFLD [109] and NASH [110].

4.4. Inflammasomes

Inflammasomes are large caspase-1 –activating multiprotein complexes that sense both endogenous and exogenous danger signals via intracellular NOD-like receptors (NLRs) [111]. Among the three prototypes of inflammasomes, NALP3 is associated with NAFLD and responds to danger signals by activating Caspase 1. Active Caspase-1 promotes cleavage and maturation of pro-inflammatory cytokines, such as IL-1β, IL-18, IL-33, which further promote inflammation [111]. Gut-derived endotoxin and free fatty acid may act as danger associated molecular pattern (DAMP) which may lead to activation of inflammasomes [112].

To validate the role of inflammasomes in NASH, it was seen that there was increased gene expression of inflammasomes in livers of patients with NASH as compared to liver of healthy controls [113]. Furthermore, LPS and saturated fatty acids amplify the expression and activation of inflammasomes, and free fatty acids sensitize the hepatocytes to LPS-induced IL-1β secretion [112]. It was seen observed that saturated fatty acids also directly induce hepatocyte apoptosis and activation of Caspase 8, which triggers the release of danger molecules from hepatocytes [112].

IL-1β induces the suppression of peroxisome proliferator activated receptor-α (PPAR-α), activates the stellate cells to promote fibrosis and promotes TNF-α-induced cell death [114].

5. Toll-like receptors and innate immunity

Toll-like receptors are sensors of microbial and endogenous danger signals which are expressed in innate immune cells and liver parenchyma and contribute towards progression of NASH [90]. Upon activation by gut microbiota-released pathogen- or damage- associated molecular pattern (PAMP and DAMP), downstream signals are activated which lead to progression of NASH. TLR2, TLR4 and TLR9 are most commonly associated with NASH [90].

The gut-derived bacterial endotoxin is brought to liver via portal circulation where they activate the kupffer cell by way of TLR4 receptor complex. This interaction leads to activation of nuclear transcription factors, leading to release of pro-inflammatory mediators such as TNFα which can induce liver injury and fibrosis [115]. The role of TLR4 in pathogenesis of NASH is further supported by study where TLR4-deficient mice, which were fed high fructose diet,were protected from formation of reactive oxygen species, induction of TNFα expression in liver and insulin resistance [116].

TLR9 is located on endoplasmic reticulum and is activated by unmethylated CpG DNA particles that are released from bacteria [90]. It is known that TLR9 is involved in steatohepatitis as TLR9-deficient mice are protected from liver inflammation [114]. In *CDAA diet*-(Choline-deficient amino acid defined diet) induced NASH, translocated bacterial DNA from gut binds to TLR9 receptor on kupffer cell to produce IL-1β which activate hepatic stellate cells to induce liver fibrosis, and also stimulate hepatocytes for lipid accumulation and cell death [114]. The induction of hepatic steatosis is independent of TLR2, however, functional TLR2 receptors are found on kupffer cells which mediate liver inflammation and fibrosis in CDAA diet-induced NASH [117].

Recently, another data that implicated TLR5 in pathogenesis of metabolic syndrome was presented. It was reported that mice deficient in TLR5 developed all features of metabolic syndrome including, hyperphagia, obesity, insulin resistance, pancreatic inflammation and hepatic steatosis. It was proposed that TLR5 altered the gut microbiota and the finding were reproducible when microbiota from TLR5 $^{-/-}$ mice was transferred to healthy mice [118]. However, another study did not find any such results in TLR5-deficient mice [119]. Indeed, more studies are needed to elicit role of TLR5 in steatohepatitis.

6. Endoplasmic reticulum (ER) stress

Endoplasmic reticulum (ER) is an important intracellular organelle involved in production, folding, post-translational modification and trafficking of secretory and membrane proteins. Also present in the ER is endoplasmic reticulum-associated degradation (ERAD) machinery that ensures that misfolded proteins are re-translocated back to cytoplasm for degradation by proteasomes [120]. Thus, ER serves as a quality control checkpoint, allowing only properly folded proteins to be transported to Golgi apparatus [121, 122] (**Figure 3**).

Any event that disturbs ER protein folding capacity- be it due to excessive protein synthesis, accumulation of misfolded proteins, depletion of calcium in ER, disturbance in redox regulation, glucose depletion, viral infection or high-fat diet (saturated fatty acid such as palmitic acid and stearic acid) [123] - leads to induction of evolutionarily conserved ER stress response, known as Unfolded protein response (UPR). The role of sensing ER stress and activating UPR is performed by three ER transmembrane proteins, mentioned as following:

1. RNA-dependent Protein kinase-like ER eukaryotic initiation factor-2α Kinase (PERK)

2. Inositol-requiring ER-to-nucleus signaling protein1 (IRE1) and,

3. Transcription factor 6 (ATF6)

Each of these transmembrane proteins has an ER luminal domain to sense unfolded protein, a transfolded domain for targeting to the ER membrane, and a cytosolic domain to transmit signals to the transcriptional and/or translational apparatus [124]. In an unstressed cell, these ER proteins are maintained in an inactive state via their association with the ER chaperon protein, glucose-regulated protein 78 (GRP78)/Bip [125] and upon ER stress, unfolded/ misfolded proteins accumulation enhances the release of GRP78 from these stress-sensing proteins, leading to respective activation of PERK, ATF6 and IRE1 [126].

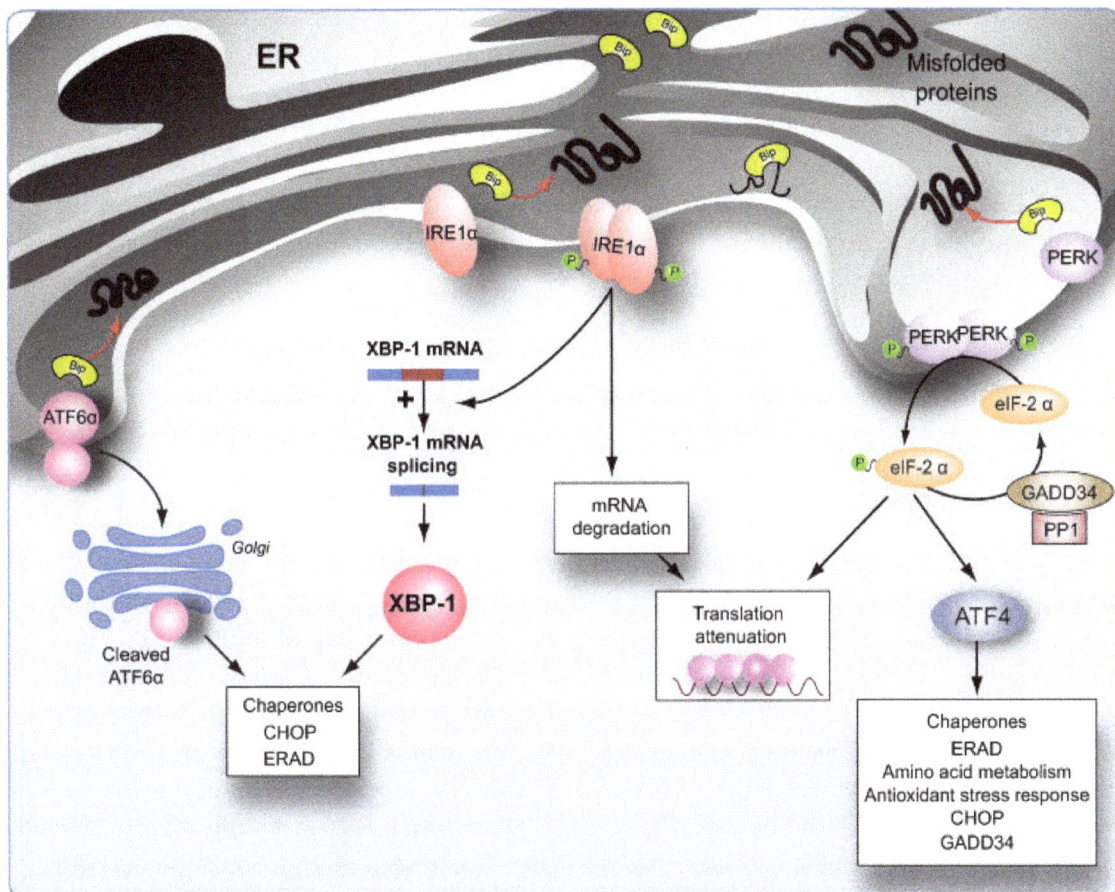

Figure 3. The figure demonstrating the three different pathways of unfolded protein response [135].

Upon activation, PERK, IRE1α and ATF6 induce signal transduction events that attenuate the accumulation of misfolded proteins in the ER by increasing expression of ER chaperons, inhibiting protein load on ER by decreasing mRNA translation, and stimulating retrograde transport of misfolded proteins from ER into cytosol for ubiquination and destruction by a process named ERAD [127]. However, under conditions where ER stress is chronically prolonged and the cell fails to restore homeostatsis in ER, the UPR will initiate cell apoptosis [126].

6.1. Protein kinase RNA-like endoplasmic reticulum kinase (PERK)

Activation of PERK leads to phosphorylation of α-subunit of eukaryotic Initiation Factor 2α (eIF-2α), leading to its inactivation and hence, attenuation of mRNA translation and decreased protein load on the ER [128]. The phosphorylated eIF-2α also causes preferential translation of UPR-dependent genes, such as activation transcription factor 4 (ATF 4). Further, ATF4 induces expression of several genes, including amino acid transporter, chaperons and CHOP [129] (*"C/EBP homologous protein"*, also known *as 'growth arrest and DNA damage (GADD 15)*).

CHOP is an ER-derived transcription factor which is an important mediator of ER stress-induced apoptosis, as evident from studies where deletion of CHOP lead to attenuation of hepatocellular apoptosis in alcohol- and cholestasis-induced liver disease [130]. Apoptosis-relevant targets of the CHOP transcription factor include:

1. *GADD34* [131]: promotes dephosphorylation of eIF2α,thus reversing translation inhibition. This leads to accumulation of unfolded proteins in ER compartment, and, simultaneously, permits translation of mRNA encoding pro-apoptotic genes,

2. *DR5*: a caspase activating cell-surface death receptor, and

3. *Ero 1 α* (Endoplasmic Reticulum Oxidoreductase-1): hyperoxdises the ER and also activates the inositol triphosphate receptor (IP_3R), causing excessive transport of Calcium from ER to the mitochondria and thus causing cell death) [132].

CHOP also induces apoptosis via direct inhibition of Bcl-2 transcription [133] and induction of Bim expression [134]. Bcl-2 proteins are localized within the ER membrane and are protective (*anti-apoptotic*) against ER stress. This cytoprotective function is mainly due to the ability of Bcl-2 to lower steady-state levels of ER Ca^{2+} via IP_3Rs. The protective role of Bcl-2 in regulating ER Ca^{2+} can be inhibited by JNK-mediated phosphorylation of Bcl-2. The Phosphorylated Bcl-2 loses its anti-apoptotic function by being unable to bind *pro-apoptotic* "BH_3-only" members of Bcl-2 family (i.e. Bim), leading to increasing calcium release from ER, which is associated with mitochondrial calcium uptake. This leads to increased mitochondrial permeabilization, release of cytochrome C, and hence apoptosis [127]. Calcium release from ER can also activate Caplains, which may further proteolytically activate Caspase-12 to induce apoptosis [135].

6.2. Inositol-requiring ER-to-nucleus signaling protein1 (IRE1)

Accumulation of unfolded proteins in ER leads to activation of IRE1, which further processes an intron from X-box binding protein-1 (XBP-1) mRNA and permits synthesis of XBP-1 protein. XBP-1 binds to promoters of genes involved in UPR (encoding ER chaperons) and ERAD to restore homeostasis and prevent cellular toxicity [127]. Apart from cytoprotective effects, IRE1 can also recruits inflammatory factors (JNK and NF-κB) which induce inflammatory response signaling [136], and apoptotic signal kinase-1 (ASK1) which causes downstream activation of stress kinases Jun-N-terminal Kinase (JNK) and p38 MAPK, that promotes apoptosis [137].

Activated JNK translocate to mitochondria and causes activation of Bim and Inhibition of Bcl-2. Activated JNK also induces the expression of pro-inflammatory genes by phosphorylating transcription factor activating protein-1(AP-1) [138]. Activated p38 MAPK phosphorylates and activates CHOP [127] to causes apoptosis.

6.3. Transcription factor 6 (ATF6)

ATF6 belongs to CREB family of transcription factors. Activation of ATF6 leads to its release from ER membrane, processing in the Golgi and entry into the nucleus. It trans-activates ER stress related genes such as ER chaperones, XBP-1, foldases and CHOP [124].

6.4. Endoplasmic reticulum stress and Steatosis

Hepatocytes, being rich in both smooth and rough EPR, perform diverse metabolic functions, including lipoprotein and very-low-density lipoprotein (VLDL) assembly and secretion, cholesterol biosynthesis and xenobiotic metabolism [121]. The Sterol regulatory element-binding protein (SREBPs) are key regulators of lipid homoeostasis and play crucial role in *de novo* lipogenesis [139], where SREBP-1 regulates fatty acid and triglycerides (TG) metabolism and SREBP-2 controls cholesterol metabolism and low density lipoprotein (LDL) receptor expression [140]. SREBP are transcription factors bound to ER membrane in inactive form and their activity is controlled within ER by interaction of *SREBP-Cleavage Activating Protein* (SCAP) and *Insulin regulated proteins* (Insigs). Insigs cause SREBP-SCAP complex to be retained within the ER and prevents SREBP-1 activation [141]. Under conditions of low sterols, Insigs are dissociated with SCAP, leading to migration of SREBP-SCAP complex to Golgi apparatus, where SREBP is processed to its active form by S1P and S2P [142]. Activated SREBP translocate to nucleus and regulates the various genes involved in lipid metabolism.

However, under ER Stress, rapid activation of precursor form of SREBP-1c and SREBP-1c target genes takes place, even in absence of Insulin [143]. Furthermore, ER stress induces proteolytic activation of SREBPs by increasing turnover of Insigs [142]. Hence, the recent data suggests that ER stress leads to hepatic steatosis by increasing de novo lipogenesis and upregulating the transcription of genes encoding for key lipogenic trans-activators and enzymes [121, 144].

Due to its high capacity for protein synthesis, ER stress plays an important part in mediating pathological changes in various liver diseases [135]. The signaling pathway activated by ER stress are implicated in lipotoxicity, Insulin Resistance, Inflammation and apoptotic cell death which are common to both NAFLD and NASH [123]. The presence of ER stress and activation of UPR in chronic disease (such as NAFLD) suggests that ability to resolve ER stress has been compromised. Inducing ER stress in individuals with genetically ablated eIF2α, IRE1α or ATF6α leads to hepatic steatosis [145], suggesting that steatosis results from impairment in the capacity to oxidize fatty acids and augmented by impaired lipoprotein secretion. Thus, initially UPR aims to prevent steatosis and re-establish *ER homeostasis* after ER stress but selective impairment to the UPR that reduce the ability of UPR to resolve ER stress leads to development and exacerbation of hepatic steatosis. However, further work is needed to investigate this Homeostatic Model hypothesis.

It is now well-established that various arms of UPR and its downstream signaling molecules play role in regulation of lipid metabolism and induction of various hepatic pathologies.

6.4.1. PERK-eIF2α-ATF4 pathway

The PERK-eIF2α-ATF4 pathway is reported to regulate lipogenesis and hepatic steatosis. PERK-dependent signaling has been crucial to sustained expression of lipogenic enzymes such as fatty acid synthase (FAS), ATP-citrate Lyase, and stearoyl-CoA Desaturase-1(SCD1) [146]. Phosphorylated eIF2α (activated form) is associated with enhanced expression of adipogenic nuclear receptor peroxisome proliferator activated receptor γ (PPAR γ) and its upstream regulators, and dephosphorylation of eIF2α using GADD34 leads to diminished hepatosteatosis in animals fed high-fat diet [147]. Furthermore, activated ATF4 increases expression of lipogenic genes, such as PPAR γ, sterol regulatory element-binding protein-1c (SREBP-1c), acetyl-CoA carboxylase (ACC), and FAS, in liver and white adipose tissue. Similarly, ATF4 knockout mice are protected from diet-induced hepatic steatosis [148, 149]. Thus, the current evidence suggests that PERK-eIF2α-ATF4 pathway plays an important role in promoting lipogenesis.

6.4.2. IRE1α-XBP1 pathway

The IRE1α-XBP1 pathway plays an important part in maintenance of hepatic lipid homeostatsis under ER stress and regulation of hepatic VLDL assembly and secretion [150]. IRE1α is also required for efficient synthesis of ApoB-containing lipoproteins [151]. Mice with hepatocyte specific deletion of IREIα show increased hepatic steatosis and reduced plasma lipids under ER stress condition due to altered expression of key metabolic players (such as PPARγ and C/EBPβ) and of enzymes involved in Triglycerides biosynthesis [151]. Thus, these results indicate IRE1α represses lipid accumulation in liver, especially under ER stress condition. However, the deletion of IRE1α leads to loss of this protective role of IRE1α, resulting in unresolved ER stress and hence, hepatic steatosis.

The role of XBP1 in lipogenesis is emphasized in a study where conditional disruption of XBP-1 in the liver of mice lead to reduced plasma level of triglycerides, cholesterol and free fatty acids, possibly due to decreased de novo lipogenesis [152]. XBP1 regulates lipogenesis in hepatocytes by directly binding to promotors of lipogenic genes such as SCD1 (Stearoyl-CoA Desaturase 1), DGAT2 (Diacylglycerol Transferase 2) and ACC2 (Acetyl-CoA carboxylase),thereby activating their transcription [152]. Thus under appropriate conditions, XBP1 promotes lipogenesis and contributes to hepatic lipogenesis.

6.4.3. Transcription factor 6 (ATF6)

ATF6 and SREBP are both ER membrane bound transcription factors, and nuclear ATF6 interacts with nuclear SREBP 2, antagonizing the SREBP2- regulated transcription of lipogenic genes and preventing lipid accumulation in cultures of liver cell [153]. Moreover, ATF2α-knockout mice develop hepatic steatosis in response to ER stress, due to reduced fatty acid oxidation and decreased VLDL secretion [154].

Thus, taken together, all three proximal UPR sensors including PERK, IRE1α and ATF6α, regulate lipid stores in liver but the degree to which the UPR contributes to hepatic steatosis may depend on activation of three proximal UPR sensors relative to each other, coupled with appropriate downstream protein–protein and/or protein-DNA interaction [120].

6.5. Endoplasmic reticulum stress and progression towards NASH

Multiple factors, including but not limited to, insulin action, oxidative stress, cytokine mediated signaling, inflammation, bacterial endotoxin, and excess fatty acids function in concert and interact with UPR to provoke disease progression of NAFLD towards NASH.

6.5.1. ER stress and hepatic inflammation

Several Signaling pathways connect ER stress to hepatic inflammation:

- Reactive oxygen species (ROS)

  Protein folding in ER is intimately linked to generation of ROS, such that each disulfide bond formation during oxidative protein folding leads to production of 1 ROS [155]. An elevated protein folding load, as in ER stress, leads to accumulation of ROS, which may lead to inflammation. In turn, the oxidative stress from ROS can disrupt ER homeostasis and induce ER stress [156].

  However, in an unsurprising adaptive pathway, UPR activates an antioxidant program via transcription factor *Nrf2* (nuclear factor erythroid-derived 2-related factor 2) to prevent accumulation of ROS [157]. *Nrf2* is activated after phosphorylation by PERK pathway of UPR and it regulates the inducible expression of anti-oxidant response element-containing genes [157]. Importantly, Nrf2 deletion results in rapid onset and progression of steato-hepatitis in mice provided a methionine choline-deficient (MCD) diet [158]. ATF4, one of the other terminal player of PERK pathway, has also been an important transcription factor in maintenance of adequate Glutathione levels in cells [159]. Thus, PERK arm of UPR and its downstream players are directly related to regulation of anti-oxidant effects. In a recent study, IRE1α-XBP1 branch of UPR was also found linked to anti-oxidant effect, where XBP1 deficiency leads to reduced catalase expression [160].

- NF-κB and JNK

  In response to ER stress, IRE1α binds to adaptor protein tumor-necrosis factor α (TNF-α) receptor-associated factor 2 (TRAF2). IRE1α-TRAF2 complex activates NF-κB and JNK, both of which induce production of Pro-inflammatory cytokines, such as C-reactive protein (CRP), amyloid P-component, fibrinogen, and interleukin-6 (IL-6) [161].

  The UPR-mediated signaling can lead to activation of NF-κB not only via IRE1α but also via PERK [162] and/or ATF6 pathway [163]. Activation of NF-κB has been detected in steatohepatitis induced by MCD diet, however, the exact mechanism about how ER stress-induced signaling involving NK-κB and JNK might regulate inflammation, cell survival and apoptosis in NAFLD is still unknown.

- PKR (double-stranded RNA-activated Protein Kinase)

  PKR is an interferon-induced Serine/threonine protein kinase, activated by dsRNA, and is capable of activating NF-κB and eIF2α in response to dsRNA and oxidative stress, respectively [164]. PKR activity is increased in adipose tissue and liver of murine model of obesity [165]. With its ability to respond to pathogens, nutrients and organelle stress, PKR appears to be core component of inflammatory and immune pathways. However, depending on which key factor is activated downstream, that is, either NF-κB (pro-apoptotic) or eIF2α (anti-apoptotic), PKR may "serve as molecular clock to time the sequential events of survival and death" [166]. In summary, PKR affirms the complexity of UPR signaling and its downstream outcomes [120].

- CREBH

    CREBH is a transcription factor belonging to CREB/ATF family of transcription factor and is required for liver synthesis of Amyloid P-component and CRP [167]. CREBH is activated via RIP process (Regulated Intramembrane Proteolysis: release and transport of ER resident protein from the ER membrane to Golgi for processing) upon ER stress. Other than ER stress, TNFα, Interleukin 6 (IL6) and lipoprotein LPS also induce expression of CREBH [168]. This makes room for another revelation: ER stress in the liver may be linked to systemic inflammation via the RIP- mediated mobilization of CREBH [120].

6.5.2. ER stress and apoptosis

Apoptosis is an important component of disease progression in NAFLD [169] and is positively correlated with disease severity in NASH [24]. The failure of UPR in mitigating the ER stress leads to cell death via several mechanisms (**Figure 4**).

CHOP is one of the best characterized UPR-regulated pro-apoptotic protein [120]. CHOP is an ER-derived transcription factor activated downstream from PKR- and ATF6-pathway of UPR. Significance of CHOP in inducing apoptosis can be emphasized from results of study where silencing CHOP lead to decreased hepatocyte apoptosis in alcohol-induced liver disease [130] and attenuated cholestasis-induced liver fibrosis [170]. However, the role of CHOP is paradoxical in NAFLD, as demonstrated in study where CHOP deletion can reduce palmitate-induced apoptosis in hepatocyte cell line, whereas MCD diet-induced apoptosis was not reduced in CHOP knockout mice [171, 172].

CHOP has been described as an unstable protein compared to other protein chaperons like GRP78 [120]. Above described paradoxical role of CHOP in NAFLD makes way for observation: role of CHOP as a pro-apoptotic protein may be dependent on level of CHOP expression, the presence of factors which increase stability and/or protein–protein interactions that direct cell specific effects [173, 174]. Hence, future studies regarding role of CHOP in mice model are needed to elicit exact contributions of CHOP towards disease progression in NAFLD and NASH.

Furthermore, The IRE1 branch of the UPR, via its activation of JNK and Caspase 12 [175], and its interaction with Bax and Bak (two pro-apoptotic Bcl2 family members) [176], can also activate path towards apoptosis.

Additionally, another mechanism proposed for hepatic cell apoptosis is dysregulation in ER calcium flux. The ER calcium flux is regulated by ER stress, ER-localized protein and BCL-2 proteins interacting with other ER-localized proteins [177, 178]. The ERO1α-mediated activation of IP$_3$, as mentioned earlier, can lead to disruption of ER calcium homeostasis [132]. This disruption inhibits sarco-endoplasmic reticulum Ca^{2+}-ATPase uptake pump, decreasing the folding capacity of ER, and hence, can induce ER stress and apoptosis [179]. Truncated variants of sarco-endoplasmic reticulum Ca^{2+}-ATPase have also been implicated in dysregulation

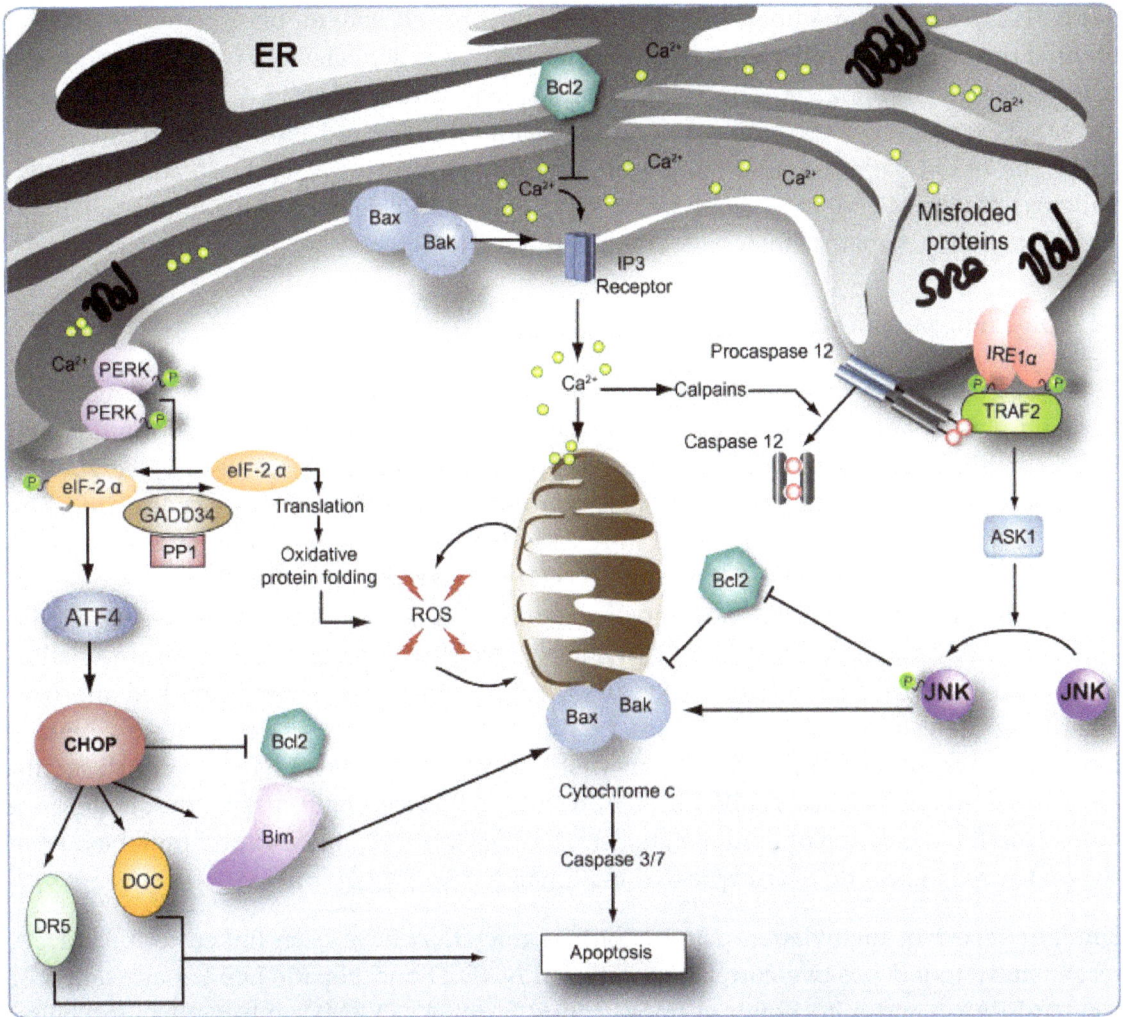

Figure 4. Different mechanisms for ER stress-induced apoptosis [135].

of Calcium flux [180]. Subsequently, the release of ER calcium and its uptake in mitochondria leads to mitochondrial membrane permeabilization, and activation of intrinsic apoptotic pathway. Recent studies also suggest that Smooth and Rough ER may be physically and functionally interacting with mitochondria via tethers and reduction in lengths of these tethers in response to pro-apoptotic agents might be one mechanism for apoptosis [181, 182].

7. Genetic factors

A possible explanation for observed inter-individual variability in susceptibility to NAFLD and progressive NASH is provided by genetics. *Patatin-like phospholipase domain-containing*

3 (PNPLA3), also called adiponutrin, is a protein expressed on endoplasmic reticulum, and on lipid droplets in hepatocytes and adipocytes [183]. It is activated after feeding and is the master regulator of lipogenesis by SREBP-1c. The 148 M variant of PNPLA3 is associated with increased expression of lipogenic transcription factor SREBP1c and alters the lipid catabolism [184]. The 148 M variant is associated with increased severity of NAFLD. In another study, patients with 148 M variant in genotype developed increased steatosis, with augmented lobular inflammation, hepatocellular ballooning and NASH [185].

7.1. Epigenetic modifications

Epigenetic modifications, mainly including microRNA, DNA methylation, histone modification and ubiquination, refers to phenotypic changes irrespective of changes to underlying DNA. "miRNA" are small single stranded RNA molecules regulating mRNA degradation or translation inhibition, subsequently altering protein expression of target genes [186]. The miR-122, which accounts for 70% of all miRNA in the liver, is significantly under-expressed in NASH subjects compared to normal subjects [187]. Inhibition of miR-122 via antisense oligonucleotide in diet-induced obesity mouse models resulted in decreased mRNA expression of acetyl-CoA carboxylase-2, fatty acid synthase, SREBP1c, Stearoyl-CoA desaturase, all of which are key lipogenic factors in human NASH, and the histology showed marked improvement in liver steatosis [188]. In another study in mice, the plasma cholesterol level, hepatic fatty acid and cholesterol synthesis rate as well as HMG CoA reductase level were all significantly reduced after silencing miR-122 [189]. These findings strongly suggest the significance miR-122 in the regulation of lipid metabolism. Besides miR-122, miR-34a and miR-146b were shown to be significantly over-expressed in human NASH [187].

Similarly, aberrant methylation patterns of genomic DNA have been linked to NAFLD. A recent study found positive correlation between NAFLD and hepatic DNA methylation of GpC in PPAR-δ and mitochondrial transcription factor A (TFAM), with methylation being higher in NAFLD liver as compared to control [190]. In conclusion, genetic and epigenetic factors interact with other determinants to produce NAFLD phenotype and determine the rate of its progression [187].

8. Conclusion

The above laborious and detailed discussion on complex molecular mechanisms associated with disease progression in NAFLD does point towards the fact: The pathogenesis and progression of disease in NAFLD is complex interplay of different hormonal, immunological, metabolic, genetic and environmental components. Each component can act on its own or act in concert with other culprits to causes augmented damage to liver. However, more studies are needed to uncover the still unknown players, and to understand the interactions between the different players of multiple-hit model.

Appendix

ACC	acetyl-CoA carboxylase
AhR	aryl hydrocarbon receptor
AMPK	cyclin AMP dependent protein kinase
AP-1	activating protein-1
ASK1	apoptotic signal kinase-1
ATF6	activating transcription factor 6
CDAA diet	choline-deficient, amino acid defined diet
CHOP	CCAAT-enhancer-binding protein homologous protein
ChREBP	carbohydrate response element-binding protein
CREB	cAMP response element-binding protein
DAMP	danger associated molecular pattern
DGAT	diacylglycerol transferase
DR5	death receptor 5
eIF-2α	eukaryotic initiation factor-2α
ER	endoplasmic reticulum
Ero 1 α	endoplasmic reticulum oxidoreductase 1
Fiaf	fasting-induced adipocyte factor
FXR	farnesoid X receptor
GADD	growth arrest and DNA damage
HNE	4-hydroxy-2-noneal
IKKb	Inhibitor of nuclear factor kappa-B kinase subunit beta
Insigs	insulin regulated proteins
IRE 1	inositol-requiring ER-to-nucleus signaling protein1
IRS	insulin receptor substrate
JNK	Jun N-terminal Kinase

LPS	lipopolysaccharide
MAP	mitogen-activated protein
MAPK	mitogen-activated protein kinase
mTOR	mechanistic target of rapamycin
NAFLD	nonalcoholic fatty liver disease
NALP	NACHT, LRR and PYD domains-containing protein 3
NF-κB	nuclear factor κ beta
NLR	nod-like receptor
NLRP	NLR family, pyrin domain-containing 3 inflammasomes
Nrf2	nuclear factor-erythroid-derived 2-related factor 2
PERK	protein kinase RNA- like endoplasmic reticulum kinase
PKC-γ	protein kinase C-gamma
PKR	RNA activated protein kinase
PNPLA3	patatin-like phospholipase domain-containing 3
PPAR	peroxisome proliferator activated receptor
ROS	reactive oxygen species
SCAP	SREBP-cleavage activating proteins
SCD1	stearoyl-CoA desaturase-1
SCFA	short chain fatty acid
SOCS	suppressor of cytokine signaling
SREBP	sterol regulatory element-binding protein
TBARS	thiobarbituric acid reacting substrate
TFAM	mitochondrial transcription factor A
TGF-β1	transforming growth factor-β1
TLR	toll-like receptor
TNF	tumor necrosis factor

TNFR	tumor necrosis factor receptor
TRAIL	TNF-related apoptosis-inducing ligand
UPR	unfolded protein response
XBP1	X-box binding protein-1

Author details

Om Parkash[1]* and Subha Saeed[2]

*Address all correspondence to: om.parkash@aku.edu

1 Section of Gastroenterology/Hepatology, Department of Medicine, The Aga Khan University Hospital, Pakistan

2 The Aga Khan University Hospital, Pakistan

References

[1] AS Y, Keeffe EB. Nonalcoholic fatty liver disease. Reviews in Gastroenterological Disorders. 2002;**2**(1):11-19

[2] Vernon G, Baranova A, Younossi ZM. Systematic review: The epidemiology and natural history of non-alcoholic fatty liver disease and non-alcoholic steatohepatitis in adults. Alimentary Pharmacology & Therapeutics. 2011;**34**(3):274-285

[3] de Alwis NM, Day CP. Non-alcoholic fatty liver disease: The mist gradually clears. Journal of Hepatology. 2008;**48**(Suppl 1):S104-S112

[4] Law K, Brunt EM. Nonalcoholic fatty liver disease. Clinics in Liver Disease. 2010;**14**(4): 591-604

[5] Ekstedt M, Franzen LE, Mathiesen UL, Thorelius L, Holmqvist M, Bodemar G, et al. Long-term follow-up of patients with NAFLD and elevated liver enzymes. Hepatology (Baltimore, Md). 2006;**44**(4):865, 73

[6] Teli MR, James OF, Burt AD, Bennett MK, Day CP. The natural history of nonalcoholic fatty liver: A follow-up study. Hepatology (Baltimore, Md). 1995;**22**(6):1714, 9

[7] Day CP, James OF. Steatohepatitis: A tale of two "hits"? Gastroenterology. 1998;**114**(4): 842-845

[8] Buzzetti E, Pinzani M, Tsochatzis EA. The multiple-hit pathogenesis of non-alcoholic fatty liver disease (NAFLD). Metabolism, Clinical and Experimental. 2016;**65**(8):1038-1048

[9]   Tilg H, Moschen AR. Evolution of inflammation in nonalcoholic fatty liver disease: The multiple parallel hits hypothesis. Hepatology (Baltimore, Md). 2010;**52**(5):1836-1846

[10] Fabbrini E, Mohammed BS, Magkos F, Korenblat KM, Patterson BW, Klein S. Alterations in adipose tissue and hepatic lipid kinetics in obese men and women with nonalcoholic fatty liver disease. Gastroenterology. 2008;**134**(2):424-431

[11] Donnelly KL, Smith CI, Schwarzenberg SJ, Jessurun J, Boldt MD, Parks EJ. Sources of fatty acids stored in liver and secreted via lipoproteins in patients with nonalcoholic fatty liver disease. The Journal of Clinical Investigation. 2005;**115**(5):1343-1351

[12] Schwarz JM, Linfoot P, Dare D, Aghajanian K. Hepatic de novo lipogenesis in nor-moinsulinemic and hyperinsulinemic subjects consuming high-fat, low-carbohydrate and low-fat, high-carbohydrate isoenergetic diets. The American Journal of Clinical Nutrition. 2003;**77**(1):43-50

[13] Lambert JE, Ramos-Roman MA, Browning JD, Parks EJ. Increased de novo lipogenesis is a distinct characteristic of individuals with nonalcoholic fatty liver disease. Gastroenterology. 2014;**146**(3):726-735

[14] Nehra V, Angulo P, Buchman AL, Lindor KD. Nutritional and metabolic considerations in the etiology of nonalcoholic steatohepatitis. Digestive Diseases and Sciences. 2001;**46**(11):2347-2352

[15] Malhi H, Gores GJ. Molecular mechanisms of lipotoxicity in nonalcoholic fatty liver disease. Seminars in Liver Disease. 2008;**28**(4):360-369

[16] Malhi H, Bronk SF, Werneburg NW, Gores GJ. Free fatty acids induce JNK-dependent hepatocyte lipoapoptosis. The Journal of Biological Chemistry. 2006;**281**(17):12093-12101

[17] Barreyro FJ, Kobayashi S, Bronk SF, Werneburg NW, Malhi H, Gores GJ. Transcriptional regulation of Bim by FoxO3A mediates hepatocyte lipoapoptosis. The Journal of Biological Chemistry. 2007;**282**(37):27141-27154

[18] Guicciardi ME, Leist M, Gores GJ. Lysosomes in cell death. Oncogene. 2004;**23**(16): 2881-2890

[19] Feldstein AE, Werneburg NW, Canbay A, Guicciardi ME, Bronk SF, Rydzewski R, et al. Free fatty acids promote hepatic lipotoxicity by stimulating TNF-alpha expression via a lysosomal pathway. Hepatology (Baltimore, Md). 2004;**40**(1):185-194

[20] Wei Y, Wang D, Topczewski F, Pagliassotti MJ. Saturated fatty acids induce endoplasmic reticulum stress and apoptosis independently of ceramide in liver cells. American Journal of Physiology. Endocrinology and Metabolism. 2006;**291**(2):E275-E281

[21] Hirosumi J, Tuncman G, Chang L, Gorgun CZ, Uysal KT, Maeda K, et al. A central role for JNK in obesity and insulin resistance. Nature. 2002;**420**(6913):333-336

[22] Kim BJ, Ryu SW, Song BJ. JNK- and p38 kinase-mediated phosphorylation of Bax leads to its activation and mitochondrial translocation and to apoptosis of human hepatoma HepG2 cells. The Journal of Biological Chemistry. 2006;**281**(30):21256-21265

[23] Yamamoto T, Nakade Y, Yamauchi T, Kobayashi Y, Ishii N, Ohashi T, et al. Glucagon-like peptide-1 analogue prevents nonalcoholic steatohepatitis in non-obese mice. World Journal of Gastroenterology. 2016;**22**(8):2512-2523

[24] Feldstein AE, Canbay A, Angulo P, Taniai M, Burgart LJ, Lindor KD, et al. Hepatocyte apoptosis and fas expression are prominent features of human nonalcoholic steatohepa-titis. Gastroenterology. 2003;**125**(2):437-443

[25] Weisberg SP, McCann D, Desai M, Rosenbaum M, Leibel RL, Ferrante AW Jr. Obesity is associated with macrophage accumulation in adipose tissue. The Journal of Clinical Investigation. 2003;**112**(12):1796-1808

[26] Hotamisligil GS, Arner P, Caro JF, Atkinson RL, Spiegelman BM. Increased adipose tis-sue expression of tumor necrosis factor-alpha in human obesity and insulin resistance. The Journal of Clinical Investigation. 1995;**95**(5):2409-2415

[27] Feldstein AE, Canbay A, Guicciardi ME, Higuchi H, Bronk SF, Gores GJ. Diet associated hepatic steatosis sensitizes to Fas mediated liver injury in mice. Journal of Hepatology. 2003;**39**(6):978-983

[28] Mari M, Fernandez-Checa JC. Sphingolipid signalling and liver diseases. Liver inter-national : official journal of the International Association for the Study of the Liver. 2007;**27**(4):440-450

[29] Paumen MB, Ishida Y, Muramatsu M, Yamamoto M, Honjo T. Inhibition of carnitine pal-mitoyltransferase I augments sphingolipid synthesis and palmitate-induced apoptosis. The Journal of Biological Chemistry. 1997;**272**(6):3324-3329

[30] Suganami T, Nishida J, Ogawa Y. A paracrine loop between adipocytes and macro-phages aggravates inflammatory changes: Role of free fatty acids and tumor necrosis factor alpha. Arteriosclerosis, Thrombosis, and Vascular Biology. 2005;**25**(10):2062-2068

[31] Shi H, Kokoeva MV, Inouye K, Tzameli I, Yin H, Flier JS. TLR4 links innate immu-nity and fatty acid-induced insulin resistance. The Journal of Clinical Investigation. 2006;**116**(11):3015-3025

[32] Chalasani N, Deeg MA, Crabb DW. Systemic levels of lipid peroxidation and its meta-bolic and dietary correlates in patients with nonalcoholic steatohepatitis. The American Journal of Gastroenterology. 2004;**99**(8):1497-1502

[33] Seki S, Kitada T, Sakaguchi H. Clinicopathological significance of oxidative cellular damage in non-alcoholic fatty liver diseases. Hepatology Research: The Official Journal of the Japan Society of Hepatology. 2005;**33**(2):132-134

[34] Yesilova Z, Yaman H, Oktenli C, Ozcan A, Uygun A, Cakir E, et al. Systemic markers of lipid peroxidation and antioxidants in patients with nonalcoholic fatty liver disease. The American Journal of Gastroenterology. 2005;**100**(4):850-855

[35] Valenzuela R, Videla LA. The importance of the long-chain polyunsaturated fatty acid n-6/n-3 ratio in development of non-alcoholic fatty liver associated with obesity. Food & Function. 2011;**2**(11):644-648

[36] Lombardo YB, Chicco AG. Effects of dietary polyunsaturated n-3 fatty acids on dyslipidemia and insulin resistance in rodents and humans. A review. The Journal of Nutritional Biochemistry. 2006;**17**(1):1-13

[37] Valenzuela R, Barrera C, Espinosa A, Llanos P, Orellana P, Videla LA. Reduction in the desaturation capacity of the liver in mice subjected to high fat diet: Relation to LCPUFA depletion in liver and extrahepatic tissues. Prostaglandins, Leukotrienes and Essential Fatty Acids (PLEFA). 2015;**98**:7-14

[38] Puri P, Baillie RA, Wiest MM, Mirshahi F, Choudhury J, Cheung O, et al. A lipidomic analysis of nonalcoholic fatty liver disease. Hepatology (Baltimore, Md). 2007;**46**(4):1081-1090

[39] Mari M, Caballero F, Colell A, Morales A, Caballeria J, Fernandez A, et al. Mitochondrial free cholesterol loading sensitizes to TNF- and Fas-mediated steatohepatitis. Cell Metabolism. 2006;**4**(3):185-198

[40] Koliwad SK, Streeper RS, Monetti M, Cornelissen I, Chan L, Terayama K, et al. DGAT1-dependent triacylglycerol storage by macrophages protects mice from diet-induced insulin resistance and inflammation. The Journal of Clinical Investigation. 2010;**120**(3):756-767

[41] Yamaguchi K, Yang L, McCall S, Huang J, Yu XX, Pandey SK, et al. Inhibiting triglyceride synthesis improves hepatic steatosis but exacerbates liver damage and fibrosis in obese mice with nonalcoholic steatohepatitis. Hepatology (Baltimore, Md). 2007;**45**(6): 1366-1374

[42] Unger RH, Scherer PE. Gluttony, sloth and the metabolic syndrome: A roadmap to lipotoxicity. Trends in Endocrinology and Metabolism: TEM. 2010;**21**(6):345-352

[43] Lin HZ, Yang SQ, Chuckaree C, Kuhajda F, Ronnet G, Diehl AM. Metformin reverses fatty liver disease in obese, leptin-deficient mice. Nature Medicine. 2000;**6**(9):998-1003

[44] Li Z, Yang S, Lin H, Huang J, Watkins PA, Moser AB, et al. Probiotics and antibodies to TNF inhibit inflammatory activity and improve nonalcoholic fatty liver disease. Hepatology (Baltimore, Md). 2003;**37**(2):343-350

[45] Tilg H, Jalan R, Kaser A, Davies NA, Offner FA, Hodges SJ, et al. Anti-tumor necrosis factor-alpha monoclonal antibody therapy in severe alcoholic hepatitis. Journal of Hepatology. 2003;**38**(4):419-425

[46] Clementi AH, Gaudy AM, van Rooijen N, Pierce RH, Mooney RA. Loss of Kupffer cells in diet-induced obesity is associated with increased hepatic steatosis, STAT3

signaling, and further decreases in insulin signaling. Biochimica et Biophysica Acta. 2009; **1792**(11):1062-1072

[47] Bugianesi E, Gastaldelli A, Vanni E, Gambino R, Cassader M, Baldi S, et al. Insulin resistance in non-diabetic patients with non-alcoholic fatty liver disease: Sites and mechanisms. Diabetologia. 2005;**48**(4):634-642

[48] Sabio G, Das M, Mora A, Zhang Z, Jun JY, Ko HJ, et al. A stress signaling pathway in adipose tissue regulates hepatic insulin resistance. Science (New York, N.Y.). 2008; **322**(5907):1539-1543

[49] Taniguchi CM, Emanuelli B, Kahn CR. Critical nodes in signalling pathways: Insights into insulin action. Nature Reviews. Molecular Cell Biology. 2006;**7**(2):85-96

[50] Luyckx F, Lefebvre P, Scheen A. Non-alcoholic steatohepatitis: Association with obesity and insulin resistance, and influence of weight loss. Diabetes & Metabolism. 2000; **26**(2):98-106

[51] Lam TK, Carpentier A, Lewis GF, van de Werve G, Fantus IG, Giacca A. Mechanisms of the free fatty acid-induced increase in hepatic glucose production. American Journal of Physiology-Endocrinology and Metabolism. 2003;**284**(5):E863-EE73

[52] Videla LA, Rodrigo R, Araya J, Poniachik J. Insulin resistance and oxidative stress interdependency in non-alcoholic fatty liver disease. Trends in Molecular Medicine. 2006; **12**(12):555-558

[53] Houstis N, Rosen E, Lander E. Reactive oxygen species have a causal role in multiple forms of insulin resistance. Nature. 2006;**440**:944-948. Find this article online

[54] Woodcroft KJ, Hafner MS, Novak RF. Insulin signaling in the transcriptional and post-transcriptional regulation of CYP2E1 expression. Hepatology. 2002;**35**(2):263-273

[55] Stefan N, Kantartzis K, Häring H-U. Causes and metabolic consequences of fatty liver. Endocrine Reviews. 2008;**29**(7):939-960

[56] Peverill W, Powell LW, Skoien R. Evolving concepts in the pathogenesis of NASH: Beyond steatosis and inflammation. International Journal of Molecular Sciences. 2014; **15**(5):8591-8638

[57] Arumugam M, Raes J, Pelletier E, Le Paslier D, Yamada T, Mende DR, et al. Enterotypes of the human gut microbiome. Nature. 2011;**473**(7346):174-180

[58] Turnbaugh PJ, Ley RE, Mahowald MA, Magrini V, Mardis ER, Gordon JI. An obesity-associated gut microbiome with increased capacity for energy harvest. Nature. 2006; **444**(7122):1027-1131

[59] Miele L, Valenza V, La Torre G, Montalto M, Cammarota G, Ricci R, et al. Increased intestinal permeability and tight junction alterations in nonalcoholic fatty liver disease. Hepatology (Baltimore, Md). 2009;**49**(6):1877-1887

[60] Brun P, Castagliuolo I, Di Leo V, Buda A, Pinzani M, Palù G, et al. Increased intestinal permeability in obese mice: New evidence in the pathogenesis of nonalcoholic steatohepatitis. American Journal of Physiology. Gastrointestinal and Liver Physiology. 2007;**292**(2):G518-GG25

[61] Cani PD, Bibiloni R, Knauf C, Waget A, Neyrinck AM, Delzenne NM, et al. Changes in gut microbiota control metabolic endotoxemia-induced inflammation in high-fat diet-induced obesity and diabetes in mice. Diabetes. 2008;**57**(6):1470-1481

[62] Cani PD, Amar J, Iglesias MA, Poggi M, Knauf C, Bastelica D, et al. Metabolic endotoxemia initiates obesity and insulin resistance. Diabetes. 2007;**56**(7):1761-1772

[63] Noverr MC, Huffnagle GB. Does the microbiota regulate immune responses outside the gut? Trends in Microbiology. 2004;**12**(12):562-568

[64] Rivera CA, Adegboyega P, van Rooijen N, Tagalicud A, Allman M, Wallace M. Toll-like receptor-4 signaling and Kupffer cells play pivotal roles in the pathogenesis of nonalcoholic steatohepatitis. Journal of Hepatology. 2007;**47**(4):571-579

[65] Pappo I, Becovier H, Berry EM, Freund HR. Polymyxin B reduces cecal flora, TNF production and hepatic steatosis during total parenteral nutrition in the rat. The Journal of Surgical Research. 1991;**51**(2):106-112

[66] Topping DL, Clifton PM. Short-chain fatty acids and human colonic function: Roles of resistant starch and nonstarch polysaccharides. Physiological Reviews. 2001; **81**(3):1031-1064

[67] Vernia P, Marcheggiano A, Caprilli R, Frieri G, Corrao G, Valpiani D, et al. Short-chain fatty acid topical treatment in distal ulcerative colitis. Alimentary Pharmacology & Therapeutics. 1995;**9**(3):309-313

[68] Maslowski KM, Vieira AT, Ng A, Kranich J, Sierro F, Yu D, et al. Regulation of inflammatory responses by gut microbiota and chemoattractant receptor GPR43. Nature. 2009;**461**(7268):1282-1286

[69] Zeisel SH, Wishnok JS, Blusztajn J. Formation of methylamines from ingested choline and lecithin. The Journal of Pharmacology and Experimental Therapeutics. 1983; **225**(2):320-324

[70] Abu-Shanab A, Quigley EM. The role of the gut microbiota in nonalcoholic fatty liver disease. Nature Reviews Gastroenterology & Hepatology. 2010;**7**(12):691-701

[71] Zhu L, Baker SS, Gill C, Liu W, Alkhouri R, Baker RD, et al. Characterization of gut microbiomes in nonalcoholic steatohepatitis (NASH) patients: A connection between endogenous alcohol and NASH. Hepatology (Baltimore, Md). 2013;**57**(2):601-609

[72] Lieber CS. Role of S-adenosyl-L-methionine in the treatment of liver diseases. Journal of Hepatology. 1999;**30**(6):1155-1159

[73] Henao-Mejia J, Elinav E, Jin C, Hao L, Mehal WZ, Strowig T, et al. Inflammasome-mediated dysbiosis regulates progression of NAFLD and obesity. Nature. 2012;**482**(7384):179-185

[74] Tremaroli V, Bäckhed F. Functional interactions between the gut microbiota and host metabolism. Nature. 2012;**489**(7415):242-249

[75] Sinal CJ, Tohkin M, Miyata M, Ward JM, Lambert G, Gonzalez FJ. Targeted disruption of the nuclear receptor FXR/BAR impairs bile acid and lipid homeostasis. Cell. 2000;**102**(6):731-744

[76] Cariou B. The farnesoid X receptor (FXR) as a new target in non-alcoholic steatohepatitis. Diabetes & Metabolism. 2008;**34**(6):685-691

[77] Tetri LH, Basaranoglu M, Brunt EM, Yerian LM, Neuschwander-Tetri BA. Severe NAFLD with hepatic necroinflammatory changes in mice fed trans fats and a high-fructose corn syrup equivalent. American Journal of Physiology. Gastrointestinal and Liver Physiology. 2008;**295**(5):G987-G995

[78] Bergheim I, Weber S, Vos M, Krämer S, Volynets V, Kaserouni S, et al. Antibiotics protect against fructose-induced hepatic lipid accumulation in mice: Role of endotoxin. Journal of Hepatology. 2008;**48**(6):983-992

[79] Abdelmalek MF, Suzuki A, Guy C, Unalp-Arida A, Colvin R, Johnson RJ, et al. Increased fructose consumption is associated with fibrosis severity in patients with nonalcoholic fatty liver disease. Hepatology. 2010;**51**(6):1961-1971

[80] Lim JS, Mietus-Snyder M, Valente A, Schwarz J-M, Lustig RH. The role of fructose in the pathogenesis of NAFLD and the metabolic syndrome. Nature Reviews. Gastroenterology & Hepatology. 2010;**7**(5):251-264

[81] Lanaspa MA, Sanchez-Lozada LG, Choi Y-J, Cicerchi C, Kanbay M, Roncal-Jimenez CA, et al. Uric acid induces hepatic steatosis by generation of mitochondrial oxidative stress potential role in fructose-dependent and -independent fatty liver. The Journal of Biological Chemistry. 2012;**287**(48):40732-40744

[82] Pérez-Carreras M, Del Hoyo P, Martín MA, Rubio JC, Martín A, Castellano G, et al. Defective hepatic mitochondrial respiratory chain in patients with nonalcoholic steatohepatitis. Hepatology. 2003;**38**(4):999-1007

[83] Jegatheesan P, De Bandt JP. Fructose and NAFLD: The multifaceted aspects of fructose metabolism. Nutrients. 2017;**9**(3):230

[84] Stevens EA, Mezrich JD, Bradfield CA. The aryl hydrocarbon receptor: A perspective on potential roles in the immune system. Immunology. 2009;**127**(3):299-311

[85] Lee JH, Wada T, Febbraio M, He J, Matsubara T, Lee MJ, et al. A novel role for the dioxin receptor in fatty acid metabolism and hepatic steatosis. Gastroenterology. 2010;**139**(2):653-663

[86] Hernandez-Rodas MC, Valenzuela R, Videla LA. Relevant aspects of nutritional and dietary interventions in non-alcoholic fatty liver disease. International Journal of Molecular Sciences. 2015;**16**(10):25168-25198

[87] Xu A. The fat-derived hormone adiponectin alleviates alcoholic and nonalcoholic fatty liver diseases in mice. Journal of Clinical Investigation. 2003;**112**(1):91-100

[88] Arita Y, Kihara S, Ouchi N, Takahashi M, Maeda K, Miyagawa J, et al. Paradoxical decrease of an adipose-specific protein, adiponectin, in obesity. Biochemical and Biophysical Research Communications. 1999;**257**(1):79-83

[89] Weyer C, Funahashi T, Tanaka S, Hotta K, Matsuzawa Y, Pratley RE, et al. Hypoadiponectinemia in obesity and type 2 diabetes: Close association with insulin resistance and hyperinsulinemia. The Journal of Clinical Endocrinology and Metabolism. 2001;**86**(5):1930-1935

[90] Takaki A, Kawai D, Yamamoto K. Multiple hits, including oxidative stress, as pathogenesis and treatment target in non-alcoholic steatohepatitis (NASH). International Journal of Molecular Sciences. 2013;**14**(10):20704-20728

[91] Kaser S, Moschen A, Cayon A, Kaser A, Crespo J, Pons-Romero F, et al. Adiponectin and its receptors in non-alcoholic steatohepatitis. Gut. 2005;**54**(1):117-121

[92] Yamauchi T, Kamon J, Minokoshi YA, Ito Y, Waki H, Uchida S, et al. Adiponectin stimulates glucose utilization and fatty-acid oxidation by activating AMP-activated protein kinase. Nature Medicine. 2002;**8**(11):1288-1295

[93] Tilg H, Moschen AR. Adipocytokines: Mediators linking adipose tissue, inflammation and immunity. Nature Reviews Immunology. 2006;**6**(10):772-783

[94] Yamauchi T, Kamon J, Ito Y, Tsuchida A, Yokomizo T, Kita S, et al. Cloning of adiponectin receptors that mediate antidiabetic metabolic effects. Nature. 2003;**423**(6941):762-769

[95] Maeda N, Takahashi M, Funahashi T, Kihara S, Nishizawa H, Kishida K, et al. PPARγ ligands increase expression and plasma concentrations of adiponectin, an adipose-derived protein. Diabetes. 2001;**50**(9):2094-2099

[96] Friedman JM, Leibel R, Siegel D, Walsh J, Bahary N. Molecular mapping of the mouse ob mutation. Genomics. 1991;**11**(4):1054-1062

[97] Carbone F, La Rocca C, Matarese G. Immunological functions of leptin and adiponectin. Biochimie. 2012;**94**(10):2082-2088

[98] Polyzos SA, Kountouras J, Mantzoros CS. Leptin in nonalcoholic fatty liver disease: A narrative review. Metabolism, Clinical and Experimental. 2015;**64**(1):60-78

[99] Choi SS, Syn W-K, Karaca GF, Omenetti A, Moylan CA, Witek RP, et al. Leptin promotes the myofibroblastic phenotype in hepatic stellate cells by activating the hedgehog pathway. The Journal of Biological Chemistry. 2010;**285**(47):36551-36560

[100] Aleffi S, Navari N, Delogu W, Galastri S, Novo E, Rombouts K, et al. Mammalian target of rapamycin mediates the angiogenic effects of leptin in human hepatic stellate cells. American Journal of Physiology. Gastrointestinal and Liver Physiology. 2011;**301**(2):G210-G2G9

[101] Wang J, Leclercq I, Brymora JM, Xu N, Ramezani-Moghadam M, London RM, et al. Kupffer cells mediate leptin-induced liver fibrosis. Gastroenterology. 2009;**137**(2):713-723. e1

[102] Imajo K, Fujita K, Yoneda M, Nozaki Y, Ogawa Y, Shinohara Y, et al. Hyperresponsivity to low-dose endotoxin during progression to nonalcoholic steatohepatitis is regulated by leptin-mediated signaling. Cell Metabolism. 2012;**16**(1):44-54

[103] Polyzos SA, Aronis KN, Kountouras J, Raptis DD, Vasiloglou MF, Mantzoros CS. Circulating Leptin in Non-alcoholic Fatty Liver Disease: A Systematic Review and Meta-Analysis. Springer; 2016

[104] Poniachik J, Csendes A, Díaz JC, Rojas J, Burdiles P, Maluenda F, Videla LA. Increased production of IL-1α and TNF-α in lipopolysaccharide-stimulated blood from obese patients with non-alcoholic fatty liver disease. Santiago, Chile: Cytokine; 2006;**33**(5): 252-257

[105] Hotamisligil GS, Shargill NS, Spiegelman BM. Adipose expression of tumor necrosis factor-alpha: Direct role in obesity-linked insulin resistance. Science (New York, N.Y.). 1993;**259**(5091):87-91

[106] Fernandez-Real JM, Vayreda M, Richart C, Gutierrez C, Broch M, Vendrell J, et al. Circulating interleukin 6 levels, blood pressure, and insulin sensitivity in apparently healthy men and women. The Journal of Clinical Endocrinology and Metabolism. 2001;**86**(3):1154-1159

[107] Tomita K, Tamiya G, Ando S, Ohsumi K, Chiyo T, Mizutani A, et al. Tumour necrosis factor α signalling through activation of Kupffer cells plays an essential role in liver fibrosis of non-alcoholic steatohepatitis in mice. Gut. 2006;**55**(3):415-424

[108] Senn JJ, Klover PJ, Nowak IA, Zimmers TA, Koniaris LG, Furlanetto RW, et al. Suppressor of cytokine signaling-3 (SOCS-3), a potential mediator of interleukin-6-dependent insulin resistance in hepatocytes. The Journal of Biological Chemistry. 2003; **278**(16):13740-13746

[109] Cai D, Yuan M, Frantz DF, Melendez PA, Hansen L, Lee J, et al. Local and systemic insulin resistance resulting from hepatic activation of IKK-β and NF-κB. Nature Medicine. 2005;**11**(2):183-190

[110] Ribeiro PS, Cortez-Pinto H, Solá S, Castro RE, Ramalho RM, Baptista A, et al. Hepatocyte apoptosis, expression of death receptors, and activation of NF-κB in the liver of nonalcoholic and alcoholic steatohepatitis patients. The American Journal of Gastroenterology. 2004;**99**(9):1708-1717

[111] Yu HB, Finlay BB. The caspase-1 inflammasome: A pilot of innate immune responses. Cell Host & Microbe. 2008;**4**(3):198-208

[112] Csak T, Ganz M, Pespisa J, Kodys K, Dolganiuc A, Szabo G. Fatty acid and endotoxin activate inflammasomes in mouse hepatocytes that release danger signals to stimulate immune cells. Hepatology (Baltimore, Md). 2011;**54**(1):133-144

[113] Wree A, McGeough MD, Peña CA, Schlattjan M, Li H, Inzaugarat ME, et al. NLRP3 inflammasome activation is required for fibrosis development in NAFLD. Journal of Molecular Medicine. 2014;**92**(10):1069-1082

[114] Miura K, Kodama Y, Inokuchi S, Schnabl B, Aoyama T, Ohnishi H, et al. Toll-like receptor 9 promotes steatohepatitis by induction of interleukin-1beta in mice. Gastroenterology. 2010;**139**(1):323-334. e7

[115] Nagy LE. Recent insights into the role of the innate immune system in the development of alcoholic liver disease. Experimental Biology and Medicine. 2003;**228**(8):882-890

[116] Spruss A, Kanuri G, Wagnerberger S, Haub S, Bischoff SC, Bergheim I. Toll-like receptor 4 is involved in the development of fructose-induced hepatic steatosis in mice. Hepatology (Baltimore, Md). 2009;**50**(4):1094-1104

[117] Miura K, Yang L, van Rooijen N, Brenner DA, Ohnishi H, Seki E. Toll-like receptor 2 and palmitic acid cooperatively contribute to the development of nonalcoholic steatohepatitis through inflammasome activation in mice. Hepatology (Baltimore, Md). 2013;**57**(2):577-589

[118] Vijay-Kumar M, Aitken JD, Carvalho FA, Cullender TC, Mwangi S, Srinivasan S, et al. Metabolic syndrome and altered gut microbiota in mice lacking toll-like receptor 5. Science (New York, N.Y.). 2010;**328**(5975):228-231

[119] Letran SE, Lee S-J, Atif SM, Flores-Langarica A, Uematsu S, Akira S, et al. TLR5-deficient mice lack basal inflammatory and metabolic defects but exhibit impaired CD4 T cell responses to a flagellated pathogen. The Journal of Immunology. 2011;**186**(9):5406-5412

[120] Gentile CL, Frye M, Pagliassotti MJ. Endoplasmic reticulum stress and the unfolded protein response in nonalcoholic fatty liver disease. Antioxidants & Redox Signaling. 2011;**15**(2):505-521

[121] Ashraf NU, Sheikh TA. Endoplasmic reticulum stress and oxidative stress in the pathogenesis of non-alcoholic fatty liver disease. Free Radical Research. 2015;**49**(12):1405-1418

[122] Schroder M, Kaufman RJ. ER stress and the unfolded protein response. Mutation Research. 2005;**569**(1-2):29-63

[123] Ozcan U, Cao Q, Yilmaz E, Lee AH, Iwakoshi NN, Ozdelen E, et al. Endoplasmic reticulum stress links obesity, insulin action, and type 2 diabetes. Science (New York, N.Y.). 2004;**306**(5695):457-461

[124] Wu J, Kaufman RJ. From acute ER stress to physiological roles of the unfolded protein response. Cell Death and Differentiation. 2006;**13**(3):374-384

[125] Zhang K, Kaufman RJ. From endoplasmic-reticulum stress to the inflammatory response. Nature. 2008;**454**(7203):455-462

[126] Ron D, Walter P. Signal integration in the endoplasmic reticulum unfolded protein response. Nature Reviews. Molecular Cell Biology. 2007;**8**(7):519-529

[127] Sano R, Reed JCER. Stress-induced cell death mechanisms. Biochimica et Biophysica Acta. 2013;**1833**(12):3460-3470

[128] Sozen E, Ozer NK. Impact of high cholesterol and endoplasmic reticulum stress on metabolic diseases: An updated mini-review. Redox Biology. 2017;**12**:456-461

[129] Harding HP, Zhang Y, Zeng H, Novoa I, Lu PD, Calfon M, et al. An integrated stress response regulates amino acid metabolism and resistance to oxidative stress. Molecular Cell. 2003;**11**(3):619-633

[130] Ji C, Mehrian-Shai R, Chan C, Hsu YH, Kaplowitz N. Role of CHOP in hepatic apoptosis in the murine model of intragastric ethanol feeding. Alcoholism, Clinical and Experimental Research. 2005;**29**(8):1496-1503

[131] Novoa I, Zeng H, Harding HP, Ron D. Feedback inhibition of the unfolded protein response by GADD34-mediated dephosphorylation of eIF2alpha. The Journal of Cell Biology. 2001;**153**(5):1011-1022

[132] Li G, Mongillo M, Chin KT, Harding H, Ron D, Marks AR, et al. Role of ERO1-alpha-mediated stimulation of inositol 1,4,5-triphosphate receptor activity in endoplasmic reticulum stress-induced apoptosis. The Journal of Cell Biology. 2009;**186**(6):783-792

[133] McCullough KD, Martindale JL, Klotz LO, Aw TY, Holbrook NJ. Gadd153 sensitizes cells to endoplasmic reticulum stress by down-regulating Bcl2 and perturbing the cellular redox state. Molecular and Cellular Biology. 2001;**21**(4):1249-1259

[134] Wang XZ, Ron D. Stress-induced phosphorylation and activation of the transcription factor CHOP (GADD153) by p38 MAP kinase. Science (New York, N.Y.). 1996; **272**(5266):1347-1349

[135] Malhi H, Kaufman RJ. Endoplasmic reticulum stress in liver disease. Journal of Hepatology. 2011;**54**(4):795-809

[136] Hu P, Han Z, Couvillon AD, Kaufman RJ, Exton JH. Autocrine tumor necrosis factor alpha links endoplasmic reticulum stress to the membrane death receptor pathway through IRE1alpha-mediated NF-kappaB activation and down-regulation of TRAF2 expression. Molecular and Cellular Biology. 2006;**26**(8):3071-3084

[137] Ron D, Hubbard SR. How IRE1 reacts to ER stress. Cell. 2008;**132**(1):24-26

[138] Davis RJ. Signal transduction by the JNK group of MAP kinases. Cell. 2000;**103**(2):239-252

[139] Amemiya-Kudo M, Shimano H, Hasty AH, Yahagi N, Yoshikawa T, Matsuzaka T, et al. Transcriptional activities of nuclear SREBP-1a, −1c, and −2 to different target promoters of lipogenic and cholesterogenic genes. The Journal of Lipid Research. 2002; **43**(8):1220-1235

[140] Brown MS, Goldstein JL. The SREBP pathway: Regulation of cholesterol metabolism by proteolysis of a membrane-bound transcription factor. Cell. 1997;**89**(3):331-340

[141] Yang T, Espenshade PJ, Wright ME, Yabe D, Gong Y, Aebersold R, et al. Crucial step in cholesterol homeostasis: Sterols promote binding of SCAP to INSIG-1, a membrane protein that facilitates retention of SREBPs in ER. Cell. 2002;**110**(4):489-500

[142] Lee JN, Ye J. Proteolytic activation of sterol regulatory element-binding protein induced by cellular stress through depletion of Insig-1. The Journal of Biological Chemistry. 2004;**279**(43):45257-45265

[143] Kammoun HL, Chabanon H, Hainault I, Luquet S, Magnan C, Koike T, et al. GRP78 expression inhibits insulin and ER stress-induced SREBP-1c activation and reduces hepatic steatosis in mice. The Journal of Clinical Investigation. 2009;**119**(5):1201-1215

[144] Lee JS, Zheng Z, Mendez R, Ha SW, Xie Y, Zhang K. Pharmacologic ER stress induces non-alcoholic steatohepatitis in an animal model. Toxicology Letters. 2012;**211**(1):29-38

[145] Rutkowski DT, Wu J, Back SH, Callaghan MU, Ferris SP, Iqbal J, et al. UPR pathways combine to prevent hepatic steatosis caused by ER stress-mediated suppression of transcriptional master regulators. Developmental Cell. 2008;**15**(6):829-840

[146] Bobrovnikova-Marjon E, Hatzivassiliou G, Grigoriadou C, Romero M, Cavener DR, Thompson CB, et al. PERK-dependent regulation of lipogenesis during mouse mammary gland development and adipocyte differentiation. Proceedings of the National Academy of Sciences of the United States of America. 2008;**105**(42):16314-16319

[147] Oyadomari S, Harding HP, Zhang Y, Oyadomari M, Ron D. Dephosphorylation of translation initiation factor 2alpha enhances glucose tolerance and attenuates hepatosteatosis in mice. Cell Metabolism. 2008;**7**(6):520-532

[148] Seo J, Fortuno ES 3rd, Suh JM, Stenesen D, Tang W, Parks EJ, et al. Atf4 regulates obesity, glucose homeostasis, and energy expenditure. Diabetes. 2009;**58**(11):2565-2573

[149] Xiao G, Zhang T, Yu S, Lee S, Calabuig-Navarro V, Yamauchi J, et al. ATF4 protein deficiency protects against high fructose-induced hypertriglyceridemia in mice. The Journal of Biological Chemistry. 2013;**288**(35):25350-25361

[150] Wang S, Chen Z, Lam V, Han J, Hassler J, Finck BN, et al. IRE1alpha-XBP1s induces PDI expression to increase MTP activity for hepatic VLDL assembly and lipid homeostasis. Cell Metabolism. 2012;**16**(4):473-486

[151] Zhang K, Wang S, Malhotra J, Hassler JR, Back SH, Wang G, et al. The unfolded protein response transducer IRE1alpha prevents ER stress-induced hepatic steatosis. The EMBO Journal. 2011;**30**(7):1357-1375

[152] Lee AH, Scapa EF, Cohen DE, Glimcher LH. Regulation of hepatic lipogenesis by the transcription factor XBP1. Science (New York, N.Y.). 2008;**320**(5882):1492-1496

[153] Zeng L, Lu M, Mori K, Luo S, Lee AS, Zhu Y, et al. ATF6 modulates SREBP2-mediated lipogenesis. The EMBO Journal. 2004;**23**(4):950-958

[154] Yamamoto K, Takahara K, Oyadomari S, Okada T, Sato T, Harada A, et al. Induction of liver steatosis and lipid droplet formation in ATF6alpha-knockout mice burdened with pharmacological endoplasmic reticulum stress. Molecular Biology of the Cell. 2010;**21**(17):2975-2986

[155] Santos CX, Tanaka LY, Wosniak J, Laurindo FR. Mechanisms and implications of reactive oxygen species generation during the unfolded protein response: Roles of endoplasmic reticulum oxidoreductases, mitochondrial electron transport, and NADPH oxidase. Antioxidants & Redox Signaling. 2009;**11**(10):2409-2427

[156] Hanada S, Harada M, Kumemura H, Bishr Omary M, Koga H, Kawaguchi T, et al. Oxidative stress induces the endoplasmic reticulum stress and facilitates inclusion formation in cultured cells. Journal of Hepatology. 2007;**47**(1):93-102

[157] Cullinan SB, Diehl JA. Coordination of ER and oxidative stress signaling: The PERK/Nrf2 signaling pathway. The International Journal of Biochemistry & Cell Biology. 2006;**38**(3):317-332

[158] Sugimoto H, Okada K, Shoda J, Warabi E, Ishige K, Ueda T, et al. Deletion of nuclear factor-E2-related factor-2 leads to rapid onset and progression of nutritional steatohepatitis in mice. American Journal of Physiology. Gastrointestinal and Liver Physiology. 2010;**298**(2):G283-G294

[159] Cullinan SB, Zhang D, Hannink M, Arvisais E, Kaufman RJ, Diehl JA. Nrf2 is a direct PERK substrate and effector of PERK-dependent cell survival. Molecular and Cellular Biology. 2003;**23**(20):7198-7209

[160] Liu Y, Adachi M, Zhao S, Hareyama M, Koong AC, Luo D, et al. Preventing oxidative stress: A new role for XBP1. Cell Death and Differentiation. 2009;**16**(6):847-857

[161] Urano F, Wang X, Bertolotti A, Zhang Y, Chung P, Harding HP, et al. Coupling of stress in the ER to activation of JNK protein kinases by transmembrane protein kinase IRE1. Science (New York, N.Y.). 2000;**287**(5453):664-666

[162] Jiang H-Y, Wek SA, McGrath BC, Scheuner D, Kaufman RJ, Cavener DR, et al. Phosphorylation of the α subunit of eukaryotic initiation factor 2 is required for activation of NF-κB in response to diverse cellular stresses. Molecular and Cellular Biology. 2003;**23**(16):5651-5663

[163] Yamazaki H, Hiramatsu N, Hayakawa K, Tagawa Y, Okamura M, Ogata R, et al. Activation of the Akt-NF-κB pathway by subtilase cytotoxin through the ATF6 branch of the unfolded protein response. The Journal of Immunology. 2009;**183**(2):1480-1487

[164] Donze O, Abbas-Terki T, Picard D. The Hsp90 chaperone complex is both a facilitator and a repressor of the dsRNA-dependent kinase PKR. The EMBO Journal. 2001;**20**(14):3771-3780

[165] Nakamura T, Furuhashi M, Li P, Cao H, Tuncman G, Sonenberg N, et al. Double-stranded RNA-dependent protein kinase links pathogen sensing with stress and meta-bolic homeostasis. Cell. 2010;**140**(3):338-348

[166] Donze O, Deng J, Curran J, Sladek R, Picard D, Sonenberg N. The protein kinase PKR: A molecular clock that sequentially activates survival and death programs. The EMBO Journal. 2004;**23**(3):564-571

[167] Luebke-Wheeler J, Zhang K, Battle M, Si-Tayeb K, Garrison W, Chhinder S, et al. Hepatocyte nuclear factor 4alpha is implicated in endoplasmic reticulum stress-induced acute phase response by regulating expression of cyclic adenosine monophosphate responsive element binding protein H. Hepatology (Baltimore, Md). 2008;**48**(4):1242-1250

[168] Zhang K, Shen X, Wu J, Sakaki K, Saunders T, Rutkowski DT, et al. Endoplasmic reticulum stress activates cleavage of CREBH to induce a systemic inflammatory response. Cell. 2006;**124**(3):587-599

[169] Wieckowska A, Zein NN, Yerian LM, Lopez AR, McCullough AJ, Feldstein AE. In vivo assessment of liver cell apoptosis as a novel biomarker of disease severity in nonalco-holic fatty liver disease. Hepatology (Baltimore, Md). 2006;**44**(1):27-33

[170] Tamaki N, Hatano E, Taura K, Tada M, Kodama Y, Nitta T, et al. CHOP deficiency atten-uates cholestasis-induced liver fibrosis by reduction of hepatocyte injury. American Journal of Physiology. Gastrointestinal and Liver Physiology. 2008;**294**(2):G498-G505

[171] Pfaffenbach KT, Gentile CL, Nivala AM, Wang D, Wei Y, Pagliassotti MJ. Linking endo-plasmic reticulum stress to cell death in hepatocytes: Roles of C/EBP homologous pro-tein and chemical chaperones in palmitate-mediated cell death. American Journal of Physiology - Endocrinology and Metabolism. 2010;**298**(5):E1027-E1E35

[172] Zhang XQ, CF X, CH Y, Chen WX, Li YM. Role of endoplasmic reticulum stress in the pathogenesis of nonalcoholic fatty liver disease. World Journal of Gastroenterology. 2014;**20**(7):1768-1776

[173] Rutkowski DT, Arnold SM, Miller CN, Wu J, Li J, Gunnison KM, et al. Adaptation to ER stress is mediated by differential stabilities of pro-survival and pro-apoptotic mRNAs and proteins. PLoS Biology. 2006;**4**(11):e374

[174] Masciarelli S, Fra AM, Pengo N, Bertolotti M, Cenci S, Fagioli C, et al. CHOP-independent apoptosis and pathway-selective induction of the UPR in developing plasma cells. Molecular Immunology. 2010;**47**(6):1356-1365

[175] Yoneda T, Imaizumi K, Oono K, Yui D, Gomi F, Katayama T, et al. Activation of cas-pase-12, an endoplastic reticulum (ER) resident caspase, through tumor necrosis factor receptor-associated factor 2-dependent mechanism in response to the ER stress. The Journal of Biological Chemistry. 2001;**276**(17):13935-13940

[176] Hetz C, Bernasconi P, Fisher J, Lee A-H, Bassik MC, Antonsson B, et al. Proapoptotic BAX and BAK modulate the unfolded protein response by a direct interaction with IRE1α. Science (New York, N.Y.). 2006;**312**(5773):572-576

[177] Oakes SA, Scorrano L, Opferman JT, Bassik MC, Nishino M, Pozzan T, et al. Proapoptotic BAX and BAK regulate the type 1 inositol trisphosphate receptor and calcium leak from the endoplasmic reticulum. Proceedings of the National Academy of Sciences of the United States of America. 2005;**102**(1):105-110

[178] Deniaud A, Sharaf el dein O, Maillier E, Poncet D, Kroemer G, Lemaire C, et al. Endoplasmic reticulum stress induces calcium-dependent permeability transition, mitochondrial outer membrane permeabilization and apoptosis. Oncogene. 2008;**27**(3):285-299

[179] Luciani DS, Gwiazda KS, T-LB Y, Kalynyak TB, Bychkivska Y, Frey MH, et al. Roles of IP 3 R and RyR Ca 2+ channels in endoplasmic reticulum stress and β-cell death. Diabetes. 2009;**58**(2):422-432

[180] Chami M, Oulès B, Szabadkai G, Tacine R, Rizzuto R, Paterlini-Bréchot P. Role of SERCA1 truncated isoform in the proapoptotic calcium transfer from ER to mitochondria during ER stress. Molecular Cell. 2008;**32**(5):641-651

[181] Csordas G, Renken C, Varnai P, Walter L, Weaver D, Buttle KF, et al. Structural and functional features and significance of the physical linkage between ER and mitochondria. The Journal of Cell Biology. 2006;**174**(7):915-921

[182] Rizzuto R, Pinton P, Carrington W, Fay FS, Fogarty KE, Lifshitz LM, et al. Close contacts with the endoplasmic reticulum as determinants of mitochondrial Ca2+ responses. Science (New York, N.Y.). 1998;**280**(5370):1763-1766

[183] Huang Y, He S, Li JZ, Seo Y-K, Osborne TF, Cohen JC, et al. A feed-forward loop amplifies nutritional regulation of PNPLA3. Proceedings of the National Academy of Sciences. 2010;**107**(17):7892-7897

[184] He S, McPhaul C, Li JZ, Garuti R, Kinch L, Grishin NV, et al. A sequence variation (I148M) in PNPLA3 associated with nonalcoholic fatty liver disease disrupts triglyceride hydrolysis. The Journal of Biological Chemistry. 2010;**285**(9):6706-6715

[185] Valenti L, Alisi A, Galmozzi E, Bartuli A, Del Menico B, Alterio A, et al. I148M patatin-like phospholipase domain-containing 3 gene variant and severity of pediatric nonalcoholic fatty liver disease. Hepatology (Baltimore, Md). 2010;**52**(4):1274-1280

[186] Li YY. Genetic and epigenetic variants influencing the development of nonalcoholic fatty liver disease. World journal of gastroenterology: WJG. 2012;**18**(45):6546

[187] Cheung O, Puri P, Eicken C, Contos MJ, Mirshahi F, Maher JW, et al. Nonalcoholic steatohepatitis is associated with altered hepatic MicroRNA expression. Hepatology. 2008;**48**(6):1810-1820

[188] Esau C, Davis S, Murray SF, XX Y, Pandey SK, Pear M, et al. miR-122 regulation of lipid metabolism revealed by in vivo antisense targeting. Cell Metabolism. 2006;**3**(2):87-98

[189] Krutzfeldt J, Rajewsky N, Braich R, Rajeev KG, Tuschl T, Manoharan M, et al. Silencing of microRNAs in vivo with 'antagomirs. Nature. 2005;**438**(7068):685-689

[190] Sookoian S, Rosselli MS, Gemma C, Burgueno AL, Fernandez Gianotti T, Castano GO, et al. Epigenetic regulation of insulin resistance in nonalcoholic fatty liver disease: Impact of liver methylation of the peroxisome proliferator-activated receptor gamma coactivator 1alpha promoter. Hepatology (Baltimore, Md). 2010;**52**(6):1992-2000

12

Imaging Evaluation of Liver Tumors in Pediatric Patients

Chengzhan Zhu, Bingzi Dong and Qian Dong

Abstract

Imaging plays crucial roles in the management of pediatric patients with suspected liver malignant tumors. Three-dimensional (3D) imaging could significantly improve the resection rate of pediatric tumors and increase the safety of the surgery. With the development of medical imaging, 3D reconstruction technology, the innovation of liver surgery and the proposal of precise hepatectomy, the intrahepatic vascular anatomy of the liver and liver segmentectomy based on that vascular anatomy have become well developed. With the analysis of 3D digital liver, we proposed a new type of liver classification system: Dong's digital liver classification system. And we measured the normal total liver volume from neonate to aging making a reference for surgeons all around the world. And the Human Digital Liver Database was established by the Affiliated Hospital of Qingdao University and Hisense Company, aiming to collect digital liver from neonates, children, adults, and the elderly, from normal livers, livers with cancer, and simulated livers resected using Hisense CAS. Then we showed one case report of patient with giant liver tumor. With the application of Hisense CAS and our data, we successfully removed the tumor. We believe that the new techniques in imaging will help surgeons to accomplish better operations.

Keywords: three-dimensional imaging, liver tumor, digital liver classification, total liver volume, Human Digital Liver Database

1. Introduction

Liver tumors constitute 1–4% of all solid tumors in children, of which 40% are benign. They mainly include hemangioma, liver hamartoma, and liver cell adenoma. Malignant tumors mainly include hepatoblastoma (HB), hepatocellular carcinoma (HCC), malignant liver mesothelioma, and rhabdomyosarcoma [1]. For most hepatic malignancies, hepatectomy or liver transplantation is optimal for cure. Resectability can be limited by multifocality, bilobar involvement, vascular thrombus or vascular invasion, extension to hepatic hilum, and distant metastasis [2]. If the tumor cannot be resected at initial imaging evaluation, the child is usually first treated with chemotherapy and/or radiation, and then re-imaged. For this reason, proper imaging evaluation of the liver is necessary which will shorten the surgical waiting duration and increase the success of the resection. In the cases where liver resection has high morbidity and high incidence, liver transplantation is recommended.

Imaging plays crucial roles in the management of pediatric patients with suspected liver tumors. MR imaging is recommended for children than computed tomography (CT) because of less radiation [3, 4]. However, CT could clearly show the liver anatomy and be helpful in staging, which is widely used in preoperative evaluation in the pediatric patients [3, 5]. Moreover, if the CT or MR imaging indicates a malignant mass, CT of the chest should be performed to assess the presence of lung metastasis [6].

In our experience, three-dimensional imaging can significantly improve the resection rate of pediatric tumors and increase the safety of the surgery [7]. In our center, we prefer CT scans for preoperative evaluation of pediatric liver tumors. However, it is very important to avoid non-contrast and multiphase images, and use low-dose CT scan in pediatric patients. CT phase of portal venous are very useful for evaluation of primary malignant liver tumors in children.

2. Common malignant liver tumors in pediatric patients

2.1. Hepatoblastoma (HB)

HB comprises 1% of all pediatric malignancies. HB most often occurs in infants and young children between 6 months and 4 years old. The median age of occurrence is 18 months. After 5 years of age, it becomes rare but histologically more aggressive in children over 8 years old. It occurs equally in males and females [8]. Based on radiological imaging, preoperative staging system (Pretreatment Extent of Disease or PRETEXT) which define extent of liver parenchyma involvement is an important guideline for treatment selection [9]. The new international surgical guidelines, which are being developed for the upcoming Pediatric Hepatic International Tumor Trial, will recommend primary surgical resection at diagnosis for PRETEXT I and II tumors of which the radiographic margin on the middle hepatic vein is wide [10].

As staging and treatment are mainly dependent on imaging, high-quality radiographic imaging has come to be of vital importance. For imaging assessment, both contrast-enhanced CT and MRI are recommended. Non-contrast CT typically shows a relatively well-defined, heterogeneous mass, slightly hypodense compared with liver tissue, with or without calcifications. On contrast-enhanced CT (**Figure 1**), the tumor reveals a heterogeneous enhancement, which may be hyperdense relative to liver parenchyma in the early arterial postcontrast phase and usually appears iso- or hypodense on delayed images (11). Invasion of the portal vein and its subsequent thrombosis must be evaluated in all suspected cases of hepatoblastoma. The tumor thrombus can even spread along IVC and encroach in the lumen of right atrium.

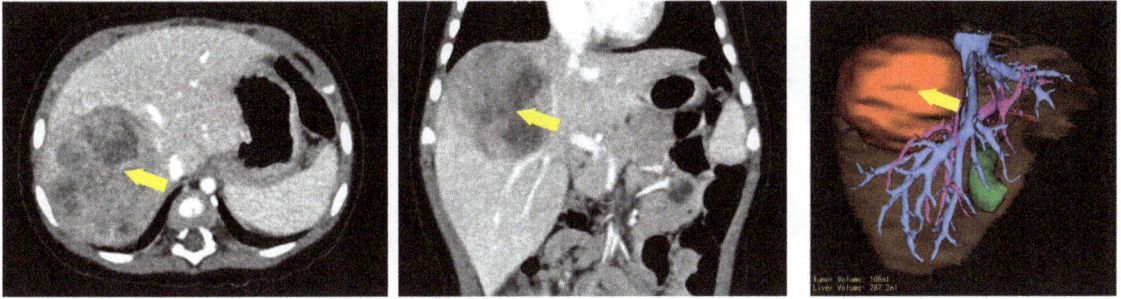

Figure 1. CT and three-dimensional reconstructed liver of PRETEXT II hepatoblastoma resectable at diagnosis (white arrow).

Metastasis may be seen in lymph nodes and lung parenchyma; it is rare in the brain and bones [11]. Twenty percent of HBs present with metastasis and most of them are in the lungs; therefore CT chest is necessary for staging.

2.2. Hepatocellular carcinoma (HCC)

The incidence of HCC in children was 0.5–1.0 cases per million children [12]. Different from HB, the median age of occurrence in children with HCC is 10 to 11.2 years [3]. The male to female ratio is 2:1 in young children, but it increases with age. Unlike adults, in whom HCC usually accompanies underlying liver disease, only 20–35% of children with HCC children have underlying liver disease [13]. HCC in children is now considered a distinct tumor family consisting of adult type HCC and variants, fibrolamellar HCC, and transitional liver cell tumor [14]. HCC is usually multifocal and may present with a variable number and distribution of tumor nodules. Recognizing HCC lesions smaller than 1.0 cm is still difficult.

In fibrolamellar HCCs, tumor cells are circumscribed by bundles of acellular collagen. This form is seen more frequently in adolescents than in adults and has better prognosis. HCCs are highly variable and show non-characteristic features on CT imaging: the tumors may be homogeneous or heterogeneous, solitary or multifocal, well- or ill-defined. On unenhanced CT images, HCCs typically appear isodense or slightly hypodense relative to liver parenchyma. On enhanced CT, they show early arterial contrast enhancement and rapid washout. HCCs are often inconspicuous on delayed scans. HCC sometimes invades the vasculature in the liver, and even the inferior vena cava may be seen [11]. The diagnosis of underlying cirrhosis may help during differential diagnosis, but it is rare in children. Three-dimensional CT image (**Figure 2**) analysis techniques are now available to estimate tumor volume and provide detailed information regarding the intrahepatic anatomy that resembles the actual intraoperative findings [15]. CT volumetry may permit calculation of resected tumor volume and anticipated size of the remnant liver in planning resection [16]. Plain CT of the chest should be performed to rule out the lung metastases. As for HB, tumor staging is an important consideration in determining the plan of treatment and prognosis. The PRETEXT staging system is recommended because it is currently the only staging system that allows surgical planning [9]. HCC is relatively chemoresistant. Complete resection or liver transplantation of localized tumor is the best option. In the SIOPEL-1 report, the overall resection rate was 36% and the 5 y OS and EFS was 28 and 17% respectively [13]. For liver transplantation, patient survival was

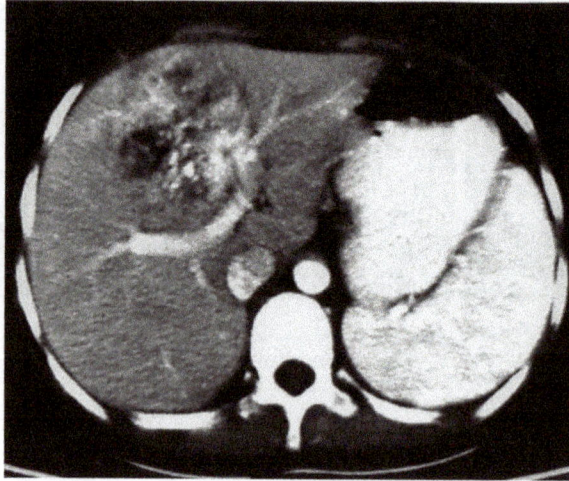

Figure 2. CT of hepatocellular carcinoma in pediatric patient.

63% at 5 years and 58% at 10 years in a study of orthotopic liver transplantation in 41 HCC children <18 years. Recurrence was the primary cause of death in 86% [17]. The outcomes of liver transplantation in HCC are not as good as that for HB.

2.3. Pediatric hepatic sarcomas

Pediatric hepatic sarcomas include undifferentiated embryonal sarcoma (UES), biliary rhabdo-myosarcoma, and angiosarcoma [5]. UES is a rare malignant neoplasm, and its the incidence is higher than the other two types of sarcoma. UES was recently shown to share genetic features with mesenchymal harmatoma. Diagnosis of UES is usually between 6 and 10 years but some studies report presentation in young teenagers [18]. The tumor appears on ultrasound as a hetero-echoic mass, and a hypodense multicystic lesion on CT scan or MRI (**Figure 3**), usually exceeding 10 cm in size, with a predominance for involving the right hepatic lobe [19].

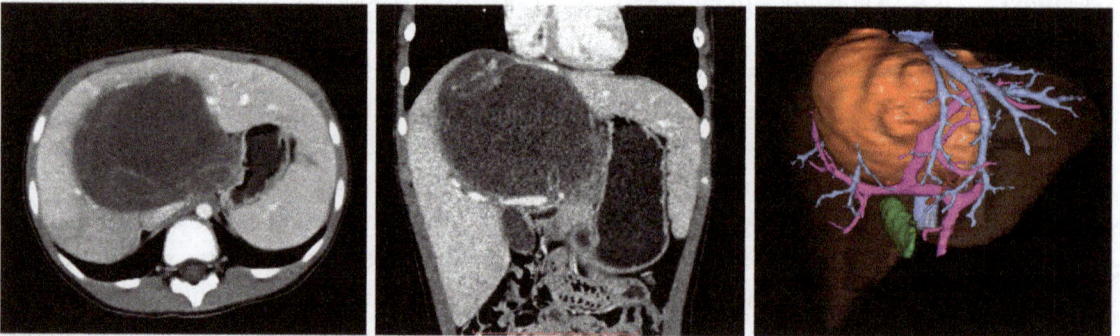

Figure 3. CT and three-dimensional reconstructed liver of undifferentiated embryonal sarcoma.

3. Value of CT scan in guiding the surgical treatment

The objective of surgery is to achieve complete resection of the tumor, both macro- and microscopically, which is paramount for cure of malignant liver cancers. The liver resection strategy is based on pre-operative understanding of liver segmentation, vascular occlusion techniques, and experience in performing different types of hepatectomy, including extensive resection (left and right trisegmentectomies). Although abdominal CT should only be considered if MR imaging is not available or contraindicated, there are some limitations of MRI in some hospitals at developing countries. In our experience, MRI is the best available technique for diagnosing liver tumors, but its value is less clear in preoperatively evaluating the resectability of liver tumors especially in pediatric patients. The development and rapid clinical acceptance of single-detector helical CT during the last decade and, more recently, the introduction of multidetector CT (MDCT) have resulted in significant improvements in the study of the liver. MDCT makes it possible to precisely image the vascular anatomy, including the anomalous branches, feeding arteries, or drainage veins. Moreover, each image phase could be independently and simultaneously extracted or combined. In addition to technical advances, such as shorter scanning times, multiplanar imaging, and improved ability to perform multiphasic contrast-enhanced studies, newer and better intravenous contrast media and advances in post-acquisition data processing techniques have renewed researchers' enthusiasm for using hepatic CT scanning [11].

Furthermore, the software program for volumetry provides a proposed remnant liver volume and an optimal cut line of the liver. Various preoperative simulations can thus be considered. This volumetric analysis positively contributes to the safety of the procedure by assisting in the selection of the optimal operations. Preoperative evaluation of the relationship between the tumor and surrounding vasculature was simulated to perform liver resection with 3D software (**Figure 4**).

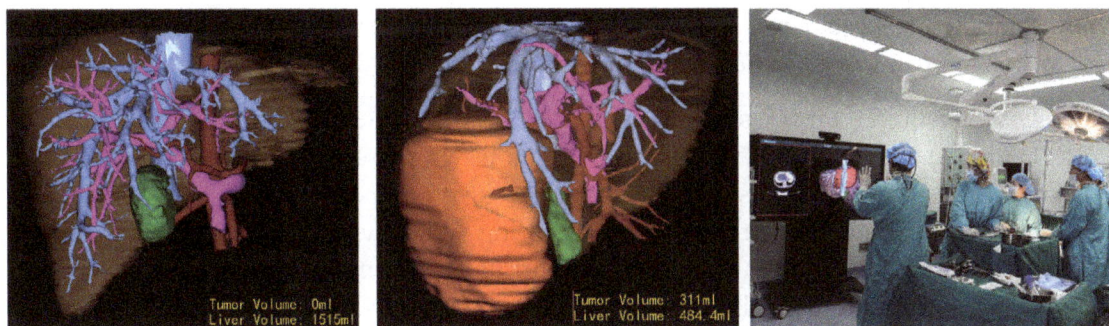

Figure 4. Three-dimensional reconstructed liver indicating total liver volume, liver tumor volume, and intraoperative navigation system.

4. 3D simulation software and Hisense Computer Assisted Surgery System (Hisense CAS)

With the development of three-dimensional simulation software, it is possible to achieve virtual hepatectomy, which can assist the surgeons planning the operation. The development of three-dimensional simulation software makes it possible to achieve virtual hepatectomy, which can assist surgeons to plan the operation, especially the complicated one. The history of 3D simulation software as it relates to hepatectomy can be divided into three stages: [1] successful 3D rendering of liver structures due to the introduction of multidetector row CT in the 1990s [20, 2] virtual hepatectomy depending on the reconstruction of the liver using 3D simulation software since 2000 [21, 3] the clinical practice and popularization of virtual hepatectomy using software packages since 2005, such as operation planning and operative navigation [22]. In some developed countries, such as Japan, virtual hepatectomy has routinely been performed in adult patients undergoing anatomic liver resection. It helps surgeons to plan the operative approach precisely, accurately position the lesion range, and be familiar with the operative route. Hisense Computer Assisted Surgery System (Hisense CAS) is a 3D simulation software package specifically developed for pediatric patients. It can provide precise and exquisite 3D visualization of pediatric liver structures using DICOM data from conventional CT. Considering that children have more refined anatomical structures, the accuracy of Hisense CAS was improved. Hepatectomy can be simulated on a personal computer, and the results can be shared with anyone in the cooperative team. Hisense CAS allows a surgeon to instantaneously manipulate the liver simulation in the operating room using a gesture-controlled display (**Figure 4**).

CT imaging can be performed using a 64-row-MDCT Scanner (Sensation64; Siemens, Erlangen, Germany) with the following parameters: kVp 120, mAs 100, slice collimation 0.625 mm, feed/rotation 12 mm, and rotation time 0.5 s. Patients received 2.0 ml/kg of an iodinated contrast agent (Ultravist; Bayer HealthCare LLC, Germany) to delineate the hepatic vasculature, which was administered intravenously using an automated injector system (CT 9000; Liebel-Flarsheim, Cincinnati, OH) at a rate of 2.0 ml/s. Automated bolus tracking with bolus detection on the level of the ascending aorta assured accurate timing of the arterial phase. For display of the portal and hepatic venous anatomy, third and fourth CT image sets were acquired at 10 and 40 s after the arterial imaging [23].

Four steps are required for transferring the CT DICOM file into 3D digital liver using Hisense CAS: [1] upload the primary CT DICOM data into the Hisense CAS; [2] auto or semi-automatically reconstruct the liver structures (liver parenchyma, portal vein, hepatic veins, and tumors) in a 3D context by extraction of neighboring voxels with a similar CT density, and automatically calculate the total liver volume and tumor volume; [3] virtual liver resection using the software (automatically calculating the remnant liver volume); and [4] assessment of the optimal surgical procedures based on the virtual hepatectomy. The surgical team could communicate and discuss the surgical liver anatomy with radiologists or pediatricians based on 3D reconstruction, such as the tumor locations, the appearance of the vessel branches, or approach of liver resection. Various virtual surgical strategies could be explored in the Hisense CAS. Finally, the surgical team could develop the optimal plan of operation [7].

5. Dong's digital liver classification

With the development of medical imaging, 3D reconstruction technology, the innovation of liver surgery and the proposal of precision hepatectomy, the intrahepatic vascular anatomy of the liver and liver segmentectomy based on that vascular anatomy have become well developed. With the analysis of 3D digital liver, we proposed a new type of liver classification system: Dong's digital liver classification system. Professor Dong Qian of the Affiliated Hospital of Qingdao University analyzed the anatomy of thousands of digital human livers from newborns to the elderly to build a new system of liver classification based on intrahepatic vascular anatomy [24].

1260 cases of normal human liver were rendered into 3D digital livers using their DICOM files. Based on the anatomical variation of the portal branches supplying liver segments, we built our Dong's digital liver classification system.

We divided the digital liver into four groups based on the type of segmentation and the variations in portal vein anatomy. Type A livers are similar to Couinaud or Cho's segmentation, containing eight segments (**Figure 5**). Type B livers have nine segments because there are three subdivisions of right-anterior portal vein (**Figure 6**). The defining characteristic of Type C is the variation in the right-posterior portal vein, which is arcuate-shaped (**Figure 7**). Type C-a livers have arcuate-shaped right-posterior portal veins and right-anterior portal veins like those in Type A livers. Type C-b livers have arcuate-shaped right-posterior portal veins and right-anterior portal veins like those in Type B livers. Type D livers have anomalous portal vein variations, which require three-dimensional simulation and individualized liver resection plan (**Figure 8**).

Type A: Similar to Couinaud [25] or Cho's segmentation [26], containing eight segments (**Figure 5**).

Segment I (3–6 P1 branches): Caudate lobe. There are 3–6 small branches (P1) originating from the back of right and left portal vein, surrounded by 5–8 tiny short hepatic veins.

Segments II and III: The left portal vein divides into the third-grade portal vein (P2 and P3) and perfuses the upper and lower outer sides of the left liver, which contains segments II and III.

Segment IV: Portal veins divided from the left portal vein perfuse the inner part of the left liver.

Segments V and VIII: The right portal vein divides into the right anterior and posterior branches, and then the anterior trunk further divides into several branches. (**Figure 5**).

Segments VI and VII: The right posterior portal vein further divides into right anterior (P6) and posterior branches (P7). The anterior branches perfuse segment VI, the lower outer area of the right liver.

Type B: Nine segments due to three subdivisions of right-anterior portal vein (**Figure 6**).

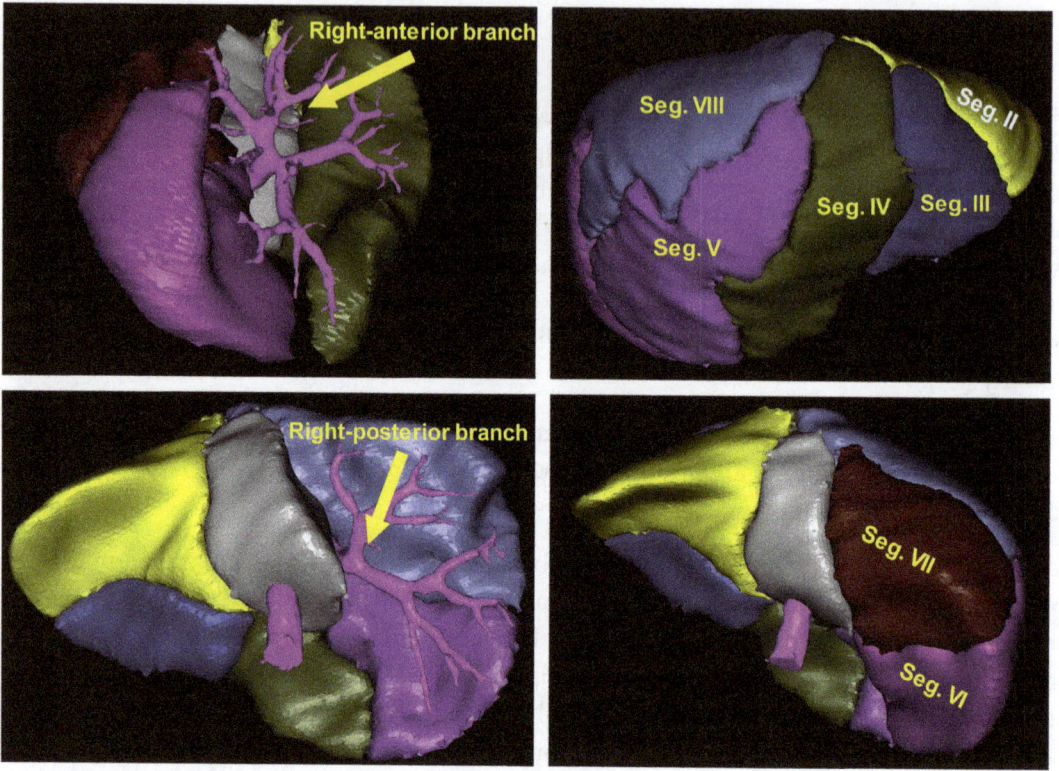

Figure 5. Right-anterior and right-posterior part of liver anatomy indicating Type A segmentation of Dong's digital liver classification system, similar to Couinaud or Cho's segmentation.

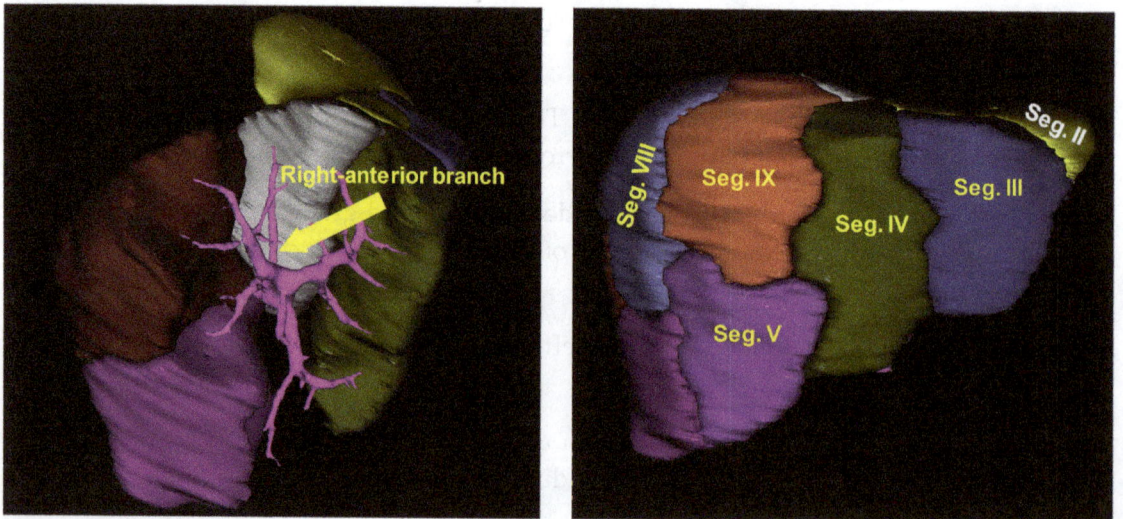

Figure 6. Right-anterior part of liver anatomy indicating Type B segmentation of Dong's digital liver classification system.

Type C: The right posterior portal vein does not divide into main branches as in Type A or B livers, whose portal veins separate into 5–11 branches from an arcuate trunk. During precise hepatectomy, it is difficult to resect only segments VI or VII as in Type A and Type B. The prevalence of Type C livers is not high, but it makes a considerable difference in precise surgery. Cases in which the right posterior portal vein is arcuate type and the right anterior portal vein separates into only P8 and P5 are defined as Type C-a (**Figure 7**). When the right posterior portal vein is arcuate type and the right anterior portal vein separate to P5, P8, and P9, we define it as Type C-b.

Type D: This is a catchall category, appearing in about 12.43% of all livers. It includes all variations that cannot be classified into any of the previous three types (**Figure 8**).

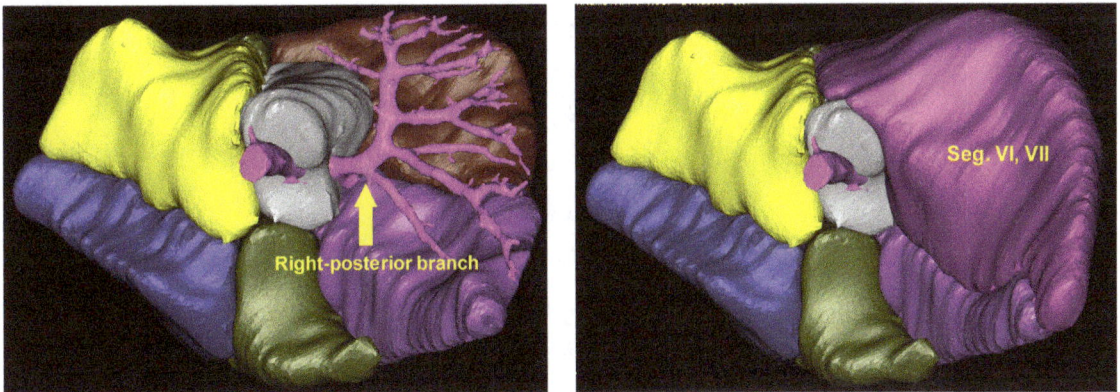

Figure 7. Type C livers have arcuate-shaped right-posterior portal veins.

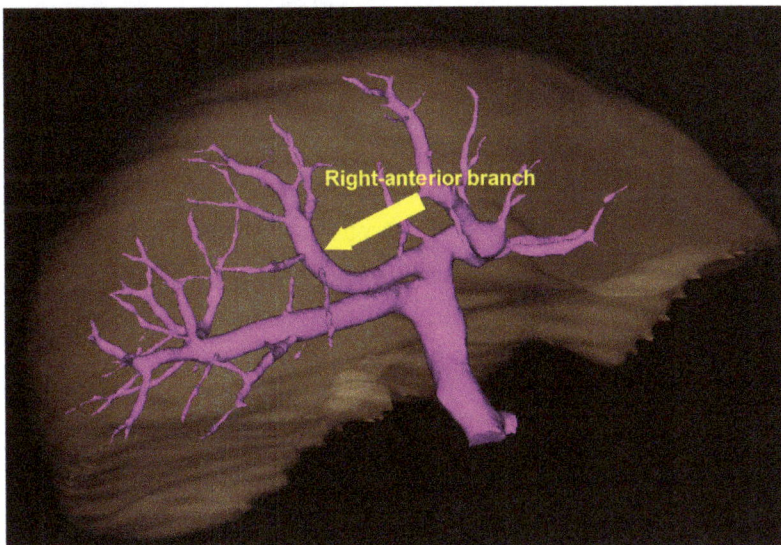

Figure 8. Rare variation of portal vein which is classified into Type D segmentation.

6. Measurement of liver volume from neonates to the elderly

Total liver volume, the basic unit of liver function, is an important factor to evaluate the resectability of liver cancer. There have been many studies of the total liver volume and necessary remnant liver volume in adult patients but only a few reports regarding liver volume in children. Because measured total liver volume has been proposed as the golden standard of liver volume for preoperative surgical plan, we tried to summarize the average total liver volume of Chinese patients of different ages, from neonates to the elderly.

Age	N	Liver volume (cm³)
<1 Month	28	140.0339 ± 50.0707
1–3 Months	26	191.1462 ± 38.9132
4–6 Months	31	261.5065 ± 70.9437
7–9 Months	22	273.1917 ± 50.0732
10–12 Months	33	305.4692 ± 36.3323
1–2 Years	56	374.3617 ± 65.8447
2–3 Years	66	440.8111 ± 71.4779
3–4 Years	58	500.0037 ± 103.2837
4–5 Years	49	549.4533 ± 84.6325
5–6 Years	33	639.4677 ± 126.7067
6–7 Years	44	722.0357 ± 140.8796
7–8 Years	44	824.6372 ± 137.9766
8–9 Years	32	844.4633 ± 93.6353
9–10 Years	37	935.8571 ± 189.1018
10–11 Years	29	985.0464 ± 121.0802
11–12 Years	27	1048.9250 ± 167.5279
12–13 Years	29	1118.4593 ± 155.2817
13–14 Years	22	1125.0250 ± 147.9899
14–18 Years	30	1323.8862 ± 226.3454
18–30 Years	42	1361.8682 ± 205.3783
30–40 Years	74	1381.1037 ± 300.3834
40–50 Years	139	1423.7647 ± 216.9305
50–60 Years	197	1343.2768 ± 246.6878
60–70 Years	181	1284.4183 ± 190.7129
70–80 Years	106	1263.1282 ± 170.2464
80–100 Years	21	1089.3429 ± 199.0259
Total	1456	

Table 1. Standard liver volume range (X ± S, cm³).

Upper abdominal CT films from 1456 children (enhanced CT 837, plain CT 619) aged 1 day to 100 years were selected. None had any history of liver disease, and CT had been performed for other clinical purposes. The patients were divided into 26 groups by age (**Table 1**).

7. Human Digital Liver Database

The Human Digital Liver Database (HDLD) was established by the Affiliated Hospital of Qingdao University and Hisense Company, aiming to collect digital liver from neonates, children, adults, and the elderly, from normal livers, livers with cancer, and simulated livers resected using Hisense CAS. The link of the HDLD is http://www.hdldb.net, which now is only available in Chinese (the English version is being translated now). The HDLD will show the digital liver in image and video form. All visitors could study the updated clinical cases at any angle of reconstructed 3D digital liver, including the vascular system, anatomical differences in the liver, and the correlation between vascular and liver tumors. The HDLD will also provide the intra-operation video comparing to the preoperative surgical plan, to help doctors and medical students better understand the anatomy and surgical procedure of pediatric liver resection, especially for patients with giant liver tumors (**Figure 9**).

7.1. Normal children and adult digital liver database

Vascular anatomical variation and total liver volume are two of the more important factors that surgeons consider when making surgical plans. We have collected thousands of CT scan data from across the nation. We would like to establish a digital liver database showing the reconstructed digital liver and separate these digital livers into different groups according to the anatomical variations in liver vasculature and liver volume (**Figure 9**). The Dong's Digital Liver Classification was established based on our collection of digital livers. We believe that a normal digital liver database may serve as an important reference for surgeons all around world.

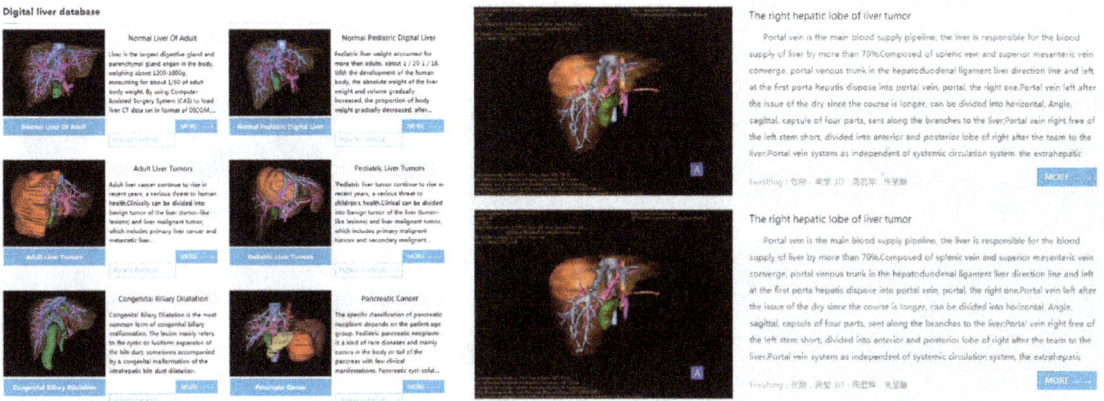

Figure 9. The Human Digital Liver Database.

7.2. Liver tumor database and simulated liver surgery

The liver tumor database shows the reconstructed digital liver image and simulated liver resection according to the surgeon's preoperative plan, and the intraoperative video of clinical cases, aiming to share the experience gained by staff at our center freely around the world. With the help of Hisense CAS, the successful surgical resection of liver tumors in pediatric patients has improved in our center. With the 3D simulation, we have found that we can clearly understand the anatomical variation in intrahepatic vasculature, the correlation of vasculature with liver tumors, and calculate the remnant liver volume of the simulated liver easily. In the database, we would like to show some difficult cases, such as those with very large liver tumors and those with vascular variation.

8. Clinical application of Hisense CAS for diagnosis and surgical plans in children with large liver tumors

An 11-month-old male infant was referred with abdominal distension and loss of appetite for the past 2 months [27]. Upon examination, a firm, non-tender mass with a smooth surface was evident arising from the right lobe of the liver, which filled the abdominal cavity. Serum ALT, AST, GGT, ALP, and Alb were normal. Both serum α-fetoprotein (AFP) and carcinoembryonic antigen (CEA) levels were within normal ranges. Ultrasound (US) revealed a well-defined, multicystic mass involving the liver. Enhanced CT images similarly showed a giant cystic mass with minimally enhanced septation and peripheral solid components (**Figure 10**).

The DICOM data obtained from the CT images were uploaded to 3D simulation software, the Hisense Computer Assisted Surgery System (Hisense, China) to simulate the liver. The relationship between HMH and the intrahepatic vasculature was revealed in a 3D context (**Figure 11**). The right hepatic vein (RHV), the middle hepatic vein (MHV), and the left hepatic vein (LHV) were confluent with a common trunk. The hepatic veins (HVs), the portal veins (PVs), and the inferior vena cava (IVC) were displaced, with no obvious infiltration or encasement. The volume of both the functional liver and the HMH was automatically calculated. The positional relationship between the vessels and HMH could be confirmed from any angle instantaneously in the computer. Various virtual hepatectomies were performed to predict the risk and the difficulty of the actual hepatectomy. Finally, an optimal surgical

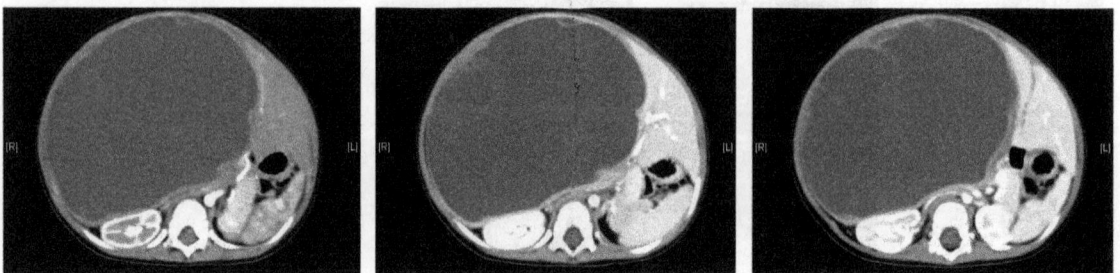

Figure 10. Preoperative enhanced CT scan.

plan was developed using 3D simulation software to safeguard RHV. The enucleation of HMH for the case was performed after adequate preoperative preparation.

After laparotomy, the fluid was aspirated using a 20 G needle from the cystic components of HMH to reduce its volume, thereby facilitating surgical resection. The resection line at the rim of HMH, which was indicated by virtual hepatectomy was made using the electrotome. The hepatic portal occlusion was used to reduce the risk of bleeding. The hepatic parenchyma was dissected using the CUSA system. The intrahepatic vessels were dissected to be safeguarded or else ligated and divided, a matter that had been assessed by the virtual hepatectomy. After 20 min, the HMH was removed with surrounding rim of normal liver tissue. The right hepatic vein was successfully safeguarded. The remnant liver volume was about 210 ml, which approximately equaled the automatically calculated remnant liver volume (230.1 ml). There was no anatomical discrepancy between the operation and the 3D simulation. The convalescence was uneventful. Histopathology confirmed the diagnosis of mesenchymal hamartoma (**Figure 12**).

In summary, three-dimensional (3D) imaging could significantly improve the resection rate of pediatric tumors and increase the safety of the surgery. Dong's digital liver classification system and human digital liver classification system will be useful for surgeons all around the world.

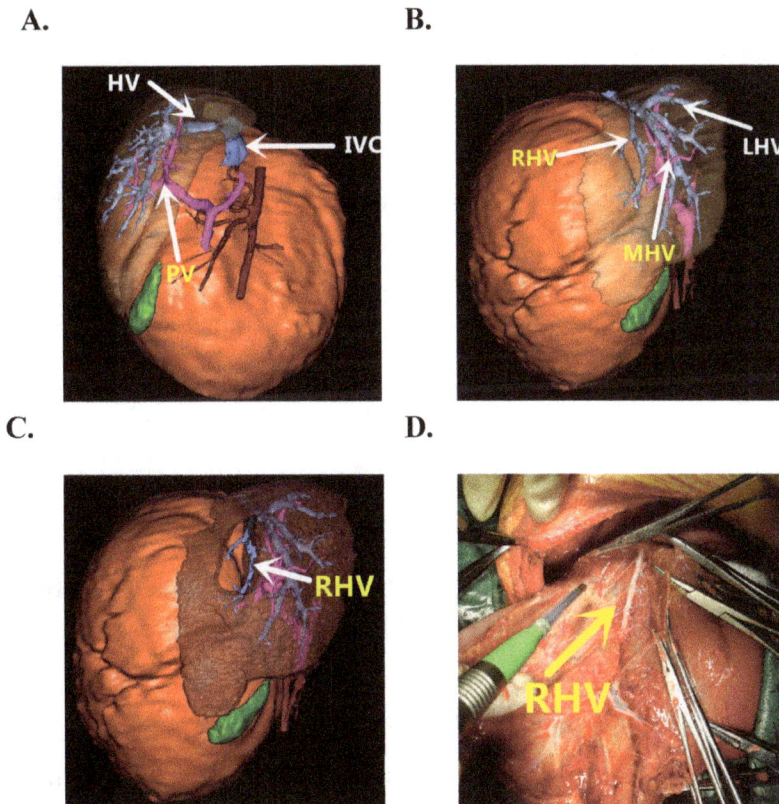

Figure 11. Comparison of 3D simulation and intraoperative liver anatomy.

A.   B.

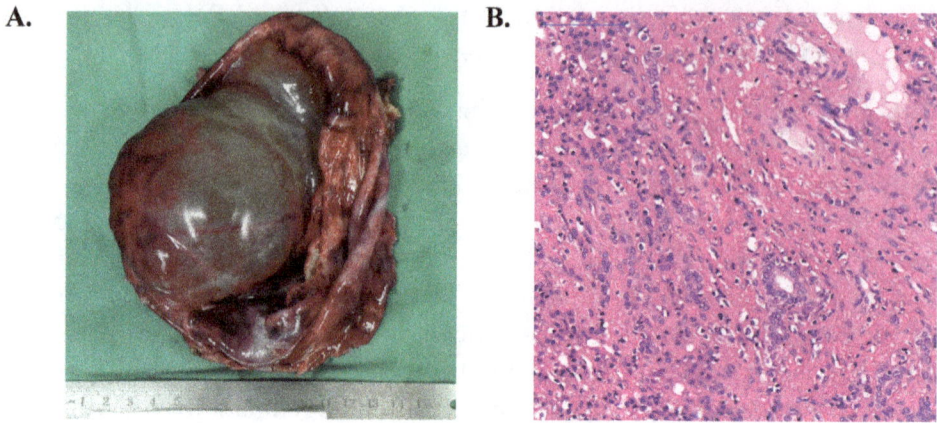

Figure 12. Resected HMH tumor and pathology.

Author details

Chengzhan Zhu[1,4], Bingzi Dong[2] and Qian Dong[3,4]*

*Address all correspondence to: 13608968352@163.com

1 Department of Hepatobiliary and Pancreatic Surgery, The Affiliated Hospital of Qingdao University, Qingdao, China

2 Department of Endocrinology and Metabolism, The Affiliated Hospital of Qingdao University, Qingdao, China

3 Pediatric Surgery Department, The Affiliated Hospital of Qingdao University, Qingdao, China

4 Shandong Key Laboratory of Digital Medicine and Computer Assisted Surgery, The Affiliated Hospital of Qingdao University, Qingdao, China

References

[1] Stocker JT. Hepatic tumors in children. Clinics in Liver Disease. 2001;**5**(1):259-281 viii-ix

[2] LaBerge JM. Liver tumors. In: O'Neill JA Jr, Grosfeld JL, Fonkalsrud EW, et al., editors. Principles of Pediatric Surgery. 2nd ed. St Louis: Mosby; 2003

[3] Yikilmaz A, George M, Lee EY. Pediatric hepatobiliary neoplasms: An overview and update. Radiologic Clinics of North America. 2017;**55**(4):741-766

[4] De Ugarte DA, Atkinson J. Liver tumors. In: Grosfeld JL, O'Neill JA Jr, Fonkalsrud AG, Coran AG, editors. Pediatric Surgery. 6th ed. Philadelphia: Mosby-Elsevier; 2006. pp. 502-505

[5] Aronson DC, Meyers RL. Malignant tumors of the liver in children. Seminars in Pediatric Surgery. 2016;**25**(5):265-275

[6] Roebuck DJ. Assessment of malignant liver tumors in children. Cancer Imaging. 2009; **9 Spec No A**:S98-S103

[7] Zhang G, Zhou XJ, Zhu CZ, Dong Q, Su L. Usefulness of three-dimensional(3D) simulation software in hepatectomy for pediatric hepatoblastoma. Surgical Oncology. 2016;**25**(3):236-243

[8] Czauderna P, Haeberle B, Hiyama E, Rangaswami A, Krailo M, Maibach R, et al. Novel global rare tumor database yields new prognostic factors in hepatoblastoma and becomes a research model. European Journal of Cancer. 2016;**52**:92-101

[9] Brown J, Perilongo G, Shafford E, Keeling J, Pritchard J, Brock P, et al. Pretreatment prognostic factors for children with hepatoblastoma-- results from the International Society of Paediatric Oncology (SIOP) study SIOPEL 1. European Journal of Cancer. 2000;**36**(11):1418-1425

[10] Czauderna P, Otte JB, Aronson DC, Gauthier F, Mackinlay G, Roebuck D, et al. Guidelines for surgical treatment of hepatoblastoma in the modern era--recommendations from the Childhood Liver Tumour Strategy Group of the International Society of Paediatric Oncology (SIOPEL). European Journal of Cancer. 2005;**41**(7):1031-1036

[11] Dong Q, Chen J. CT scan of pediatric liver tumors. In: Subburaj K, editor. CT Scanning Techniques and Applications. Intech; 2011

[12] Darbari A, Sabin KM, Shapiro CN, Schwarz KB. Epidemiology of primary hepatic malignancies in U.S. children. Hepatology. 2003;**38**(3):560-566

[13] Czauderna P, Mackinlay G, Perilongo G, Brown J, Shafford E, Aronson D, et al. Hepatocellular carcinoma in children: Results of the first prospective study of the International Society of Pediatric Oncology group. Journal of Clinical Oncology. 2002;**20**(12): 2798-2804

[14] Agarwala S. Primary malignant liver tumors in children. The Indian Journal of Pediatrics. 2012;**79**(6):793-800

[15] Su L, Dong Q, Zhang H, Zhou X, Chen Y, Hao X, et al. Clinical application of a three-dimensional imaging technique in infants and young children with complex liver tumors. Pediatric Surgery International. 2016;**32**(4):387-395

[16] Shoup M, Gonen M, D'Angelica M, Jarnagin WR, DeMatteo RP, Schwartz LH, et al. Volumetric analysis predicts hepatic dysfunction in patients undergoing major liver resection. Journal of Gastrointestinal Surgery. 2003;**7**(3):325-330

[17] Austin MT, Leys CM, Feurer ID, Lovvorn HN 3rd, O'Neill JA Jr, Pinson CW, et al. Liver transplantation for childhood hepatic malignancy: A review of the United Network for Organ Sharing (UNOS) database. Journal of Pediatric Surgery. 2006;**41**(1):182-186

[18] Plant AS, Busuttil RW, Rana A, Nelson SD, Auerbach M, Federman NC. A single-insti-
      tution retrospective cases series of childhood undifferentiated embryonal liver sarcoma
      (UELS): Success of combined therapy and the use of orthotopic liver transplant. Journal
      of Pediatric Hematology/Oncology. 2013;**35**(6):451-455

[19] Cao Q, Ye Z, Chen S, Liu N, Li S, Liu F. Undifferentiated embryonal sarcoma of liver:
      A multi-institutional experience with 9 cases. International Journal of Clinical and
      Experimental Pathology. 2014;**7**(12):8647-8656

[20] Hashimoto D, Dohi T, Tsuzuki M, Horiuchi T, Ohta Y, Chinzei K, et al. Development of
      a computer-aided surgery system: Three-dimensional graphic reconstruction for treat-
      ment of liver cancer. Surgery. 1991;**109**(5):589-596

[21] Lamade W, Glombitza G, Fischer L, Chiu P, Cardenas CE Sr, Thorn M, et al. The impact
      of 3-dimensional reconstructions on operation planning in liver surgery. Archives of
      Surgery. 2000;**135**(11):1256-1261

[22] Souzaki R, Ieiri S, Uemura M, Ohuchida K, Tomikawa M, Kinoshita Y, et al. An aug-
      mented reality navigation system for pediatric oncologic surgery based on preoperative
      CT and MRI images. Journal of Pediatric Surgery. 2013;**48**(12):2479-2483

[23] Fuchs J, Warmann SW, Szavay P, Kirschner HJ, Schafer JF, Hennemuth A, et al. Three-
      dimensional visualization and virtual simulation of resections in pediatric solid tumors.
      Journal of Pediatric Surgery. 2005;**40**(2):364-370

[24] Zhou X, Dong Q, Zhu C, Chen X, Wei B, Duan Y, et al. The role and significance of digi-
      tal reconstruction technique in liver segments based on portal vein structure. Chinese
      Journal of Surgery. 2018;**56**(1):61-67

[25] Couinaud C. The anatomy of the liver. Annali Italiani di Chirurgia. 1992;**63**(6):693-697

[26] Cho A, Okazumi S, Miyazawa Y, Makino H, Miura F, Ohira G, et al. Proposal for a reclas-
      sification of liver based anatomy on portal ramifications. American Journal of Surgery.
      2005;**189**(2):195-199

[27] Zhao J, Zhou XJ, Zhu CZ, Wu Y, Wei B, Zhang G, et al. 3D simulation assisted resec-
      tion of giant hepatic mesenchymal hamartoma in children. Computer Assisted Surgery
      (Abingdon). 2017;**22**(1):54-59

Permissions

All chapters in this book were first published in NAFLD&LRCM, by InTech Open; hereby published with permission under the Creative Commons Attribution License or equivalent. Every chapter published in this book has been scrutinized by our experts. Their significance has been extensively debated. The topics covered herein carry significant findings which will fuel the growth of the discipline. They may even be implemented as practical applications or may be referred to as a beginning point for another development.

The contributors of this book come from diverse backgrounds, making this book a truly international effort. This book will bring forth new frontiers with its revolutionizing research information and detailed analysis of the nascent developments around the world.

We would like to thank all the contributing authors for lending their expertise to make the book truly unique. They have played a crucial role in the development of this book. Without their invaluable contributions this book wouldn't have been possible. They have made vital efforts to compile up to date information on the varied aspects of this subject to make this book a valuable addition to the collection of many professionals and students.

This book was conceptualized with the vision of imparting up-to-date information and advanced data in this field. To ensure the same, a matchless editorial board was set up. Every individual on the board went through rigorous rounds of assessment to prove their worth. After which they invested a large part of their time researching and compiling the most relevant data for our readers.

The editorial board has been involved in producing this book since its inception. They have spent rigorous hours researching and exploring the diverse topics which have resulted in the successful publishing of this book. They have passed on their knowledge of decades through this book. To expedite this challenging task, the publisher supported the team at every step. A small team of assistant editors was also appointed to further simplify the editing procedure and attain best results for the readers.

Apart from the editorial board, the designing team has also invested a significant amount of their time in understanding the subject and creating the most relevant covers. They scrutinized every image to scout for the most suitable representation of the subject and create an appropriate cover for the book.

The publishing team has been an ardent support to the editorial, designing and production team. Their endless efforts to recruit the best for this project, has resulted in the accomplishment of this book. They are a veteran in the field of academics and their pool of knowledge is as vast as their experience in printing. Their expertise and guidance has proved useful at every step. Their uncompromising quality standards have made this book an exceptional effort. Their encouragement from time to time has been an inspiration for everyone.

The publisher and the editorial board hope that this book will prove to be a valuable piece of knowledge for researchers, students, practitioners and scholars across the globe.

List of Contributors

Rocío González Grande and Miguel Jiménez Pérez
Department of Gastroenterology and Hepatology, Liver Transplantation Unit, Regional University Hospital, Málaga, Spain

Shuai Xue, Peisong Wang, Hui Han and Guang Chen
The General Surgery Center, The First Hospital of Jilin University, Changchun, Jilin, China

Ian James Martins
Centre of Excellence in Alzheimer's Disease Research and Care, School of Medical and Health Sciences, Edith Cowan University, Joondalup, Australia
School of Psychiatry and Clinical Neurosciences, The University of Western Australia, Nedlands, Australia
McCusker Alzheimer's Research Foundation, Hollywood Medical Centre, Nedlands, Australia

Xiao-Ying Huang, Jin-Guang Yao, Qun-Ying Su, Xue-Min Wu, Juan Wang and Bing-Chen Huang
Department of Pathology, the Affiliated Hospital of Youjiang Medical University for Nationalities, Baise, China

Xi-Dai Long
Department of Pathology, the Affiliated Hospital of Youjiang Medical University for Nationalities, Baise, China
Department of Liver Surgery, Ren Ji Hospital, School of Medicine, Shanghai Jiao Tong University, Shanghai, China
Guangxi Clinic Research Center of Hepatobiliary Diseases, Baise, China

Qiang Xia
Department of Liver Surgery, Ren Ji Hospital, School of Medicine, Shanghai Jiao Tong University, Shanghai, China

Qun-Qing Xu and Xiao-Ying Zhu
Guangxi Clinic Research Center of Hepatobiliary Diseases, Baise, China

Yan Deng
Department of Epidemiology, Youjiang Medical University for Nationalities, Baise, China

Chao Wang
Department of Medicine, the Affiliated Hospital of Youjiang Medical University for Nationalities, Baise, China

Andra Iulia Suceveanu, Roxana Popoiag, Laura Mazilu, Irinel Raluca Parepa, Andreea Gheorghe, Felix Voinea, Claudia Voinea and Adrian Paul Suceveanu
Ovidius University, Faculty of Medicine, Constanta, Romania

Anca Stoian
Carol Davila University, Bucharest, Romania

Kingsley Asare Kwadwo Pereko
School of Medical Sciences, University of Cape Coast, Cape Coast, Ghana

Jacob Setorglo
School of Allied Health Sciences, University of Cape Coast, Cape Coast, Ghana

Matilda Steiner-Asiedu
Department of Nutrition and Food Science, University of Ghana, Legon, Ghana

Joyce Bayebanona Maaweh Tiweh
Eye Unit, Manhyia Government Hospital, Kumasi, Ghana

Mihaela Fadgyas Stanculete
Department of Neurosciences, Psychiatry, Iuliu Hatieganu University of Medicine and Pharmacy, Cluj Napoca, Romania

Chinmaya Kumar Bal, Ripu Daman and Vikram Bhatia
Department of Hepatology, Institute of Liver and Biliary Science, New Delhi, India

Monica Lupsor-Platon
Department of Medical Imaging, Iuliu Hatieganu University of Medicine and Pharmacy, Regional Institute of Gastroenterology and Hepatology "Prof. Dr. Octavian Fodor", Cluj-Napoca, Romania

Kurt Grüngreiff
Clinic of Gastroenterology Klinikum Magdeburg, Germany

Om Parkash
Section of Gastroenterology/Hepatology, Department of Medicine, The Aga Khan University Hospital, Pakistan

Subha Saeed
The Aga Khan University Hospital, Pakistan

Chengzhan Zhu
Department of Hepatobiliary and Pancreatic Surgery, The Affiliated Hospital of Qingdao University, Qingdao, China
Shandong Key Laboratory of Digital Medicine and Computer Assisted Surgery, The Affiliated Hospital of Qingdao University, Qingdao, China

Bingzi Dong
Department of Endocrinology and Metabolism, The Affiliated Hospital of Qingdao University, Qingdao, China

Qian Dong
Pediatric Surgery Department, The Affiliated Hospital of Qingdao University, Qingdao, China
Shandong Key Laboratory of Digital Medicine and Computer Assisted Surgery, The Affiliated Hospital of Qingdao University, Qingdao, China

Index

www.ingramcontent.com/pod-product-compliance
Lightning Source LLC
Chambersburg PA
CBHW061947190326
41458CB00009B/2812